BIOLOGICAL MODELS IN RADIOPHARMACEUTICAL DEVELOPMENT

Developments in Nuclear Medicine

VOLUME 27

Series Editor: Peter H. Cox

The titles published in this series are listed at the end of this volume.

Biological Models in Radiopharmaceutical Development

by

RICHARD M. LAMBRECHT

PET-Zentrum des Universitätsklinikums,
Eberhard-Karls-Universität Tübingen,
Tübingen, Germany

KLUWER ACADEMIC PUBLISHERS

DORDRECHT / BOSTON / LONDON

Library of Congress Cataloging-in-Publication Data

Lambrecht, Richard M., 1943-
    Biological models in radiopharmaceutical development / Richard M.
  Lambrecht.
        p.   cm. -- (Developments in nuclear medicine ; 27)
    Includes bibliographical references and index.
     ISBN-13: 978-94-010-6558-0 (HB : alk. paper)
    1. Radiopharmaceuticals--Research--Methodology. 2. Pharmacology-
  -Animal models.   I. Title. II. Series.
  RM833.L36   1996
  616.07'575--dc20   95-43931

ISBN-13: 978-94-010-6558-0   e-ISBN-13: 978-94-009-0159-9
DOI: 10.1007/978-94-009-0159-9

Published by Kluwer Academic Publishers,
P.O. Box 17, 3300 AA Dordrecht, The Netherlands.

Kluwer Academic Publishers incorporates
the publishing programmes of
D. Reidel, Martinus Nijhoff, Dr W. Junk and MTP Press.

Sold and distributed in the U.S.A. and Canada
by Kluwer Academic Publishers,
101 Philip Drive, Norwell, MA 02061, U.S.A.

In all other countries, sold and distributed
by Kluwer Academic Publishers Group,
P.O. Box 322, 3300 AH Dordrecht, The Netherlands.

Printed on acid-free paper

DEDICATION

to my mother
Eulina Elizabeth Neal Lambrecht

and
to my father
Bernard Henry Lambrecht

TABLE OF CONTENTS

PREFACE

Radiopharmaceuticals labeled with short-lived radionuclides are utilized to unravel biochemical processes, and to diagnosis and treat diseases of the living body are developed through extensive evaluation in biological models. The first attempt to compile information was a volume entitled *ANIMAL MODELS IN RADIOTRACER DESIGN* that was edited by William C. Eckelman and myself in 1983. The volume had a focus on the animal models that investigators were using in order to design radiotracers that displayed *in vivo* selectivity as measured by biodistribution and pharmacokinetic studies. A concern in the early days of nuclear medicine was species differences. Often a series of labeled compounds were evaluated in a several different animal models in order to gain confidence that the selected radiotracer would behave appropriately in humans. During the past 12 years there have been remarkable advances in molecular genetics, molecular biology, synthetic radiopharmaceutical chemistry, molecular modeling and visualization, and emission tomography. Biological models can now be selected that are better defined in terms of molecular aspects of the disease process. The development of high resolution PET and SPET for clinical applications facilitates the development of new radiopharmaceuticals by the use of models to quantitatively evaluate drug effects, and progression of disease, and hence to arrive at better diagnosis and treatments for animals and humans. With these advances there is an effective use of biological models, and the refinement of alternatives for the development of new radiopharmaceuticals.

This comprehensive resource guide reflects an analysis of the world literature, for the period between 1983 and June, 1995. It is intended to provide a succinct overview of the current status of biological models that can facilitate advances in the development of drugs and radiopharmaceuticals. This book is written primarily for scientists, physicians, post-graduate students, members of animal care and ethics committees, and other professionals involved in biomedical research, drug and radiopharmaceutical development.

Richard M. Lambrecht
Tübingen
28 July, 1995

ACKNOWLEDGEMENTS

The images and illustrations were provided through the kind cooperation of Professor Dr. W.-D. Heiss of the Max-Plank-Institut für Neurologische Forschung, Köln; Professor Michael R. Zalutsky of Department of Radiology, Duke University Medical Center, Durham, NC; Dr. R. J. Hicks of Nuclear Medicine Department, Heidelberg Hospital, Melbourne; Dr. J. Clerc of Hopital Neckar-Enfants Malades, Service de Radioisotopes, Paris; and Associate Professor A.J. Simusas of Yale University - Section of Cardiovascular Medicine, New Haven, CT.

I am pleased to express my appreciation for the assistance of Mr. Suliman Bakr and Ms. Sandra Gorringe in the literature search, and Mr. Tayfun Oezen in the retrieval of original literature. Ms. Filomina Mattner assisted in some of the tabulations and classifications. The cooperative assistance of the staff of the Research Library at the King Faisal Specialist Hospital, Riyadh, Kingdom of Saudi Arabia; the Research Library of the Australian Nuclear Science & Technology Organization, Sydney; and the Libraries at the Eberhard-Karls-Universität Tübingen is acknowledged. Continuing discussions with Prof. H.-J. Machulla on PET radiopharmaceuticals for clinical needs, and his telephone call in April 1993 are acknowledged. Mr Hans-Jörg Rahm demonstrated extraordinary computer skills, and attention to details in preparation of the camera-ready-copy for publication. The presentation is a reflection of his interest in the project. I thank Shirley Cacho Aglibut, meine Lebengefährtin, for her supportive understanding and assistance throught-out the time this volume was in preparation.

INTRODUCTION

In 1865 Claude Bernard stated in his *Introduction to the Study of Experimental Medicine* that

> "I not only conclude that experiments made on animals from the physiological, pathological and therapeutic points of view have results that are applicable to theoretical medicine, but I think that without such comparative study of animals, practical medicine can never acquire a scientific character."

The second Nobel price in medicine and physiology was given to Emil Adolf von Behring for the first successful application of molecular biology a short time after Röntgen discovered the X-rays in 1895 - for his discovery of a cure for diphtheria by the injection of the serum of immunized horses. The integration of radioisotopes into tracers for physiological measurements in animal models gave raise to many important discoveries , such as radioiodine treatment of thyroid carcinoma, and the development of the Anger camera for non-invasive in vivo imaging.

In the 1960's the term "biomedical reseach" referred to comparative studies with animal models and humans. Until about 1985 biomedical research with animals was characterized by discovery, description and characterization of new models. The medical and behavioral benefits of biomedical research are many and varied (King and Yarbrough, 1985; Hass, 1993; Proceedings, 1987). In a few instances studies of animal diseases preceeded those of the equivalent human disease (Prieur, 1983).

As we approach the year 2000, it is appropriate to consider biomedical research in terms of research with animal species, humans, and alternatives (such as tissue culture and molecular modeling), as research with "biological models."

A first attempt at the definition of *Animal Models in Radiotracer Design* (Lambrecht and Eckelman, Eds., 1983) was described by experts in the field with emphasis placed heavily upon studies with labeled compounds, screening, structure-activity-relationship, tumor uptake, the ratio of target to non-target uptake, bio-distribution, and pharmacokinetics.

The results of radiopharmaceutical developments since the 1980's has been a change from diagnosis to prognosis and better patient management. The rapid developments in the fields of molecular genetics and molecular biology have lead to new opportunities for the design and the development of radiopharmaceuticals targeted to cancer, and human genetic diseases, such as in-born errors of metabolism. These advances were only possible through research that required the use of biological models prior to applications to humans. There are ethical, legal and practical constraints that limit experimentation in humans. Many of the concerns facing the radiopharmaceutical scientist in selection of appropriate biological models in which to evaluate potential radiopharmaceuticals has moved from a semi-empirical or screening approach to a basis for rational selection of appropriate models. The use of animals in biomedical research provides a scientifically valid and moral approach to the development of knowledge. Radiopharmaceuticals are used to measure *in situ* biochemical processes and their responses to drugs or stimuli. Radiopharmaceutical development and research benefits both human and animal welfare (Kotz, 1995).

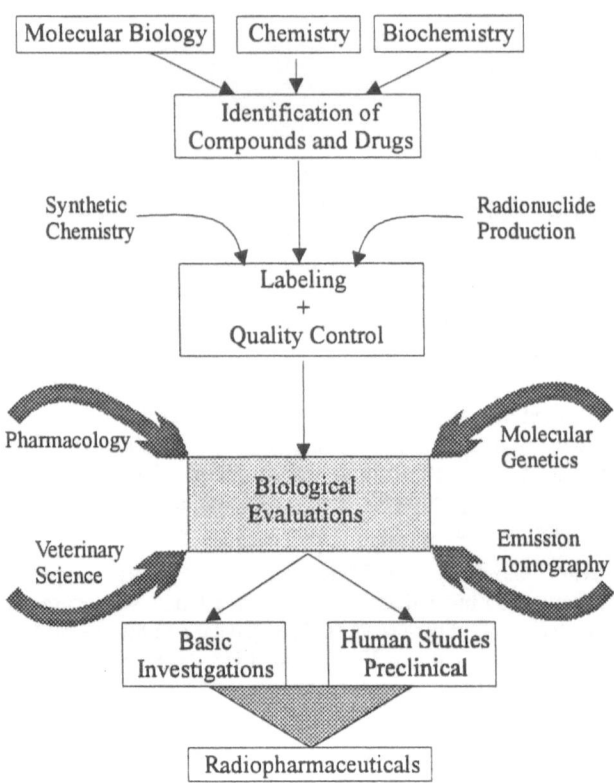

Figure 1. Interdisciplinary relationships in the development of diagnostic and therapeutic radiopharmaceuticals

Figure 1 depicts the interdisciplinary relationships of chemistry, biochemistry, molecular biology, molecular genetics and related disciplines on the design and evaluation of labeled compounds as potential radiopharmaceuticals. The cross-interactions of chemistry, molecular biology and genetics in collaboration with nuclear medicine specialists and emission tomography give rise to the development of new and improved diagnostic and therapeutic radiopharmaceuticals for improved health care and better patient management.

The development of radiopharmaceuticals applied to medical diagnosis and treatment has evolved from ATOMIC MEDICINE (1950's - 1960's) which involved atomic cocktails, such as iodine-131 iodide. The field became known as NUCLEAR MEDICINE (1970's - 1980's) and was characterized by the introduction of technetium-99m compounds that allowed physicians to image organs and relate radiotracer pharmacodynamics to physiologic function of the living body. Sub-specialities in the practice of nuclear medicine are recognized by learned organizations; such as the European Society of Nuclear Medicine, and the Society of Nuclear Medicine. In 1991 the discipline was proclaimed as MOLECULAR NUCLEAR MEDICINE by Henry N. Wagner, Jr. as a result of the significant advances that had been made in the development of specifically labeled molecular compounds with a high specificity for specific biochemical processes (Wagner, 1991).

Hundreds of small molecule radiopharmaceuticals have been labeled with short-lived radionuclides such as carbon-11 ($T_{1/2}$ = 20 min.), fluorine-18 ($T_{1/2}$ = 110 min), oxygen ($T_{1/2}$ = 122 sec.), and copper-62 ($T_{1/2}$ = 9.78 min) (Kilbourn, 1989). Following extensive evaluations only about 35 are presently considered to be of major interest in Europe for clinical applications with positron emission tomography (Stöcklin and Pike, 1993). The radionuclides such as iodine-123 ($T_{1/2}$ = 13.1 hr), technetium-99m ($T_{1/2}$ = 6.02 hr), and indium-111 ($T_{1/2}$ = 2.83 d) are applied to single photon emission tomographic (SPET) imaging (Nunn, 1992).

We are now in an era evolving to therapeutic nuclear oncology as a sub-speciality of molecular nuclear medicine. Studies with SPET and quantitative PET using radiopharmaceuticals such as radiolabeled monoclonal antibodies, FDG, and pain palliation agents are a focus. Through the use of PET and iodine-124 ($T_{1/2}$ = 4.12 da), copper-64 ($T_{1/2}$ = 12.4 hr), and ytterium-86 ($T_{1/2}$ = 14.74 hr) as positron-emitting radionuclidic labels, it becomes feasible to estimate uptake and appropriate dosage of therapeutic radiopharmaceuticals administered in patient treatments with high doses of iodine-131 ($T_{1/2}$ = 8.04 da), copper-67 ($T_{1/2}$ = 61.7 hr), and ytterium-90 ($T_{1/2}$ = 64.0 hr). (Lambrecht et al, 1988; Qureshi et al, 1987; Pentlow et al, 1991; Wilson, et al, 1991; Larson et al., 1992; Ott et al, 1992; Herzog et al, 1993; Anderson et al, 1995; Pentlow et al, 1994). Rhenium-186 ($T_{1/2}$ = 90.6 hr). Rhenium-188 ($T_{1/2}$ = 17.0 hr), and holmium-166 ($T_{1/2}$ = 26.8 hr) are examples of radionuclides for therapy that can also be imaged by SPET (Turner et al., 1994).

For a contemporary introduction to the *Principles of Nuclear Medicine* and the clinical applications of radiopharmaceuticals, see Wagner, Szabo and Buchanan (1995).

SCOPE OF THE WORK

This volume is intended to provide researchers with a compilation of data and information to allow rationale choices of appropriate biological models for investigations of the development of drugs and radiopharmaceuticals specific to understanding disease processes and the development of treatments for diseases afflicting society and its members. Selection criteria included the world literature for the period 1983 until June, 1995. The searches utilized all available data bases. The searches conducted through research library services in Germany, the Kingdom of Saudi Arabia, and Australia resulted in 3865 citations. These were evaluated and screened to the listing of 2884 references cited in this volume.

The references cited may mention the language of the report, and indicate cases where an English translation of the abstract was published. If an investigator has a series of publications on a particular topic, then in the interest of brevity, only the most recent or directly relevant citations are given. Further details can usually be found within the references of the given citations.

Table I cites examples of 44 representative physiological states involving the use of biological models, radiopharmaceuticals and state-of-the-art medical imaging instrumentation.

Table II is comprised of selected books and reviews that highlight collections of works on 143 specific topics related to biological models of human disease, and extended summaries on the use of specific models such as non-human primates and swine.

Guidelines for the use of animals in research are necessarily re-stated in this monograph, as well as brief remarks concerning alternatives. A brief review of philosophical, ethical and moral arguments concerning the use of animals in research and testing is provided as background on the past and current situation in the use of animals.

Examples of the utility of PET, SPET, SIMS, and Autoradiography for physiologic studies in drug and radiopharmaceutical development are illustrated.

Table III is a keyword guide of 1909 disease states and/or biochemical processes that are alphabetically classified by disease state. The compilation is intended as a convenience for researchers in the process of selection of the appropriate biological model. The entries are arranged in alphabetical order according to the physiological process or disease state.

This volume is intended to identify choices in the selection and use of appropriate biological models. It is not intended to classify the thousands of radiotracers that have been studied in biological models. It was not practical to detail the large number of tumors that have been induced or transplanted into rodents. For example, virtually every organ and tissue of mice and humans is disposed to neoplastic processes (Jonas, 1984), and the reader is referred to comprehensive bibliography of the mesotheliomas of mice (Ilgren, 1993). The uptake of radiotracers as potential radiopharmaceuticals in experimental tumor models has been tabulated (Wiebe et al, 1983; 1991; Shah and Sands, 1990). Nor was it within the scope to detail the use of genetically defined mice, see for example the bibliography of 1916 references of mammalian behavior studies sorted by categories such as cognitive and convulsive disorders, maturity and pharmacologic agents (Sprott and Staats, 1975, 1978, 1980). The radiopharmacology of labeled compounds is extensive, and the current literature should be consulted (Nunn, 1992).

Exclusion criteria were applied to use of animals in studies that induce pain and suffering, or cause lasting harm - such as burns and traumatic head injury. There is an opinion that biomedical research is necessary within these areas in order to obliterate human pain and suffering. In some instances research in humans can proceed ethically, where the studies are directly relevant to the human subject. For example, it is well-documented that the evaluation scales and criteria for evaluation of the efficiency of radiopharmaceuticals for palliation of bone pain due to cancer vary depending on the patient's thresholds for pain, and the psychological evaluations. It is even more difficult to evaluate pain and its relief in animal subjects.

This comprehensive reference is intended as a resource for radiopharmaceutical scientists, pharmacists, physicians, veterinarians, post-graduate researchers, members of animal care and ethics committees and other professionals involved in biomedical research, drug and radiopharmaceutical development.

GUIDELINES FOR RESEARCH WITH ANIMALS

A monograph facilitating the use of animals in research requires a statement of the principles for the use and care of animals. The Australian Code of Practice (1990) is cited as an example. The United States, the European Community, and Japan have debated the moral, ethical and scientific considerations, and have similar statements of principle. The guidelines encompass all aspects of the care and use of animals for scientific purposes in medicine, biology, veterinary, agriculture, industry and education.

The choice of the example code was a personal choice based upon the author's familiarity with the Australian code, having been chairperson of the Animal Care and Ethics Committee (1991 - March 1993) as well as the director of the Biomedicine and Health Program at the Australian Nuclear Science and Technology Organization (Ansto), Sydney, Australia. One achievement was the accreditation of the animal facilities for the first time in the laboratory's 40 year history. The "Shield of the Crown" of the national laboratory had seemed to prevent New South Wales state government from inspection of the practices and facilities at Ansto. A check for fees to proceed towards accreditation inspection was returned in 1991. The author and colleagues persisted and inspection occured late in 1992 resulting in accreditation early in 1993.

The Australian Code of Practice is reproduced with permission of the National Health and Medical Research Council (NHMRC):

- Experiments on animals may be performed only when they are essential to obtain and establish significant information relevant to the understanding of human or animal health and welfare, to the improvement of animal management or production, or to the achievement of educational objectives.
- People who use animals for scientific purposes have an obligation to treat the animals with respect and to consider their welfare as an essential factor when planning and conducting their experiments.
- Investigators have direct and ultimate responsibility for all matters relating to the welfare of the animals they use in experiments.
- Techniques which replace or complement animal experiments must be used wherever possible.
- Experiments using animals may be performed only after a decision has been made that they are justified, weighing the scientific or educational value of the experiment against the potential effects on the welfare of the animal.
- Animals choosen must be of an appropriate species with suitable biological characteristics, including behavioral characteristics, genetic constitution and nutritional, microbiological and general health status.
- Animals must not be taken from their natural habitats if animals bred in captivity are available and suitable.
- Experiments must be scientifically valid, and must use no more than the minimum number of animals needed.
- Experiments must use the best available scientific techniques and must be carried out only by persons competent in the procedures they perform.
- Experiments must not be repeated unnecessarily.
- Experiments must be as brief as possible.
- Experiments must be designed to avoid pain or distress to animals. If this is not possible, pain or distress must be minimised.

- Pain and distress cannot be evaluated easily in animals and therefore investigators must assume that animals experience pain in a manner similar to humans. Decisions regarding the animals' welfare must be based on this assumption unless there is evidence to the contrary.
- Experiments which may cause pain or distress of a kind and degree for which anaesthesia would normally be used in medical or veterinary practice must be carried out using anaesthesia appropriate to the species and the procedure. When it is not possible to use anaesthesia, such as in certain toxicological or animal production experiments or in animal models of disease, the end-point of the experiment must be as early as possible to avoid or minimise pain or distress to the animals.
- Investigators must avoid using death as an experimental end-point whenever possible.
- Analgesic and tranquilliser usage must be appropriate for the species and should at least parallel the usage in medical or veterinary practice.
- An animal which develops signs of pain or distress of a kind and degree not predicted in the proposal, must have the pain or distress alleviated promptly. If severe pain cannot be alleviated without delay, the animal must be killed humanely forthwith. Alleviation of such pain or distress must take precedence over finishing an experiment.
- Neuromuscular blocking agents must not be used without appropriate general anaesthesia, except in animals where sensory awareness has been eliminated. If such agents are used, continuous or frequent intermittent monitoring of paralysed animals is essential to ensure that the depth of anaesthesia is adequate to prevent pain or distress.
- Animals must be transported, housed, fed, watered, handled and used under conditions which are appropriate to the species and which ensure a high standard of care.
- Institutions using animals for scientific purposes must establish Animal Experimentation Ethics Committees (AEECs) to ensure that all animal use conforms with the standards of this Code.
- Investigators must submit written proposals for all animal experimentation to an AEEC which must take into account the expected value of the knowledge to be gained, the validity of the experiments, and all ethical and animal welfare aspects.
- Experiments must not commence until written approval has been obtained from the AEEC.
- The care and use of animals for all scientific purposes in Australia must be in accord with this Code of Practice, and with Commonwealth, State and Territory legalisation.

MORAL AND ETHICAL CONSIDERATIONS

It would be remiss not to comment on the philosophical arguments on the moral and ethical considerations for use of animals in research, development and testing. The synopsis has been expanded and in part quoted with permission from the excellent summary prepared by members of the steering committee of the Parliamentary Office of Science and Technology, U.K. (Home Office, 1992).

Ancient religions have taken different positions on the place of animals in society. Oriental creeds, particularly those involving the transmigration of souls, judged animals lives as worthy of protection, while some were viewed as sacred. Judeo-Christian doctrine appears to assign value to animals primarily for their ability to serve human purposes, as in the Biblical references to man having 'dominion' over the animals. Aristotle and Plato held similar views. The primacy of human interests over animal interests was not unrestrained. Outright cruelty has never been condoned. The parable of the good shepherd in both the Old and the New Testaments provides a role-model illustrating concern for animals welfare. As Jesus healed the possessed at Gerasa (Mk 5,1-20), he drove the demons out of the man and they went into a flock of pigs. The pigs then plunged into the lake and drowned, and the man was saved. This may be the first report about animals playing a main role in the process of healing humans.

Both Protestant and Catholic religions teach that humans are priviledged and have a rightful hegemony over other animals, but that this should be respected. People believe it is right to treat animals gently, and because it is usually in the human interest. One differentiation between human and animal was the concept of soul which made humans naturally suited to rule over other living beings.

In the 17th Century different philosophical views arose. Descartes viewed animals as basically 'machines' which lack the human 'mind' and the capacity to suffer. This view was challenged by Hume and other philosophers. As scientific evidence mounted in the 18th Century that animals were capable of experiencing pain and suffering, the debate concerning whether animal experimentation was morally justifiable intensified. Influential voices raised against vivisection included: Pope, Johnson, Addison, and the Utilitarian philosophers Jeremy Bentham and John Stewart Mill. Others including Huxley, supported animal experiments strongly, because they felt animals would benefit mankind.

As we approach the 21st century there is a very wide spectrum of attitudes concerning the use of animals to advance perceived human needs. At one extreme, animals are viewed to be entitled to have their interests considered equally with those of humans. However, others view human interests as superior to the normal interests of animals, which therefore gives an authority for placing human interests before those of animals. There are different views and interpretations of the moral standings of animals.

The animal welfare and animal rights movements have existed at least since 1831 when Marshall Hall drew up five principles of ethics for self-regulation of scientific investigations (See French, 1975). However, a book entitled "Animal Liberation" by the Australian philosopher (Peter Singer, 1975) fueled an outcry from radical animal rights groups in the U.K. and U.S.A. that advocated halting all research with animals largely based on moral and ethical arguments. Other disruptive actions included vandalized laboratories, threats to scientists and public property, and the agitation of the public through anarchic expressions in the media (Holden,1986; Eckholm, 1985; Bleiberg, 1989). Ensuing legal arguments concerning stricter regulations and compliance requirements, (Watson, 1993; Holden, 1986; Wooton and Fleckell, 1987;) lead universities and professional organizations to debate and publicize principles, policies and practices to assert continuation of biomedical research using animal models (Thomas, et al., 1988; AAAS, 1990; ASIH, 1990; Schwarz, 1990; and others).

A campaign raised the public awareness of the benefits of improvements in both human and animal health (Baum, 1990; Woolsey, 1988; Home Office, 1992; AMA, 1992).

A recent sociological account of the animal rights movement categorizes activists as welfarists, pragmatists and fundamentalists (Jasper and Nelkin, 1992). The Humane Society for the Care and Protection of Animals (ASPCA) is an animal welfare organization that strives to improve conditions for laboratory animals. Pragmatic groups advocate reduction in use of animals through political and legal protests, but would allow use of animals when the benefits outweigh other considerations. Fundamentalist or anarchic radical groups are blind to the use of animals regardless of the benefits.

There were some negative outcomes and two positive outcomes for society resulting in part from Animal Rights Groups and these are:

- Replacement of the classical LD_{50} test which is a measure of acute toxicity based upon establishing a dose at which 50% of the rodents tested die upon exposure to the substance;
- Replacement of the Draize Eye Irritancy Test which was used to test cosmetics placed directly into the eye of a restrained rabbit.

Nevertheless it is clear that the radical Animal Rights Groups for the most part fail society. They are in general extreme in their efforts because they work to impede and refuse to acknowledge that essential medical research have historically benefited both animals and humans. Efforts that adversely drive up the cost of research without benefit to either animals or society is a disruptive motivation of certain Groups that are unable to achieve legislative means to accomplish their objectives.

Biomedical research is not always attractive, but then neither is AIDS, Malaria, or Alzheimer's Disease.

One of the basic premises behind animal rights, philosophies is that if animals are sufficiently similar to humans to be useful experimental models, then animals are sufficiently similar to be afforded equal moral status. Philosophers such as Singer (1975, 1980) and Regan (1983) have argued that no morally significant features exist that are unique to humans and absent from animals. They argue it follows that there is not a moral justification for using animals in laboratory experiments. They argue that features normally associated with adult humans such as self-conciousness, language and rationality exist, at least to some degree, in other species. They observed that we attach human rights to members of society who lack some of these attributes (the severely and the mentally disabled, the infants and the senile). They further argue that it is logically inconsistent to apply different moral codes to humans and animals. In particular, most people sense that both humans and animals share a capacity of suffering.

To those who see humans as possessing no unique, morally significant features, the experimental use of animals, rather than humans, is discrimination against animals purely on the basis of species. Ryder (1975) has coined the term "speciesism" to describe this discrimination and considers it a moral injustice analogous to racism or sexism.

This line of reasoning has been challenged (Hart, 1980). Science animals are incapable of waiving their rights. Discussion of animal rights could be defined in terms of human duties. The analogy with incompetent humans is seen as misleading since most humans possess the capacity for rationality, freedom or choice and self-conciousness, whereas animals lack this ability. Even if some members lack all 'human' characteristics, it is argued that if most humans have special characteristics, then it is logical to treat them as a single group. Babies will acquire all the human characteristics in the future, whereas animals will not gain these characteristics at any time.

Humans do not have to recognise animal rights to try and avoid or minimise suffering. This is part of generally accepted 'humane' behaviour which can cover a whole spectrum of responses from a strict prohibition on inflicting suffering, to a general propensity to avoid it where no great personal sacrifice is involved. Humane behaviour would not normally require that animals be afforded the same degree of protection or attention as humans; the amount of empathy between humans and the particular species of animal could influence the moral weight that humane considerations will have

(Home Office, 1992). Cats may well attract more sympathy than damselfish. Predatory animals may not attract affection, because they are cunning and they are often seen to interfere with human activities (e.g. coyotes attacks on domestic sheep). Rodents may not be regarded sympathetically, because society usually views rodents as pests.

Some philosophers have argued that irrespective of whether or not animals have rights *per se*, humans have moral obligations towards animals. Singer (1980) argues that the ultimate test of moral conduct is whether it maximises the welfare of all the sentient organisms affected by the conduct. This Utilitarian argument allows the use of animals in laboratory experiments only if it is for the common good, and only if we are prepared to use humans in the same way. Others agreeing that sentience should be the currency of morality, have suggested that animal experiments should only be allowed if they benefit the individuals concerned - rather than being for the common good (Ryder, 1975, 1983, 1989, 1991).

Such arguments have been challenged both on their specific reference to the issue of animal use, and by the general criticism that Utilitarism, by allowing the claims of one individual to be overridden by the needs of the majority, permits violations of individual rights. However, other interpretations of utility would not view the condition to avoid suffering as absolute. A comparative Utilitarian approach would seek an action that had better consequences than any other alternative. UK and other legislation requires the weighing of the potential benefits against the suffering in making a decision. Non-Utilitarian philosophy can also accomodate both sides of the animal use debate (Home Office, 1992).

A recent Institute of Medical Ethics Working Party (see Smith and Boyd, 1991) considered in detail the ethics of animal research. The group questioned if 'individual, metaphysical visions' could yet provide a basis for decisions relating to our treatment of animals and suggested that a 'common morality' might be a better approach. The continued use of animals in biomedical research is justified by an evolving moral consensus rather than being derived from first principles. The use of animals is regarded as a 'necessary evil' until better alternatives are found, and recognises the need to consider the balance between human and animal well-being (Home Office, 1992).

The ethical framework that arises from this approach involves minimising the conflict between the moral obligations to promote both human and animal welfare. In reality, this involves balancing the costs, of probable pain, distress or suffering of the animals involved in research against the likely benefits that arise to man or animals from such activities.

The present possibilities and future prospects of the replacement, reduction and refinement of animals in biomedical research was summarized by Hendriksen and Koeter (1991). There is a concerted effort amongst many organizations to encourage and to fund scientific efforts to pursue the development, validation and use of alternative methods for testing product safety and efficacy. For example, alternatives encouraged by the Procter & Gamble Company include:

- New *in vitro* biochemical and cellular approches that could replace *in vivo* testing.
- Non-invasive *in vivo* procedures that reduce the distress imposed on animals.
- Reduction of the use of animals through the development of new models, for example computer modeling.
- Scientific validation of alternative methods.

PRINCIPLES AND TRAINING PROGRAMS

Anyone contemplating research with biological models must be aware of the fundamental and well-defined techniques for the efficient use of laboratory animals, and the guidelines for the welfare and comfort of the subjects used in research. Recommended reading and training programs include:

Essentials for Animal Research: A Primer for Research Personnel. (1990). BT Bennett, MJ Brown and JC Schofield. National Agriculture Library, U.S. Department of Agriculture, 126 pp. Available free from Animal Welfare Information Center, National Agricultural Library, 10301 Baltimore Boulevard, Room 304, Beltsville, MD 20705. Topics covered include: animal care and use; principles of aseptic techniques, anesthesia, analgesia, euthanasia, regulations, requirements and alternate methodologies.

Guide for the Care and Use of Laboratory Animals. (1985). Publication no 017-040-00498-2. Available free from the Superintendent of Documents, U. S. Government Printing Office, Washington, DC 20402.

Principles of Proper Laboratory Animal Use in Research. (1989). GR Novak and R Hityelberg, Eds. MTM Associates. The training software program ($495) is available for both PC or Mac computers, or as hard copy ($40) from MTM Associates, Inc., P. O Box 1606, Manassas, VA 22110. The program consists of a template divided into a series of modules covering wide range of topics as above plus pre- and post-operative care, disease, nutrition, models and species information.

Audiovisual Materials Concerning the Care, Use, Behavior and General Biology of Animals. (1989). W Threlfall. Atlantaic Provinces Council in the Sciences. ISSN 0702-0007. 353 pp. Available for $15 from Dr. William Threlfall, Department of Biology, Memorial University of Newfoundland, St. John's, Newfoundland A1B 3X9 Canada. The resources lists computer programs and audiovisual aids that can be used in university education laboratories to reduce the number of animals used. Subject and source listings are provided.

Guidelines on the Care of Laboratory Animals and Their Use for Scientific Purposes. IV. Planning and Design of Experiments. (1990). Laboratory Animals Science Association and Universities Federation for Animal Welfare (UFAW), Potters Bar, United Kingdom. ISBN 0-900767-68-5. 21 pp. Available for £ 2.50 from UFAW, 8 Hamilton Close, South Mimms, Potters Bar, Herts, E6 3QD, United Kingdom.

Australian Code of Practice for the Care and Use of Animals for Scientific Purposes. (1990). Australian Government Printing Service (AGPS), Canberra, ISBN 0-644-10292-6. 75 pp. Available free from the AGPS, GPO Box 84, Canberra ACT 2601. Contents include principles and responsibilities of investigators, institutions, ethics committees, and teachers; and a bibliography.

ILAR News. A quarterly publication for biomedical investigators, laboratory animal scientists, institutional officials for research and members of animal care and use committees. Available free from the Institution of Laboratory Animal Recources, 2101 Constitution Avenue NW, Washington DC 20077-5576.

DESIGN OF CANDIDATE RADIOPHARMACEUTICALS

IDENTIFICATION OF CLINICAL NEED

The first step is the identification of the fundamental questions and the clinical needs relevant to understanding physiological function and the biochemical and/or molecular basis of disease process. Ultimately the goal is development of new or improved diagnostic methods and treatment. Considerations for the assessment of new radiopharmaceuticals were recently outlined (Patterson and Sisner, 1995).

Table I presents a cross-section of 44 recent examples of the use of imaging modalities and a particular radiotracer for the study of specific biochemical processes and disease states in biological models including humans. Table I is a representative of investigations undertaken at various laboratories. Table I is not intended to be comprehensive. Further examples that focus on design and evaluations of candidate radiopharmaceuticals are the subject of several recent reviews (Maziere and Maziere, 1991; Mazoyer, Heiss and Comar, Eds, 1993; Crouzel, Guillaume, Barre', Lamaire, and Pike, 1992; and Maziere, Coenen, Halldin et al, 1992).

CHOICE OF RADIONUCLIDE

The choice of a radioisotope having appropriate nuclear decay characteristics for the intended applications, e.g. positron emission for PET; emission of 100 to 200 keV gamma radiation for SPET; beta, electron capture or alpha emission for radiotherapeutic aplications. The half life of the radionuclide should be appropriate to maximize information, and to minimize the absorbed radiation to the subject. Radionuclides having a half life of a few seconds to a few days are used depending upon the physiological process being diagnosed or treated.

- The labeled compound must be conveniently synthesized and chemically stable in vivo.
- High specific activity radiotracers are required in order to minimize pharmacological effects, and to avoid toxicological effects.
- Selection of appropriate biological models in which to screen the radiotracer in the living subject.

The process of development of a compound labeled with a radionuclide into a radiopharmaceutical involves various criteria (Schubiger and Westera, 1992).

SCREENING STUDIES

Screening studies must be performed in at least two models, such as in vitro testing and 2 or more appropriate species.

Screening data of interest to the radiopharmaceutical scientist (Pickett, 1987) includes:

- Determination of the normal bio-distribution of the radioactivity into tissues as a function of time;
- The calculation of percent uptake per gram of tissue and for the total organ;
- The determination of the target to non-target ratio's;
- The clearance times of the radioactivity of the substrate and its radioactive metabolites from the blood, etc.

The radiolabeled compound once demonstrated in biological models to meet the above criteria must be qualified through peer-review, and regulatory compliance to assure it is safe and efficious for the stated purposes before being marketed as a radiopharmaceutical for either veterinary or human use (Kristensen and Nørbygaard, 1987).

DRUG DEVELOPMENT

Another aspect of radiopharmaceuticals is their application for drug development and evaluation. An EEC Concerted Action on the investigation of cellular regeneration and degeneration resulted in a symposium addressing the communication gap between researchers and the radiopharmaceutical industry was sponsored by both the European Commission and by the European Federation for Radiopharmaceutical Sciences. The development of new drugs is a long and expensive process. Some lead compounds fail due to toxicity or adverse effects, or lack of efficacy. The development time of drugs can be shortened through either labeling the candidate compound and tracing its pharmacokinetics and metabolism with emission tomography; or through studies with established radiopharmaceuticals to ascertain biological effects of drug action, i.e. alteration on blood flow, local glucose or oxygen metabolism, tissue pH, receptor sub-type specificity, and pharmacological interactions under physiological or pathological conditions. The proceedings will appear in a future volume of the Series in Nuclear Medicine, Peter Cox, Series Editor, published by Kluwer Academic, Dordrecht.

Table I. Examples of radiotracers and imaging to study physiologic processes and human disease using biological models

Target	Model	Imaging	Tracer	Reference
5HT$_{2A}$ receptor	Baboon	SPET	^{123}I-new ligand	Terriere et al., 1995
Angiotensen-converting enzyme	Rat, human	PET	^{18}F-fluorocaptopril	Hwang et al., 1991
Antipsychotic drug action	Baboon	PET	^{18}F-BMY 14802	Ding et al., 1993
Basal ganglia visualization	Primate, human	SPET	^{77}Br-spiperone	Friedman et al., 1982
Benzodiazepine receptor	Baboon, Macaca mulatta	SPET	^{123}I-Ro16-0154	Innis et al., 1991
Beta adrenergic receptor	Rat	γ-camera	^{123}I-iodocyanopindolol	Sisson et al., 1991
	Dog	PET	^{76}Br-m-bromobenzylguanidine	Valette et al., 1993
	Human	SPET	^{123}I-m-iodobenzylguanidine	Sisson et al., 1987
C-erb2 Protein overexpression	Nude mouse	PET	^{124}I-ICR12	Bakir et al., 1993
C-myc oncogene mRNA for progression of malignancy	BALB/c mice with mammary adenocarcinoma		^{111}In-DTPAAHON	Dewanjee et al., 1995
Cardiomyopathy	CM and RB strain hamster	ARG	^{131}I-DMIPP, ^{14}C-DG, ^{201}Tl	Kubota et al., 1988
Cerebral metabolism and blood flow	Cat	PET	^{15}O-tracers	Heiss et al., 1995
	Cat	PET	^{38}K	Duncan et al., 1984
	Baboon	PET	^{62}Cu-PTSM	Mathais et al., 1990
Cocaine binding in brain	Baboon	PET	^{11}C-cocaine	Volkow et al., 1995
Cocaine-induced myocardial ischemia	Dog	SPET	^{201}Tl	Oster et al., 1991
Colorectal carcinoma	Rat, hamster, baboon	PET	^{64}Cu-1A3-F(ab')$_2$	Anderson et al., 1995
Differentiation of intratumoral granulation tissue + cancer cells	C3H/He mice with FM3A and MH134 tumors	Micro-ARG	^{18}F-FDG, ^{3}H-glucose	Kubota et al., 1995
Dopamine transporter	Baboon, ovariectomized	SPET	^{123}I-βCIT, ^{123}I-IPCIT	Scanley et al., 1995
	Rodent, monkey, human	PET	^{18}F-GBR13119	Kilbourn et al., 1989

Table I. (Continued)

Target	Model	Imaging	Tracer	Reference
Dopamine D1 receptor	Baboon	PET	^{11}C-A69024	Kassiou et al., 1995
Dopamine-D$_2$ receptor	Baboon	SPET	^{123}I-iodolisuride	Loc'h et al., 1991
	Baboon, MPTP-intoxicated	PET	^{76}Br-bromolisuride	Hantraye et al., 1992
	Beagle dog	PET	^{11}C-YM-09151-2	Hatazawa et al., 1991
	Human	PET	^{11}C-spiperone	Wagner et al., 1983
Dopaminergic, 5HT, opiate, benzodiazepine, cholinergic receptors	Non-human primates, human	PET	^{11}C-, ^{18}F-, ^{75}Br-ligands	Maziere & Maziere, 1991
Extrastriatal D$_2$ dopamine receptor	Cynomolgus monkey	PET	^{11}C-FLB 457	Halldin et al., 1995
Function of neuropeptides	Rhesus monkey	PET	^{11}C-metenkephaline	Hartvig et al., 1986
GABA neurotransmission	Normal and epileptic baboons	PET	^{11}C-flumazenil	Maziere et al., 1992
Gastrointestinal bleeding	Sheep	SPET	^{99m}Tc-DTPA	Owunwanne, 1988
Histamine H$_1$ receptor	Baboon, human	PET	^{11}C-pyrilamine	Villemagne et al. 1991
Hyperthermia-induced suppression of protein synthesis in tumors	Rat	PET	^{11}C-tyrosine	Daemen et al., 1991
Hypoxia	Dog, rabbit, swine, mice, in vitro cardiac myocites	SPET	^{123}I-, ^{99m}Tc-, ^{18}F-nitroimidazoles	Nunn et al., 1995
	Rat	ARG	^{125}I-Tisch, ^{125}I-IBZM	Zouakia et al., 1994
Inflammatory process, chronic	Rat	ARG	^{18}F-FDG	Yamada et al., 1995
Lung vascular permeability	Dog	PET	^{15}O-water	Velazquez et al., 1991
Lung water measurement	Dog	PET	^{68}Ga-transferrin	Mintum et al., 1987
Metabolism of ^{13}N-ammonia	Dog, transplant patients	PET	^{13}NH$_3$	Bormans et al., 1995
Muscarinic cholinergic receptor	Greyhound dog	SPET	^{123}I-N-methyl-4-iododexetimide	Hicks et al., 1995

Table I. (Continued)

Target	Model	Imaging	Tracer	Reference
Muscarinic cholinergic receptor	Beagle dog	PET	^{11}C-CGP 12177	Valette et al., 1995
	Rat	ARG	[125]I-(RR-IQNB) (R)-quinuclidinyl-(R)-4-Iodobenzylate	Gibson et al., 1985
	Rat, baboon (Papio anubis), pigtail monkey (Macaca nemistrine)	PET	^{11}C-TRB(+)-2α-tropanylbezitate	Mulholland et al., 1992
	Baboon (Papio papio)	PET	^{11}C-quinuclidinylbenzylate	Varastet et al., 1992
Myocardial ischaemia	Dog	SPET	^{99m}Tc-BSM-181321	Shi et al., 1995
Myocardial sympathic innervation	Cynomolgus monkey	PET	[11]C-(-)-norephinephine	Farde et al., 1994
Na$^+$/K$^+$-ATPase	Dog	PET	[38]K$^+$	Lambrecht et al., 1978
Osteosarcoma	Dog	PET	^{18}F-TP-3 Fab' fragment	Page et al., 1994
Penile bloodflow	Baboon (Papio ursinus)	SPET	^{99m}Tc-red blood cells	DeBruin et al., 1991
Presynaptic dopaminergic terminals	Baboon (Papio papio)	PET	^{18}F-fluoro-L-Dopa	Hantraye et al., 1992
Radiation synovectomy	New Zealand rabbit	γ-camera	[188]Re-colloid	Wang et al., 1995
Radioimmunotherapy planning	Mouse	PET	[124]I-3F8 MAb	Pentlow et al., 1991
Radiotherapy planning, liver	Pig	SPET	[166]Ho-microspheres	Turner et al., 1994
Septic shock	Baboon (Papio ursinus)	γ-camera	^{111}In-tropolonate platelets	Dormehl et al., 1991
Striatal uptake	Cynomolgus, Rhesus monkey	PET	^{18}F-6-fluorodopa	Pate et al., 1991
Targeted radiotherapy	Athymic rat	SPET	[211]At-astatide	Johnson et al., 1995
Thrombus detection	Baboon, rabbit	γ-camera	^{99m}Tc-DD-3B6/22 Fab'	Walker et al., 1991

CONCEPT OF BIOLOGICAL MODEL

One consideration for this volume is to provide researchers with a sourcelist of biological models as a part of the experimental design. "An animal model of a disease is only as useful as the questions we ask of it." (Reid, 1980). The selection of proper biological models is a prerequisite particularly for investigations of the pathogenesis and treatment of disease (Kawamata and Matsushita, 1987; Davidson et al., 1987).

The development of drugs and radiopharmaceuticals requires interdisciplinary cooperation and collaboration. The bridge scientists that link chemistry, biology, medicine and medical physics rely upon experimental studies in animals as the prelude to human evaluations. The choice of the biological model for which initial experimentation can influence the conclusions down from the first preliminary studies. Many chemists have worked with an enthusiastic medical specialist, who requests a particular candidate radiotracer and has then abandoned the project after one set of animal experiments not yielding anticipated results. Some feel this may happen when the radiochemist relies too heavily upon another specialist on the team to select the biological model or design the experiment. All members of the team have a responsibility in the selection of the biological model.

There are several acceptable ways to describe a biological model, all of which are intended to represent models of human disease. Figure 2 depicts the inter-relationships of the various types of biological models. The diagram is practically self-explainatory.

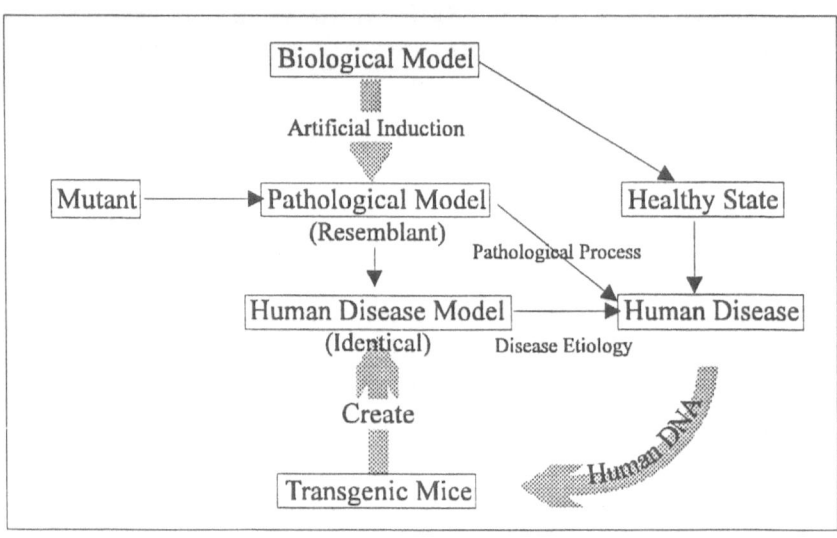

Figure 2. Concept of biological models. (Derived from Nomura et al., 1987)

A biological model arises from the comparative biological, i.e. physiological, similarities are used as the basis of the human disease condition. Resemblant pathological models arise either from chemically or surgically-induced conditions, or from naturally occuring mutants that resemble the disease in humans. The optimum biological model has an etiology of disease that is identical in mechanism to that found in humans. There are a substantial number of animal models that spontaneously arise, that are considered as good or potential models of the human condition.

Identical pathological models arise in nature, and can also be developed in transgenic mice through manipulation and transplantation of gene components into mouse embryos. The resultant transgenic mice carry the DNA molecular information and represent identical models of human disease.

With the advent of molecular genetics in the 1980's there has been a significant interest in genetic diseases. The location of 1800 genes on specific chromosomes of about 50,000 genes are known, and 4000 genetic disorders have been identified for the human genome now known to arise in humans, that are classified as "in-born errors of metabolism" or "experiments of nature".

During the time since Bradley et al (1984) demonstrated that it was possible to permanently and precisely modify genetic information by introducing foreign DNA (genes) into the genome of animals, there has been a dramatic surge in basic knowledge of pathological and physiological processes.

It is anticipated that transgenic mice will see increasing role in future radiopharmaceutical development. There are several sources of transgenic and SCID mice including the Jackson Laboratory, Bar Harbour Maine, and the Cancer Studies Unit, Queens, Medical Centre, University Hospital, Nottingham, UK. Attention: Dr. Susan Watson, Fax: 44-602-513412.

Rats and mice have contributed substantially in many areas of biomedical research such as cancer research, pharmacology, immunology, genetics, physiology, aging, cardiovascular and neurosciences (Gill et al., 1989; Jonas, 1984). Rodents are typically used in the limited biodistribution studies with labeled compounds. A reason for this is that each time point in a biodistribution study usually reflects the measurement of the radioactivity concentrations in tissues of 3-5 rodents, and generally 5 or more time points are determined. Rodents are economical to acquire and maintain and they are breed for biomedical research purposes.

Melby (1987) points out that models are analogs which possess similar or identical functions and structures as the system being studied. So biological models of closely related species are generally the best homologues, but the phylogony is not completely understood or predicted. The similarity can be genetic or evolutionary. For example, certain metabolic pathways are shared by many species at cellular and molecular levels.

Table II is intended as a succint listing of recent books and reviews that summarize the understanding of animal models and trends in their use to study specific topics. The publications make interesting and informative reading. Overviews of the development and utilization of animal models available in the United States (Melby, 1987), Australia (McNeill, 1980) and in Japan (Kawamata, 1984; Miyajima, 1984) and the prospects for new models (Nomura, 1987) complement the detailed information available to assist researches. The most significant advances have been made with genetically defined models (Smithers, 1993). Jones (1982) noted the increased number of animal models of inherited disease in which a defective enzyme was identified and found to be chemically identical to the affected enzyme. The deficient enzyme seemed always associated with a defective gene, also identified in a species in addition to humans such as gangliosidoses, specific inherited defects in blood coagulation, and several in-born errors of metabolism. The application of radiopharmaceuticals to the study of in-born errors of metabolism is predicted to be a fruitful activity. For example, Danks and Camakaris have made pioneering breakthroughs in understanding Menkes´ Disease (Kinky Hair Syndrome) which is associated with a deficiency of copper during development of the fetus. The Menkes´ gene has now been cloned in the mouse (Names, 1993). Copper-64 ($T_{1/2}$ = 12.4 h) and copper-67 ($T_{1/2}$ = 67.2 h) have been applied to study copper metabolism.

Driscoll and collaborators (1992) presented an excellent discussion of genetically defined animal models of neurobehavioral dysfunctions such as alcoholism, depression and consumption of, and addiction to, cocaine and other hallogenic drugs. Clinical investigations have only recently been initiated, although there is a considerable body of animal research literature that may lend insight to the observations made using radiolabeled cocaine in baboons (Volkow et al., 1995).

Non-human primates are used as biological models because baboons and monkeys are the nearest relatives of humans, and they share many biologic, biochemical, physiologic and immunologic similarities (King and Yarbrough, 1985; McClure, 1984). For example non-human primates and humans are susceptible to many of the same diseases such as AIDS, tuberculosis and malaria. Non-human primates are in many cases excellent models for investigation of specific diseases and drug development research with radiopharmaceuticals in combination with medical imaging techniques. For example, when radiopharmaceutical scientists have a priority to address tropical diseases such as Yellow fever, Ebola, Malaria, or complex diseases such as amyloidosis, then non-human primates have to be considered as appropriate models.

IN VITRO MODELS

Animal models have been used to develop *in vitro* assays that in turn have resulted in reduction of the use of animal models for routine testing. Two examples are cited.

The limulus amebocyte lysate (LAL) test is a method that utilizes the lysate of amebocytes from the blood of the horseshoe crab, Limulus polyphemus, as an acceptable method for the detection of endotoxins in drugs and radiopharmaceuticals. The LAL test is based on the formation of an opaque gel by pyrogens where the gelation observed is related to the endotoxin concentration. The *in vitro* kits are commercially available, can be used with a 0.1 ml of test samples, and typically yield results in 25 - 60 min. Cooper (1975, 1985) is credited for showing the sensitivity, reproducibility and advantages of the *in vitro* LAL test as an improvement over using rabbits for pyrogen testing. The rabbit test requires i.v. administration of the drug on a dose/weight basis into the marginal ear vein of 3 rabbits whose body temperature are monitored for 3 hours. In the rabbit the dose of endotoxin required to give a positive result was 0.011 g/kg of E. coli or 0.021 g/kg of Klebsiella endotoxin, while the Limulus lysate detected 0.001 g/ml of E. coli or 0.0001 g/ml of Klebsiella. The advantage of *in* vitro testing over *in vivo* testing is clear.

When the objective is to develop a radioligand that is specific to a receptor or sub-type receptor, the investigators should strive to conduct some *in vitro* assays as an early step in the biological evaluation process. In order to facilitate the rational development of drugs, the National Mental Health Institute (NIMH) Psychotherapeutic Drug Discovery & Development Program of the United States National Institute of Health (NIH) funds the project to provide IC_{50} data in both graphic and tabular form on lead compounds that are screened against a bank of receptor types. There is no charge to the investigators, and the information is confidential to the investigator for an agreed period of time. The services offered by Nova Screen are valued by investigators that do not have the facilities to conduct such assays in-house.

For information contact:

NovaScreen,   7170 Standard Drive, Hanover, MD 21076 - 1334
Attention: Scott Perschke, Manager   Fax: 410 - 712 - 4412

However, *in vitro* data does not yield sufficient information in itself to be sufficient to establish a new drug or radiopharmaceutical. *In vitro* assays are a significant aid in structure-activity such that the number of animal studies necessary can be rationally restricted to detailed *in vivo* studies only with the more promising lead compounds. In the case of radiopharmaceuticals IC_{50} may suggest that a radioligand has a high affinity for a specific receptor, but the value tells nothing about the non-specific binding of the radioligand in surrounding tissue. The use of "adjuncts" is too be encouraged, if they are found to be better or equal to animal model systems (Melby, 1987). *In vitro* assays can not replace the use of biological models, because of the complexity of the living biological system (Boobis et al., 1987; Thore, 1987).

CHOICE OF BIOLOGICAL MODELS

Figure 3 was derived by examining the abstracts dealing with the radiopharmaceutical sciences, and summarizing the frequency each type of biological model was mentioned in the abstract. Many abstracts reported that two biological models were utilized in the studies. It is significant to note that *in vitro* assays were mentioned in 17.7 % of the abstracts. Dogs, rabbits and sheep (12.8% of the abstracts) were used models, when surgery is performed in acute experiments. Non-human primates (10.5% of the abstracts) reflects a general impression that investigators with high resolution PET and SPET instruments prefer to utilize baboons and Rhesus monkey's for pharmacokinetic and bio-distribution studies where death is not an end-point.

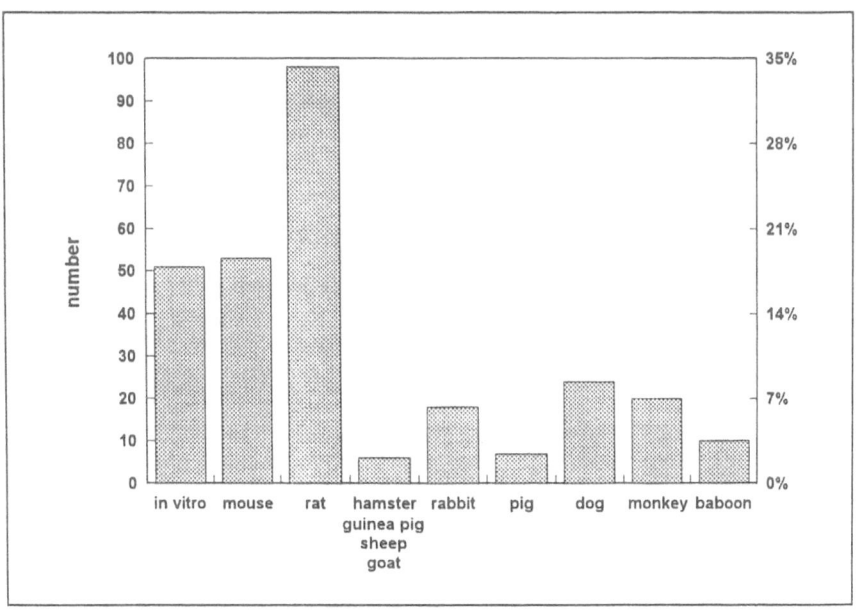

Figure 3. Choice of biological models for radiopharmaceutical development based on abstracts presented at the 42nd Annual Meeting of the Society of Nuclear Medicine, 12 - 15 June, 1995. J Nucl Med. 36:1P-328P.

Science published revised figures on primate research in the 30 March 1990 issue. For drug abuse studies involving primates the citations averaged 15.6 a year in 1977 through 1979, raising to 18 a year in 1986 to 1987, and dropping to 7.8 a year in 1988 through August 1989. The use of primates in research on depression was about 5 citations a year in the mid-1980's, but dropped to 0 between 1988 and 1990 (Holden, 1990). The *Science* report (1990) was based upon a computerized search of the National Library of Medicine, *MEDLINE*. There can be a difficulty locating all appropriate citations on a given model studied for a given purpose depending upon the choice of keywords chosen to search any given file or database. For example, our searches of multiple citation services (not just *Medline*) indicated there were several studies reported in the time frame where radiolabeled ligands in non-human primates were used for studying receptor density, eg. dopaminergic receptors thought to be associated with depression (Coenen, Wienhard, Stöcklin et al., 1988; Barrio, Satyamurthy, Huang et al., 1989; Dewey, MacGregor, Brodie et al., 1990; Fowler, Volkow, Wolf et al., 1989; Kleven, Anthony, Woolverton et al., 1990). Likewise, the unintentional omission of an important publication involving selection of biological models for radiopharmaceutical development may have occured in the finalization of this resource volume. The significant progress in development of compounds labeled with short-lived positron-emitting radionuclides, and the availability of high resolution PET instrumentation in the 1990's yields new insights in biomedical research. These factors seem to account for the increased usage of non-human primates in 1995.

Rodents are commonly used for the initial screening of labeled compounds as potential radiopharmaceuticals. Mice and rats represented 42.6 % of the abstracts in the Figure 3 survey. The frequency of citations using rodents was 49% in 4758 abstracts published in the 1981 issue of *Federation Proceedings* (Lambrecht, Rescigno and Eckelman, 1983). Rodents are often used because they are less expensive to breed, purchase and maintain than larger animal models.

Only a few examples are given, because it would require a series of volumes to illustrate all the interesting examples. The reader is referred to the extensive compilation presented in Table 3 for a classification of disease states and biological models.

SPECIES VARIATIONS

Species differences and the applicability of data from one biological model to another is not well understood (Kore, 1990; Calabrase, 1988; Fritzberg, 1995). Complex factors influence the relationship between pharmacokinetic behavior of drugs across species, and two approaches to interspecies scaling have emerged. The allometric approach involves using the pharmacokinetic profiles as described by compartmental analysis and solution of a power equation. The semi-empirical equation $Y = aW^b$ where Y is the physiologic variable of interest, W is the body weight, and log a is the y-intercept and b is the slope obtained from the graph of log Y vs log W. The power equation has been applied to demonstrate drug elimination kinetics, and is sometimes used to predict pharmacodynamic profiles in humans (Mordenti, 1986; Yates and Kugler, 1986). McAfee and Subramanian (1983) used a power equation to describe the blood or plasma disappearance and the whole body retention of renal radiopharmaceuticals to calculate the animal-base time to human-equivalent time. In the allometric approach each species is viewed in terms of physical similarity of organ size and function, body weight, and a similarity of physiological process between species. Interspecies scaling of regional drug delivery requires knowledge of the relevant inter-compartment transport parameter (Dedrick, 1986).

In the physiologic approach, a model is established by reducing the physiological, biochemical, and anatomical parameters to descriptors such as blood flow, enzyme activities, protein binding, metabolic rates, enzyme kinetics, etc. Physiologic models are preferred when the details of drug distribution (biodistribution) are important, when the central compartment is not the site of action, when protein binding is strong and/or non-linear, when tracer is lipid soluble and extensively metabolized, and when pharmacokinetic data can be obtained in only one species. Physiologic models derived from biological models are scaled to make a priori predictions to the human species (Mordetti, 1986). For details on physiologic modeling and radiopharmaceutical tracer kinetics see Lambrecht and Rescigno (1983).

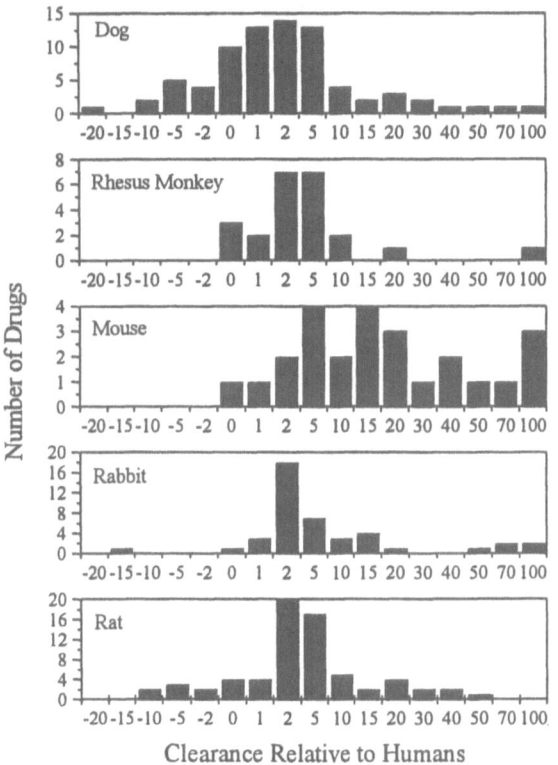

Clearance Relative to Humans

Figure 4. Systemic clearance of drugs in selected species normalized to body weight relative to humans, where 1 is the same as humans. (Derived from Smith D.A., 1987)

The clearance of drugs and radiopharmaceuticals and the uptake by specific organs are the major variables between species. In drug development compounds are studied on the basis of the physiologic chemistry in various species relative to humans. For example, Figure 4 illustrates the systemic clearance of a number of drugs in rodents, rabbits, dogs, and Rhesus monkey relative to humans. Although there are exceptions, usually drugs clear faster in all species with the drug clearance ratios of humans being 2 to 10 times greater in Rhesus monkey, rabbit and rodent; and 1 to 10 times greater in the dog. Although cardiac output and organ blood flow generally show an inverse relationship to body weight of the species - so the blood flow is in the order of mouse, rabbit, monkey, dog and man. If blood flow was the controlling factor, then one would expect a number of drugs to clear 1 to 3 times faster in the dog, and 4 to 6 times faster in the rat. With the example drugs in Figure 4 they all have a high hepatic extraction (Smith, 1987). There are large variations amongst species. Benzodiazepines are a group of drugs that usually show major differences, e.g. camazepan has a liver extraction value of 0.07 in humans, and 0.88 in the rat. The dog shows a surprising number of instances where if the drug contains a lipophilic carboxylic acid substitution clears more slowly than in humans. The class of drugs are cleared in humans by oxidation and by acyl glucuronidation. The dog depends upon acyl glucuronidation or taurine conjugation to clear the drugs. In extreme cases, such as with proxicromil, where conjugation is prevented by the pKa of the carboxylic acid, then biliary excretion is sole clearance process. (Smith, 1985). In general, due to inability to hydroxylate some carboxylic acids, the dog shows a lower relative for the drugs than does other species. The tendency, or lack thereof, to oxidize certain drugs by the cytochrome P-450 isoenzymes is dependent on a charged group, the conformation and sterochemistry of the drugs and metabolites influence the pharmacokinetics across species. Many inter-species variations and observations are not well-explained. Calabrese (1986) addressed the question of extrapolation of the specific biological model to the much more narrow spectrum of human responses.

A significant number of reports of unexplained species differences observed in the pursuit to develop radiopharmaceuticals follow specific processes in the myocardium. Bretylium had a high uptake in the heart of the rat, dog, and pig, while the uptake was nil in male stump tail monkeys and humans (Counsell et al., 1974). It was suggested that the monkey and man do not possess "uptake 2" mechanisms. Deutsch et al. (1981,1982) synthesized a ^{99m}Tc[dmpe]Cl$_2^+$ cation that exhibited a high uptake in the heart of the rat, dog, rabbit, and monkey, but that was not taken-up by the heart of swine or humans. A plausible explanation of the mechanism accounting for the species differences was developed (Deutsch et al., 1989). Although there was transient uptake of radiotracer by human heart, trapping was not observed because of a reductive mechanism that is prominent in the human myocardium. The reductive mechanism results in a neutral ^{99m}Tc(II) species from the original ^{99m}Tc(III) cation and the ^{99m}Tc(II) escapes the heart. The mechanism is probably operative in all species, but has faster kinetics in humans. The ^{99m}Tc(I) DMPE complex is not useful for human studies because the complex exhibits very high protein binding in humans. Other ^{99m}Tc-ligands were subsequently investigated. The ^{99m}Tc-isonitrile complexes seem to lack species specificity and are now used clinically (Pendleton et al, 1984). Gerundini et al. (1986) prepared 3 different cationic trimethylphosphite complexes that give good uptake in the dog myocardium, but the myocardial uptake in humans was unsatisfactory for clinical applications. The later results were correlated with the observations of binding of the complex to the plasma of human blood, but not of the plasma of dog blood. Thakur et al. (1984) obtained promising results for other ^{99m}Tc- 1,2-bis(dimethyl- and diethyl-phosphino)ethane cations, in test animals, but unacceptable myocardial images in humans.

Kronauge et al. (1992) synthesized cationic ^{99m}Tc-(2-carbomethoxy-2-isocyanopropane)$_6^+$ that contains terminal ester groups that were included to provide a pathway for its *in-vivo* metabolism. There was uptake in the heart of the rabbit, guinea pig, and chick, but not in rat or mouse. They noted that rodent serum produced complete hydrolysis at a rate 500 times greater than observed in human, rabbit, chick and guinea pig serum. These further confirmed that the neutral lipophilic monohydrolized metabolite did not accumulate in the heart of guinea pig and rabbit. The study concluded that the varying rates of enzymatic *in-vivo* hydrolysis produced the interspecies biodistribution differences.

There is not a need presently for an improved renal function radiopharmaceutical following the development of ^{99m}Tc-MAG$_3$. However in early days ^{77}Br-bromohippuran was shown to have *in vivo* pharmacokinetics similar to ^{131}I-iodohippuran in mice and rabbits, but appeared not to be useful in studies with human volunteers (Van Wijk et al., 1983; Van Aswegen et al., 1985).

Recently ^{62}Cu and ^{67}Cu - labeled copper(II) Bis(Thiosemicarbazone) (PTSM and derivatives) complexes were evaluated in dogs and appeared to be promising as radiopharmaceuticals to quantitate tissue perfusion. The cerebral extraction of Cu(PTSM) in baboons was less then anticipated, although there was retention in the brain. A mechanism was proposed that there is some type of reaction occuring between the Cu-complex and the intracellular sulfhydril groups (Green, 1987). However, species-dependent interactions were encountered in attempts to measure myocardial perfusion in humans at high flow rates (Mathias, Bergmann and Green, 1995). The authors concluded that the interspecies variations were due to variability of strength of binding to serum albumin. The importance of protein binding is widely accepted in drug development. Comparison of the binding of drugs to human plasma and that of animal species indicates that rodents and dogs tend to have a higher free fraction relative to humans (Smith, 1987).

Krohn and colleagues at the University of Washington reported a serependous observation that ^{11}C-labeled thymidine showed little retention in the heart of mice, dogs, pigs and sheep, but that the uptake by the heart in human subjects was greater than in the patient's tumor. ^{11}C-thymidine is used to measure tumor proliferation since it is readily taken up by cells and incorporated into DNA. Based upon those results they made simultaneous injections of 2-[^{14}C]-thymidine and 2-[^{11}C]-thymidine in a non-human primate (Macaca nemestrina) and saw increased retention although lower than seen in humans. The levels of labeled thymidine triphosphate (TTP) in the heart were similar to levels seen in rapidly proliferating tissues. However the TTP radioactivity was not utilized in DNA synthesis in the myocardium. Further studies are required in order to establish the physiologic role of the pathway in the heart of primates during normal and pathological states (Shields et al., 1995).

The brain imaging radiopharmaceutical ^{99m}Tc-ECD (a derivative of N,N'-Ig2-ethylenediyl-bis-2 cystine) has a satisfactory cerebral uptake in non-human primates and humans, but was nearly overlooked for commercial development because of low uptake in brain of rodents (Walovitch et al., 1994).

TRANSGENIC MICE

We are now at the beginning of a new era for cancer research (Adams and Corey, 1991). Genetic manipulation by the introduction of the transgene (i.e. foreign gene) giving rise to stable modification of the genotype results in animals that are called transgenic. The transgenic animals are being used for enhancing our understanding of gene regulation, development, pathogenesis, and other aspects of the treatment of diseases. The most important application of transgenic technology is the creation of animal models of human disease. The potential of the technology was realized by extensive characterization of gene enhancers and promoters that permit directed expression of transgenes to specific types of cells. Transgenic models can be used to unravel the molecular mechanisms contributing to the pathogenesis of each specific disease, and to identify drugs that can abrogate the onset of disease, retard its progression, or ameliorate its symptoms (Merlino,1991). Harris et al (1993) identified that transgenic animals are increasingly being utilized as research and development tools by both industry and university researchers.

Reviewing the developments of transgenic biological models is impossible herein, due to the rapid proliferation of publications on this expanding topic. Rather, the reader is referred to the topical publications (e.g. Transgenic models, SCID mice, gene therapy, genetic models, etc.) listed in Table II.

However, the new opportunities for radiopharmaceutical development in gene therapy will be highlighted.

The developments in molecular biology during the past 10 years have resulted in fascinating technology for localization of specific sequences of nucleotides was accomplished using in situ hybridization with DNA, RNA fragments or messenger RNA (mRNA) labeled with ^{125}I, ^{32}P and other labels. In DNA probing a specific nucleotide sequence reacts with a specific DNA or mRNA antisense oligodeoxynucleotide probe. Piwnica-Worms (1994), Stein and Cheng (1993) outlined strategies applicable to design antisense radiopharmaceuticals for the purpose to directly image specific genes.

Radiolabeling of antisense oligonucleotides for in situ hybridization were developed with histone4 mRNA in pig and human brain (Dewanjee et al, 1991; 1992), hematopoietic cells and mechanistic studies of membrane and intracellular retention (Dewanjee 1993; 1995).

Liu et al (1993) used a dual label of ^{32}P-antisense DNA (67 mer) complementary to ^{3}H-labeled asiolo-human alpha-1 acid glycoproteins in Sprague Dawley rats. They reported that the asiologlycoprotein may be an effective vector for delivery of antisense oligonucleotides for diagnosis and treatment of the modulation of expression of hepatic secretory proteins involved in inflammation and the inhibition of the expression of oncogens in primary liver tumors.

Dewanjee et al (1994) were the first to demonstrate the feasibility of *in vivo* imaging with radiolabeled antisense probes of c-myc oncogen mRNA in BALB/c mice bearing a transplanted mammary adenocarcinoma. The oncogen c-myc is involved in the signal transduction pathways leading to cellular proliferation.

Wiebe et al. (1995) are exploring ^{123}I-labeled antivirals with a high affinity for virus-encoded enzymes such as HSV-thymidylate kinase. Preliminary results were reported. They labeled E-5-(2-iodovinyl)-1-(2-deoxy-2-fluororibofuranosol)uracil to detect viral gene expression in Herpes simplex encephalitis.

Urbain et al (1995) concluded cancer cells which express a given oncogen are suitable targets for development of an unique class of antisense radiopharmaceuticals, and for the development of chemotherapeutic drugs, such as suggested by Ratajcak et al (1992) for the in vivo treatment of human leukemia in a SCID mouse model.

DOGS AND KANGAROOS

Dogs are usually used in cardiovascular research studies on experimental coronary artery occlusion, although pigs are used also. There are differences in coronary collateral circulation between both species. Pigs do not develop epicardial anatomoses, and the dog has limited ability to develop endocardial collaterals. Humans develop collaterals in the deep endocardial plexus as well as in the other regions of the myocardium. Flameng et al. (1986) examined the transmural distribution of myocardial infarction and collateral flow between dogs and baboons, and concluded that the dog is the better model. DeBoer et al. (1983) developed a flow-and-time-dependent index of ischemic injury after experimental coronary occlusion and reperfusion whith emphasis on the subendocardium where severe ischemic injury is anticipated during the first hours of coronary occlusion. A method for creating left-to-right shunts in infant pigs was described (Mavrouds et al., 1983). The pigs developed palpable thrills, murmurs and congestive heart failure. Improved biological models are needed to study the process of thrombus formation, infarction, and clot lysis. New physiological models are needed to study the progression of myocardial ischemic injury after coronary occlusion are needed (Hood, 1983). For example radiopharmaceutical intended for clinical evaluation for detecting of myocardial viability should include studies in an experimental model of myocardial infarction (Patterson and Eisner, 1995).

A notable demonstration of an elaborate in-vivo canine model of partial coronary occlusion and pacing induced demand ischemia was recently described (Shi, Sinusas et al., 1995). The model was selected to stimulate stress-induced ischemia as it may occur in patients with critical coronary artery disease (CAD). Uren et al. (1993) had demonstrated altered coronary vasodilator reserve and metabolism in myocardial subtended by normal coronary arteries in patients with single vessel CAD. Uren et al. (1993) noted that atrial pacing in patients with a critical coronary stenosis also produced alteration of regional metabolism in both the remote non-ischemic and ischemic regions of the heart.

Shi et al. (1995) reported for a ^{99m}Tc-labeled nitroimidazole positive imaging agent for detecting of myocardial ischemia. The investigators developed an improved biological model of myocardial ischemia in a dog with a partial coronary stenosis and proved stress-induced ischemia measured by coronary arterial pressure gradients, eg. regional venous lactate concentrations, wall thickening, and regional myocardial blood flow. The uptake of the radiotracer concentration in heart and liver was measured *in vivo* with a γ-camera, and the intact left ventricle was imaged by SPET. The study showed the relationship between the radiotracer concentration and blood flow.

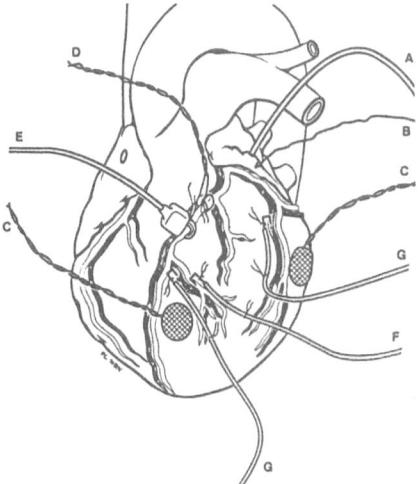

Figure 5. Illustration of heart surgical preparation and instrumentation for a model of partial coronary occlusion and pacing-induced demand ischemia. (A) Left atrial catheter, (B) atrial pacing wire, (C) Doppler thickening crystals, (D) Doppler flow probe, (E) hydraulic occluder, (F) distal coronary arterial catheter and (G) coronary venous catheters. The arterial and venous catheters were secured to the heart at two locations after vascular puncture. (Reproduced by permission of the Society of Nuclear Medicine from: Shi et al., J Nucl Med 1995;36:1079. Figure 1)

Figure 5 illustrates the surgical preparation and arrangement of the instrumentation on the heart of the anesthetized dog (Shi, Sinusas et al., 1995). The details of the apparatus are not given here. However, the salient point is that the instrumentation permitted monitoring of distal LAD pressure without compromise of distal flow. The catheter system permitted selective sampling of the distal coronary veins, and facilitated evaluation of the regional myocardial metabolism. Atrial pacing produced regional dysfunction in the central ischemic region associated with a decrease in regional lactate production and a decrease in oxygen consumption. Atrial pacing in the presence of a stenosis of the LAD also produced regional hypokinesis and altered metabolism in the remote non-ischemic left circumflex territory.

The balance of this section cites examples on the selection and preparation of biological models for studies of heart diseases. In reality, certain animal models may not be really available to a given researcher. Other investigators may have unique resources available but are not able to use them. For example, O'Rouke, Avolio and Nichols (1986) serendipitously observed in a study of 14 anaesthetized kangaroos, that 10 developed ventricular fibrillation and died. In seeking a reason for this, similarities were noted with hypertrophic cardiomyopathy in humans. The condition is the most common cause of ventricular fibrillation and sudden death in young subjects and athletes. The condition in humans is characterized by left ventricular hypertrophy powerful systolic left ventricular contraction, delayed diastolic left ventricular relaxation, decreased diastolic left ventricular compliance, and susceptibility to sudden death resulting from ventricular fibrillation. The aethiology is unknown and there is no known specific treatment. Just as with patients with this conditions, kangaroos have unexplained left ventricular hypertrophy and are known to be susceptible to sudden death with excitement and exertion. A disparity was reported between the duration of mechanical systole and electrical activation caused by a type of incomplete tetanus to develop with ventricular extrasystoles. The kangaroo may be a useful biological model for studying the fatal rhythm disturbance and abnormal ventricular dynamics in human hypertrophic cardiomyopathy.

O'Rouke et al. (1987) noted investigations of the mechanisms and relationships of ventricular hypertrophy, of ventricular vibrillation, of delayed relaxation, and of the unusually short ventricular refractory period were delayed by a state government moratorium on research with animals native to Australia. By contrast in 1992 kangaroo meat was introduced in supermarkets for human consumption in the same state.

Inbred turkeys are naturally occuring models of cardiomyopathy with inducible vetricular arrhythmias. Syrian hamsters with congestive cardiomyopathy have found some application in radiopharmaceutical development (Kubota et al., 1988; Takatsu et al., 1995).

POISON ARROW FROG

The Ecuadorian "Poison arrow" frog Epipedobates tricolor, of the Dendrobatidae family is an example of a biological model that yielded lead compounds for drug development. The skin extracts of the poison arrow frog has yielded a new class of alkaloid that has 500 times the potency of morphine in the Straub-tail analgesic assay, but the affinity for the opiate receptors in receptor binding studies was only 1/8000 of morphine (Spande et al., 1992). Natoxone, a general opiod antagonist, does not seem to reverse the analgesic effects (Qian et al., 1993). The skin extracts of 750 frogs were used to characterize the structure of epibatidine (exo-2-(2-chloropyridin-5-yl)-7-azobicyclo-[2.2.1]heptane. In view of the usual observations, several investigators successfully undertook the synthesis of epibatidine (Dehmlow, 1995). Quian et al. (1993) found that epibatidine was about 120 times more potent, and of longer duration, than nicotine in analgesia, which could be antagonized by pretreatment with mecamylamine. Also epibatidine competed for [^{3}H]-cystine binding (IC$_{50}$ = 70 pM, K$_i$ = 43 pM) in rat brain preparations. Sullivan et al. (1994) reported that epibatidine acts through nictonic acetylcholine receptors (nAChR) mechanisms in both *in vivo* and *in vitro* assays. They reported epibatidine differentiated between the two major sub-units in the neuromuscular receptor that is classically defined as a level of mentally regulated ion channel protein. The analgesic activity of epibatidine was also considered using the molecular modeling computer program SYBYL (Brandt and Barth, 1993). Epibatidine serves as novel pharmacological lead compound to probe nAChR function further. Since (+), (-) and (d,l) epibatidine can be prepared in the laboratory, and purchased from Research Biochemicals International (RBI), additional frogs are not required to further exploit the exciting possibilities suggested for analogs of epibatidine. For example, activation of nAChR's can elicit functional responses such as neurogenic control of cerebral blood flow (Linville et al., 1993) and neurotransmitter release (Wonnacott et al., 1990). Behaviorally (-) nicotine reverses impaired cognitive performance (Decker et al., 1992); has anxiolytic-like properties (Brioni et al., 1993); and improves cognitive functions such as memory and learning (Levin et al., 1992).

Radiolabeled epibatidine has been prepared and very preliminary biodistribution results in rodents have been presented at conferences that encourage potential applications of the substrate or analogs for application with PET and/or SPET imaging of the nAChR (London et al., 1995; Scheffel et al., 1995; Patt et al, 1995). Our approach has been to use molecular modeling to predict the structure of an appropriate radiolabeled analog of epibatidine prior to pursuing studies in biological models (Gündisch and Lambrecht, 1995).

GIRAFFE

The book *Animal Models in Radiotracer Design* (Lambrecht, Rescigno and Eckelman, 1983) called attention to an intriguing example of lack of understanding of the regulation of cerebral circulation in the giraffe. The animal's brain is about 8 feet above its heart, and the hydostatic equivalent of 8 feet is 200 mm Hg. Does the animal have either essential hypertension or cerebral ischemia when it is standing up. Van Citter (1973) noted even more exciting possibilitites when the giraffe bends down for a drink, or when it raises its head very suddenly.

The question was subsequently studied in detail (Hargens Millard, et at., 1987). The investigators measured blood pressures and blood flows by insertion of transducers and catheters placed into eight male and female giraffes in Africa. The models were sedated during the catherizations, and for the measurements they were stationary and upright. In addition four models were out-fitted with a radiotelemetry system mounted at the base of the giraffe's neck. Measurements were made over a day and night while the giraffes were free to move and alert. It was concluded that the tight skin and layers of connective tissue of the legs of the animal provide a type of antigravity suit that prevents pooling of blood and tissue fluids. The pressure gradient down the jugular vein was about 10% of that expected in a standing column of blood and in the opposite direction. Clearly further investigations are necessary. These results do not support a theory that the circulations above heart level depend on a siphon-like action. Other observations now available include that the giraffe's veins and lympharthatics have a one-way valve that apparently controls venous capacitance and propel blood and peripherial lymph upwards against a gravitational pressure gradient. The animal also has low-permeability capillary membranes to retain intravascular proteins. The giraffe has a novel way to adapt to the high gravitational pressure in its cardiovascular system.

Table II. Selected topical books and reviews on biological models in biomedical research

Topic	Reference
Aging	Mohr, Dungworth & Capen, 1992
AIDS	Kindt, Hirsch, Johnson et al., 1992 Letvin, Hunt & Finberg, 1984 Letvin & King, 1991 McClure et al., 1990 Racz, Letvin & Gluckman, 1993 Salzman, 1986 Spertzel, 1989
Alcoholism	Altshuler, 1981 Collins et al., 1993 Dole, 1986 Eriksson, 1980
Allergic Models and Cytokines	Bittleman & Casale, 1994
Alzheimer´s Disease	Antal & Bodis-Wollner, 1993 Smith, 1988
Amnesia and Dementia	Cohen & Eichenbaum, 1993 Dickson & Vanderwolf, 1990
Animal Models - Relevance to the Clinic	Craig, 1993
Antiviral Chemotherapy	Field & Brown, 1989 Hsiung & Chan, 1989
Anxiety	Griez, 1984 Harris, 1989
Arrhythmia Models	Cheung et al., 1993
Arteriosclerosis	Bush & Verlangieri, 1989 Fekete, 1993 Jokinen, Clarkson et al., 1985 Likar & Robinson, 1985 Prichard, 1985 Ross & Agius, 1992
Arthritis	Heymer, Spanel et al., 1982 Kerwar & Oronsky, 1989 Sokoloff, 1984
Asthma	Karol, 1994 Saetta, Fabbri, Daniel et al., 1989 Smith, 1989
Autoimmune Diseases	Druet, 1990

Table II. (Continued)

Topic	Reference
Autoimmune Diseases	Siegel, Katsumata et al., 1990
Amyotrophic Lateral Sclerosis	Appel et al., 1991
Behavior	Davey, 1983 Overmier & Burke, 1992
Biological Models	Balk, 1987 Spindleruv, 1987, 1988 Bynum, 1990 Wekerle et al., 1994
Biological Response Modifiers	Talmadge et al., 1984
Biomedical Research	Hendrikson & Koeter, 1991 Kawanta & Melby, 1985 Proceedings, 1987 Sokoloff & Smith, 1983
Blood Brain Barrier	Davson, 1993
Bone Physiology	Zallone, 1993
Brattleboro Rat Model	Valtin, 1982
Cancer	Boone, Kelloff & Malone, 1990 Hinrichs, Fontes, Bills et al., 1991 Ito & Shirai, 1986 Thompson, 1993
Cancer and Immunodeficiency Disorders	Shen, Lu & Broxmeyer, 1990
Cancer, Bladder	Raghaven et al., 1986
Cardiomyopathy	Matsumori & Kawai, 1983 Nagano, Takeda & Dhalla, 1994
Cardiovascular Research	Flameng et al., 1986 Garcia, 1984 Gross, 1994 Jokinen et al., 1985 Shi, Sinusas et al., 1995
Cartilage	Malemud, 1993
Cat Atlas	Reinoso-Suarez, 1961
Cell Transplantation	Sanberg, Wictorin & Isacson, 1994
Central Nervous System	Tauber, 1986

Table II. (Continued)

Topic	Reference
Cerebral Ischemia	Benavides et al., 1990 Hossman, 1991
Cholinergic Denervation	Smith, 1988
Colitis and Colon Carcinoma	Clapp, 1993 Newberne & Naus, 1986 Pories, Ramchurren et al, 1993 Stevens et al., 1986
Creutzfeldt-Jakob Disease	Tateishi, 1989
Degenerative Joint Disease	Adams & Billingham, 1982
Demyelination	Rodriguez et al., 1987
Depression	Harris, 1989 Richardson, 1991 Vogel, Neill, Hasler et al., 1990 Willner, 1991
Diabetes	Bach & Boitard, 1986 Sarvetnick, 1990
Diabetic Pregnancy	Baird & Aerts, 1987
Diving-related Illness	Murrison, 1993
Dog Model	Gay, 1984
Drug Addiction	Boulton, Baker & Wu, 1992 Hutchings & Dow-Edwards, 1991
Drug Development	De Lemos & Kuell, 1987 Harris, Davis, Jowett et al., 1993
Duchenne Muscular Dystrophy	Kakulas, Howell & Roses, 1992
Eating Disorders	Smith, 1989
Edemas	Zelter & Dougvet, 1986
Emphysema	Snider, Lucey & Stone, 1986
Encephalopathy	Wennberg, 1993
Epilepsy	Avanzini & Marescaux, 1991 Biriere & Chambon, 1987 Buchhalter, 1993 Le Gal, Le Salle et al., 1983 Schwartzkroin, 1993

Table II. (Continued)

Topic	Reference
Fetal Disease	Nathanielsz, 1985
Frustration	Amsel, 1992
Gene Therapy	Aguzzi et al., 1994 Briand, 1989 Kakulas et al., 1992 Yoshida & Wilson, 1992
Genetic Diseases	Clarke, 1994 Copp, 1994 Crabbe et al., 1994 Driscol, 1992 Minor et al., 1987 Smithies, 1993
Genetic Evaluation	Arnold, 1992
Glomerulonephritis	Furness & Harris, 1994 Hoedemaeker, 1991
Graft Studies	Bergqvist & Jensen, 1985
Gunn Rat Model	Chowdhury, 1993
Haemopoiteic Malignancies	Adams & Cory, 1991
Hematologic Disease, Inherited	Kaneko et al., 1987
Hemorrhage in Neonate	Kisker, 1987
HSV-Induced Petinitis	Zierhut, 1994
Human Cancer Risk, Evaluation of	D'Amato, 1992
Huntington's Disease	Anosa & Kaneko, 1983 Sanberg, Wictorin & Isacson, 1994
Hyperlipidemia	Paigen et al., 1994
Hypertension	Lovenberg, 1987 Yamori, 1991
Hypoxia	Stefanovich, 1979
Immunotherapy, Targeted	Bluethmann, 1994 Rosen & Seligmann, 1993 Ross & Steele, 1984
Immunological Process Models	Hay, 1982

Table II. (Continued)

Topic	Reference
Inherited Metabolic Disorders	Desnick & Patterson, 1982
Intrauterine Growth Retardation	Evans et al., 1983
Intestinal Disease	Pfeiffer, 1985
Ischemic Stroke	Garcia, 1984
Kidney Disease	Velasquez et al., 1990
Leprosy	Job, 1993 Johnstone, 1987 Martin, Gormus, Walf et al., 1984
Lesh-Nyhan Syndrome	Jinnah, 1990
Lysossomal Storage Disease	Alroy et al., 1989
Liver	Cornelius, 1993 Goldin, 1994 Iancu, 1993 Rojkind & Greenwel, 1993
Lung Carcinogenesis	Coggle, 1991
Memory	Amsel, 1992 Cohen & Eichenbaum, 1993
Mental Retardation	Anderson, 1994
Mesotheliomas	Ilgren, 1993
Metabolism in Newborn Infants	Mehta, 1989
Metabolism, In-born Errors of	Desnick & Patterson, 1982 Desnick et al., 1982 Gerrity & Friedman, 1982 Jones, 1982 Proceedings, 1982
Mouse Model	Jonas, 1984
Myopia Development	Achiron, 1986
Neurobehavioral Dysfunctions	Driscoll, 1992
Neurodegeneration	Benavides et al., 1990
Neurological Disorders	Aguzzi et al., 1994 Boulton, Baker et al., 1992 Woodruff & Nonneman, 1994

Table II. (Continued)

Topic		Reference
Neuropsychiatric Disorders		Proceedings, 1983
Non-Human Primates	- Brain Atlas	Riche et al., 1988
	- Benefits	King & Yarbrough, 1985
	- Chimpanzee	Eder et al., 1994
	- Cotton Top Tamarin	Clapp, 1993
	- Gorilla	Gould & Bres, 1986
	- Models	McClure, 1984
	- Monkey	Ghonien, Shoukry et al., 1994
	- Resources	National Center, 1992
NON-Mouse Model		Sakamoto, Hotta & Uchida, 1992
Numerical Compentence		Boysen & Capaldi, 1993
Nursing Research		Cunningham & Mitchell, 1982
Nutrition and Neonatal Infections		Harris & Douglas, 1990
Nutritional Dependent Disease		Workshop, 1983
Obesity		Fuller & Yen, 1987
		Proietto & Thorburn, 1994
Ocular Disease		Rank & Whitlum-Hudson, 1994
		Tabbara, 1984
Oral Candidiasis		Allen, 1994
Oral Drug Delivery		Crouthamel & Sarupu, 1983
Osmoregulary Disturbances		Van Leeuwen, 1992
Pancreatitis		Goke, 1990
		Lerch & Adler, 1994
		Working Group, 1987
Parkinson's Disease		Antal & Bodis-Wollner, 1983
		Zigmond & Stricker, 1989
Perinatal Development		Gartner & Allonso, 1993
		Rudolph, 1993
		Ruprecht, Fratazzi et al., 1993
Periodontal Disease		Boyce, 1992
		Schou et al., 1993
Pigment Gallstones		Rege, Dawes & Ostrow, 1993
Pituitary Tumor		Trouillas & Girod, 1988

Table II. (Continued)

Topic	Reference
Prostate Cancer	Bosland, 1992 Pollard & Luckert, 1984 Thompson, Truong et al., 1993
Psychiatry	Keehn, 1986 McGuire, 1983 Stein, 1994 Willner, 1984
Psychopathology	Bond, 1985
Radiation Damage	Pippin, 1992
Radiation Lung Carcinogenesis	Coggle, 1991
Radiation Therapy	Loor et al., 1988
Radioimmunotherapy	Macklis, Kaplan et al., 1989 Scheinberg & Strand, 1990
Radiolabeled Monoclonal Antibodies	Aas & Fjeld, 1993 Gallagher, 1983 Shah & Sands, 1990
Radiotracer Design	Carr, 1983 Fritzberg & Bloedow, 1983 Lambrecht & Eckelman, 1983 Mathias & Welch, 1983 McAfee & Subramanian, 1983 Nunn, 1992 Pickett, 1987 Wiebe, Turner, Franko et al., 1991
Rat Model	Gill et al., 1989
Renal Cell Carcinoma	Rangel & Pontes, 1989
Renal Cystic Disease	Resnick, 1981
Renal Failure	Ash & Thornhill, 1985 Friedman, Mehls et al., 1986 Gretz & Strauch, 1993
Reproduction	Serio & Martini, 1980
Respiratory Distress Syndrome	Lachmann, 1989 Reid, 1980
Retinal Degeneration	Hollyfield et al., 1993

Table II. (Continued)

Topic	Reference
Reye's Syndrome	Deshmukn, 1985 Kilpatrick-Smith et al., 1989
Rodent Tumors	Workshop, 1985
Schizophrenia	Feldon & Weiner, 1992
SCID Mouse Model	Hendrickson, 1993
Self Reactivity	Ferrick et al., 1994
Self-Destructive Behavior	Crawley, Sutton & Pickar, 1985
Senile Dementia	Campbell, Sananes & Gaddy, 1984
Skin	Hecker, 1993 Sundberg, 1994
Stroke	Garcia, 1984 Karpiak, Tagliavia et al., 1989
Swine Model	Swindle, Moody & Phillips, 1992
Tardive Dyskinesia	Casey, 1984 Drombowski & Kovacic, 1983
Targeted Mutagenesis	Bluethmann & Ohashi, 1994
Tinnitus	Evans, Wilson & Borerwe, 1981 Jastreboff & Sasaki, 1994
Toxicology	Calabrese, 1984 Gad & Chengelis, 1992
Tracer Kinetics and Physiologic Modeling	Lambrecht & Rescigno, 1983
Transgenic Mice Model	Adams & Cory, 1991 Basset-Seguin et al., 1992 Lathe & Mullins, 1993 Merlino, 1991 Wagner & Theuring, 1993
Transplantation research	Cramer, Podesta et al., 1994 Mueller-Sieburg, 1992 Paul, 1993
Vascular Disorders	Mathias & Welch, 1983
Vasculitis	Bishop, 1989

TOMOGRAPHIC PHYSIOLOGICAL CHEMISTRY

ARG

Autoradiography (ARG) is the classical way of measuring the deposition of carbon-14 and tritium labeled tracers in an animal. ARG has contributed significantly to our understanding of life processes and to development of radiopharmaceuticals. The most important example to radiopharmaceutical science and molecular nuclear medicine is the work of L. Sokoloff and his colleagues to develop the ^{14}C-deoxyglucose method for the measurement of local cerebral glucose utilization (Sokoloff, 1977; Sokoloff, Reivich, Kennedy, et al. 1977; Sokoloff and Smith, 1983; and others). I recall, Sokoloff advised a group of scientists including M. Reivich, D. Kuhl, A. Wolf, J. Fowler, A. Alavi and myself in a small conference room at the University of Pennsylvania on 19 December 1973, that 2-deoxyglucose would be an ideal tracer for "in vivo autoradiography" if labeled with a "gamma-emitting radioisotope". Sokoloff's prediction proved correct in August 1976 when the first tomographic image of the living brain of humans was obtained using the Mark III SPECT camera developed by D. Kuhl at Penn (Reivich, Kuhl, et al., 1979; Reivich and Alavi, 1983). Tatsu Ido (while a guest scientist in 1975 at Brookhaven National Laboratory, New York, from the National Radiological Institute, Chiba, Japan) persevered to assure the first successful synthesis of fluorine-18 labeled FDG (Ido et al., 1978) using fluorine-18 labeled molecular fluorine as the synthetic precussor which was first described by Lambrecht and Wolf (1973). FDG has subsequently been applied to 1000's of patient studies, and was approved for general marketing in the USA in August, 1994.

Table I lists some examples of ARG investigations in biological models for radiopharmaceutical development.

The time-consuming aspects of ARG is one of its limitations, but the most serious disadvantage is that each animal serves to provide information at a single time, because death is an end-point of the experiment. Recent advances in the development of Bio-imaging instrumentation facilitates rapid data collection of thin-tissue slices to measure radioactivity distribution in tissue with a resolution of 0.1 mm even with positron-emitting radionuclides.

SPET

SPET (or SPECT), i.e. Single Photon Emission (Computed) Tomography, is a non-invasive medical imaging instrument that is widely used in clinical nuclear medicine. Even though it is not yet pratical to reconstruct SPET images to give quantitative measurements of local metabolic rates in terms of mg substrate per gram of tissues; the tool does allow the pharmacodynamics of radiopharmaceuticals to be readily determined. Very high quality tomographic images can be obtained that refect the distribution of radioactivity throughout an organ, and the whole body parameters such as blood clearance, and displacement of radioactivity from receptors are easily studied.

Receptor theory can now be applied to neuroreceptor measurements through functional imaging with emission tomography (Kerwin and Pilowsky, 1995). An example is cited.

Muscarinic cholinergic receptors (mAChR) mediate the parasympathetic effects of the heart, leading decreasing the force of contraction, and to slowing in the rate of contraction. Cardiac disease associated with altered muscarine receptor density and function include diabetis mellitus and heart failure. A canine model of impaired cardiac muscarinic receptor function has been described (Vater et al., 1988). Hypersensitivity of mAChR is believed to precede the development of autonomic neuropathy in rats treated with streptozotocin to induce diabetes mellitus (Carrier and Aronstam, 1987). Biodistribution studies of [^{123}I]-N-methyl-4-iododexetimide in rats indicated a high cardiac uptake (of 2.4 % of the injected dose per gram of heart tissue), and the ratio of activity in the heart to lung was 5:1 at 10 minutes after injection. The specificity and steroselectivity of binding in the heart was demonstrated using blocking experiments in rats. Imaging studies performed in rabbits confirmed the significant uptake of the radiotracer by the heart, which was consistent with biodistribution studies in rats.

Figure 6 and 7 illustrate the applicability of SPET for dynamic imaging the myocardial muscarinic receptors of an anaesthetized greyhound dog with the novel radioligand [^{123}I]-N-methyl-4-iododexetimide (Hicks et al., 1995). The uptake by the myocardium was rapid and high while the uptake in the lungs was stable and low. Heart to lung ratios of 2.5:1.0 were observed between 10 and 30 minutes post-injection. The administration of an excess of an unlabeled muscarinic antagonist, methyl-quinuclidinyl benzylate rapidly displaced the activity in the heart to background levels (see Figure 6). The SPET images showed a clear delineation of the myocardium (Figure 7). Both the left and right ventricle was demonstrated with little blood pool or adjacent lung activity. Using three sequential cardiac short-axis images at the mid-ventricular level, the heart to lung ratio was calculated to be about 14:1.0. There was greater uptake in the inferior wall than in the anterior wall. The calculated inferior to anterior left ventricular activity ratio was 1.3:1.0. Post-mortem examination of the myocardium revealed no evidence of thinning of the anterior wall of the left ventricle or of coronary artery disease to explain the regional variation of the distribution of the radiotracer. The results urge further SPET studies to characterize the distribution of muscarinic receptors in various cardiovascular diseases known to be associated with altered parasympathetic innervation.

An imaging study was performed with the pharmacologically inactive enantiomer, [^{123}I]-*N*-methyl-4-iodolevetimide as shown in Figure 8. The experiment imaging was performed in the anterior projection with an identical acquisition protocol to that used in the studies using , [^{123}I]-*N*-methyl-4-iododexetimide. Unlike the above studies, there was no detectable myocardial uptake, indicating that the cardiac uptake of [^{123}I]-*N*-methyl-4-iododexetimide is stereoselective. The heart to lung activity ratio was calculated to be 1.1:1.0. There was apparent biliary excretion, supporting data in the rat and the rabbit for both the stereochemical isomers. There was also high renal uptake and retention of activity. The high renal uptake of [^{123}I]-*N*-methyl-4-iodolevetimide suggests that this binding is not receptor mediated.

PET

PET studies in biological models have proven very useful for quantitative measurements of the distribution of radiotracers, and tracer kinetic modeling of physiologic status, disease diagnosis and prognosis. Radiopharmaceutical scientists rose to the challenge to develop novel and specific radiotracers. As noted in Table 1 animal PET studies are presently focusing on radiotracer ligands with high-selective uptake and specificity for receptors. Other projects dealt with drug effects and inhibition. The 2nd generation PET instruments of the 1980's had a spatial resolution of 5-7 mm. This tended to limit studies to larger animals, eg. baboon, monkey, dog for heart and global brain investigations. Researchers at a few recognized institutions were fortunate to cooperate with instrumentation groups to test higher-resolution PET scanners for research with animals (Cutler et al., 1992; Watanabe et al., 1992; Rajeswaran et al., 1992; Marriott et al., 1994).

Scheuer et al. (1985) discussed animal preparation relevant for studies with PET.

The ECAT EXACT HR (Wienhard et al., 1994) has a spatial resolution of 3.6 mm in the plane of section and 4.0 mm axially at the center. The instrument consists of 24 detector rings equipped with 784 crystals each, covering an axial field of view (FOV) of 15 cm, which is divided into 47 continuous image planes. The facial dimension of the individual crystals is 5.9 x 2.9 mm^2, resulting in a resolution of 3.6 mm transaxially and 4.0 mm axially at the center of the FOV. By limiting data acquisition to straight planes, the axial resolution was improved to 3.5 mm.

The Advance GE PET (DeGrado et al., 1994) has 12,096 BGO crystals reviewed by Hamamatsu R1548 photomultiplier tubes in 18 rings. The crystal rings form 35 2-dimensional imaging planes spaced by 4.25 mm. Through an imaging FOV of 55 cm diameter and an axial FOV of 15.2 cm the transaxial resolution is 3.8 mm at the center and increases to 5.0 mm tangential and 7.3 mm radial at 20 cm from the center.

Heiss et al. (1995) noted that the resolution capacity of the ECAT EXACT HR scanner is approximately 1/10 the dimension of a cat brain averaging 40 x 30 mm transaxially and 50 mm in the axial direction. Consequently, this scanner can be utilized with the cat as the biological model, as long as tracer concentrations are sufficient for imaging. Figure 9 demonstrates four selected slices across a cat's brain. The functional images were in good agreement with the matched histological sections, permitting easy identification of specific structures in a stereotactic atlas (Reinoso-Suárez, 1961).

PET images of CBF, CBV, CMRO$_2$ and CMR$_{glc}$ were obtained in anesthetized cats. CBF and CMRO$_2$ images permitted the identification of the main anatomic, and CBV images of the main vascular structures within the cat's head. Optimum spatial resolution was afforded by the CMR$_{glc}$ images, which permitted clear distinction of caudate nucleus and olfactory bulb. Metabolism and blood flow values in gray matter (cortex or basal ganglia) are approximately 3-4 times higher than in white matter, thus permitting to distinguish gross anatomical structures: cat cerebral cortex has a thickness of only 1-2 mm, although it is folded into gyri and therefore appears thicker on images; basal ganglia and thalamus measure about 5-6 mm in diameter (Reinoso-Suárez, 1961) and was easily detected. The best anatomical detail was obtained with steady state FDG, nevertheless major structures can also be distinguished on blood flow and oxygen images. CBV images mainly show large vessels and basal structures and are useful for correcting OEF estimates. The values calculated for the physiologic variables were close to those obtained by ARG methods.

ARG studies gave values for CBF (Sakurada et al., 1978) and CMR$_{glc}$ (Ginsberg et al., 1977; Hossmann et al., 1985), comparable to the findings of Heiss et al. (1995). The autoradiographic CBF estimates were slightly higher in gray and slightly lower in white matter (cortex, 75-130; striatum, 70-110; cerebellum, 55-110; whitte matter, 15-53 ml/100g/min). CMR$_{glc}$ was almost identical, with the exeption of a lower CMR$_{glc}$ in white matter (cortex, 28-57; thalamus, 25-49; cerebellum, 45-54; whitte matter, 4-22 ml/100g/min). Those differences between methods was explained by partial volume effects, and by the lower spatial resolution of PET.

Figure 10 demonstrates that PET can be used to distinguish regional pathological change as a function of progression of time using the MCA occlusion model in the cat. Heiss et al. (1995) demonstrated for the first time the use of oxygen-15 radiotracers to achieve the correlation of matched histological sections and PET images in a medium-sized animal. Pappata et al. (1993) have investigated the changes of cerebral hemodynamics and metabolism in early stages of focal ischemia in the baboon using oxygen-15 tracers, but verification of pathoanatomical changes was not their major objective. Serial studies were performed after the lesion was fully developed - a circumstance similar to the clinical presentation of humans after acute ischemic stroke. Pappata et al. (1993) were somewhat restricted to global studies, because of the poorer resolution of the PET available to them.

Serial multi-tracer PET imaging for quantitative assessment of experimentally induced regional changes in oxygen and glucose metabolism in an animal as small as the cat brain validates Sokoloff's concept of "in vivo autoradiography" for imaging biochemical processes in biological models that can be applied to human disease.

The principles of radioimmunotherapy in experimental biological models was recently discussed (Scheinberg and Strand, 1990).

Page et al. (1994) demonstrated the feasibility of PET imaging in dogs with a ^{18}F-labeled Fab fragment of TP-3-antibody specific for human and canine osteosarcomas as a model for preclinical research with radioimmunoconjugates. Figure 11 illustrates the example of a study in an 8-yr-old male golden retriever that had undergone amputation to remove an osteosarcoma on the left distal radius. Thoracic radiographs indicated the presence of a 5-8-cm diameter extrapleural mass associated with the seventh rib. PET images collected, with time, show a gradual washout of activity from the blood pool was noted with increasing accumulation seen in a site corresponding to the rib metastasis. Figure 12 depicts the kinetics of the activity from the PET images in a region of interest set over the center of this lesion increased from 23 nCi/cc at 30 min to 45 nCi/cc at 150 min. The activity remained relatively constant at this level until the end of the 4-hr study. Assuming unit density for tumor, these values correspond to 1.5 and 3.0 x 10^{-3}% ID/g, respectively. The advantage of PET is that it is possible to non-invasively measure *in vivo* pharmacokinetiks and to utilize the results in models that describe metabolism, flow, tissue pH, receptor-ligand interactions, and drug response.

Emission tomography and specific radiopharmaceuticals are important in cancer detection and management for:

- localization of primary and metastatic sites of cancer
- differentiating malignant from benign lesions
- grading malignancy
- staging
- assessing the response to drugs and radiotherapy
- follow-up

Page et al. (1994) suggest that dogs with spontaneous tumors represent a more appropriate model for evaluation of radioimmunotherapeutic radiopharmaceuticals. Compiling arguments include:

- Quantitative measures of radiopharmaceutical biodistribution can be obtained mostly in normal and tumor tissues.
- The sensitivity of human and canine bone marrow to radiation is similar.
- Methods developed in normal dogs can be extended to clinical trials in dogs with spontaneously occurring neoplasia.
- The canine model is large enough to be used for dynamic imaging studies with either PET or SPET to develop radiation dosimetry estimates.
- Dogs have a larger body than rodent xenograft models. Therefore, SPET and PET offers the prospect of improving lesion detection and quantitative measures of physiologic responses of normal and tumor tissue to trial treatments.

The latest generation of commercial clinical PET instruments that display high spatial resolution in 3 dimensions, lead to realization of expanded opportunities to quantitatively image physiological variables, and to relate regional data to pathological and normal morphology (Wienhard et al., 1994; DeGrado et al., 1994). The results reported by Heiss et al. (1995) using the cat clearly illustrate that compared to techniques necessitating tissue sampling, brain slicing, implantation of electrodes or detector probes for clearance recording, high-resolution PET as a regional method for repeated, noninvasive measurements of physiological variables has clear advantages for experimental research in medium-sized laboratory animals. PET scanners are now a realistic, and a necessary tool to carry out significant radiopharmaceutical and drug development.

However, with the advent of high resolution PET and SPET tomographs it is no longer necessary to use non-human primate models based only on the size of the brain mass. Animals with medium-sized brains can be imaged with sufficient anatomical resolution of structures. In 1982 it was observed that baboons administered the neurotoxin MPTP (I-methyl-4-phenyl-1,2,3,6-tetrahydropyridine) developed many of the clinical and biochemical features of Parkinson's disease of the human species. There is a decrease in dopamine concentration by about 15% as a result of degeneration of the substantial nigra dopaminergic cells which lead to the caudate nucleus in the corpus stratum. Wagner (1993) illustrated that with imaging tomographs and radiopharmaceuticals one can differentiate presynaptic and postsynaptic neurons that are only 20 microns apart. In the brain of the baboon administered MPTP [^{11}C]-methyl-spiperone images show that the postsynaptic receptors are only slightly affected by the neurotoxin, while [^{11}C]-WIN-35-428 images show the presynaptic neurons are completely non-functional.

SIMS

Secondary ion mass spectrometry (SIMS) promises to be a powerful tool in biomedicine and radiotracer development (Clerc, Merdon et al., 1995; Fourré et al., 1992; Fragu et al., 1993). SIMS microscopy is a microanalytic tool based on the principles of the emission of secondary ions following bombardment of a specimen by a primary ion beam and analysis of the secondary ions by mass spectrometry. SIMS is the only method potentially capable of mapping all the elements including stable and radioactive isotopes. SIMS and ARG can be compared, but a limitation of ARG is that not all radioactive isotopes result in autoradiographs with acceptable sensitivity or lateral resolution. Due to filtering by mass spectrometry, all SIMS images have the same lateral resolution, irrespective of the physical decay processes of the analyzed ions being studied.

Clerc, Mardon et al. (1995) used meta-bromobenzylguanidine (MBBG) which can be used with either stable ^{79}Br or ^{81}Br, or radioactive ^{76}Br (T$_{1/2}$ = 16.8 h), and MIBG with non-radioactive ^{127}I to target neuroendocrine tumors, and to provide intratumor biodistribution and uptake informations needed for microdosimetry. The uptake and intratumor biodistribution of MBBG was illustrated in experimental PC12 pheochromocytoma grown in nude mice. SIMS mapping is depicted in Figure 13. Both MBBG and MIBG accumulated in the cytosal of the tumor cells, but a minute signal was also detected for iodine or bromine when these images were superimposed onto the phosphorous images, which essentially mapped cell nuclei.

Three-dimensional imaging is under development with SIMS microscope capable of parallel detection and a lateral resolution approaching 50 nm (Slodzian et al., 1992). It is anticipated that the SIMS analysis will assist in understanding heterogenecity of dose distribution of radiopharmaceuticals in development for therapeutic nuclear oncology using ^{76}Br and other therapeutic radionuclides.

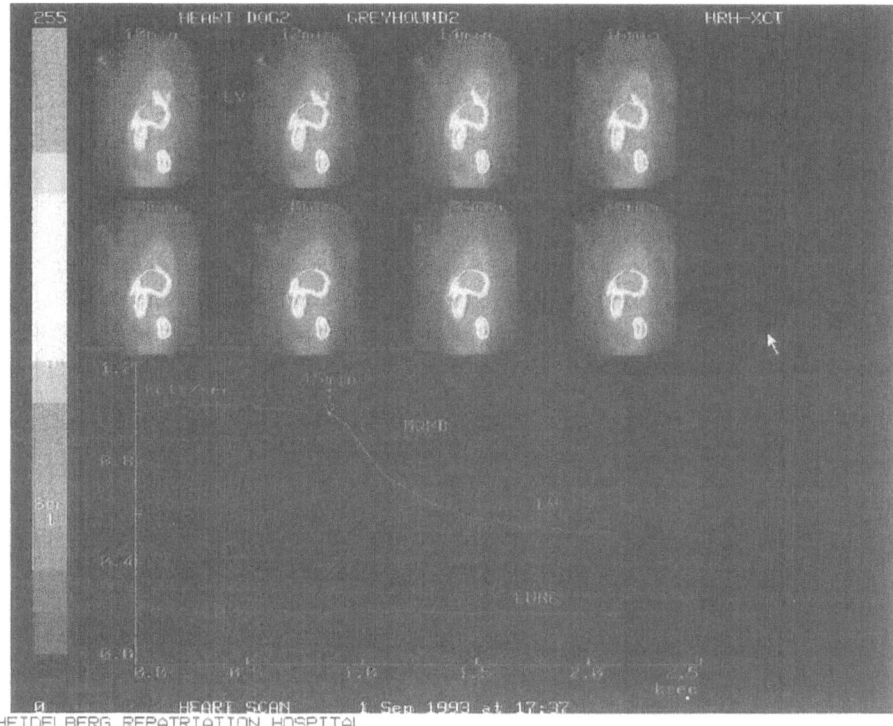

Figure 6. The administration of a muscarinic receptor antagonist methyl-quinuclidinyl benzylate (MQNB) at 15 min after injection of $[^{123}I]$-N-methyl-4-iododexetimide into the greyhound revealed rapid and qualitatively complete displacement of activity from the heart, suggesting high specific binding to muscarinic receptors. (Reproduced by premission from Hicks et al., Eur J Nucl Med. 1995;22:343, Figure 3. © Springer Verlag)

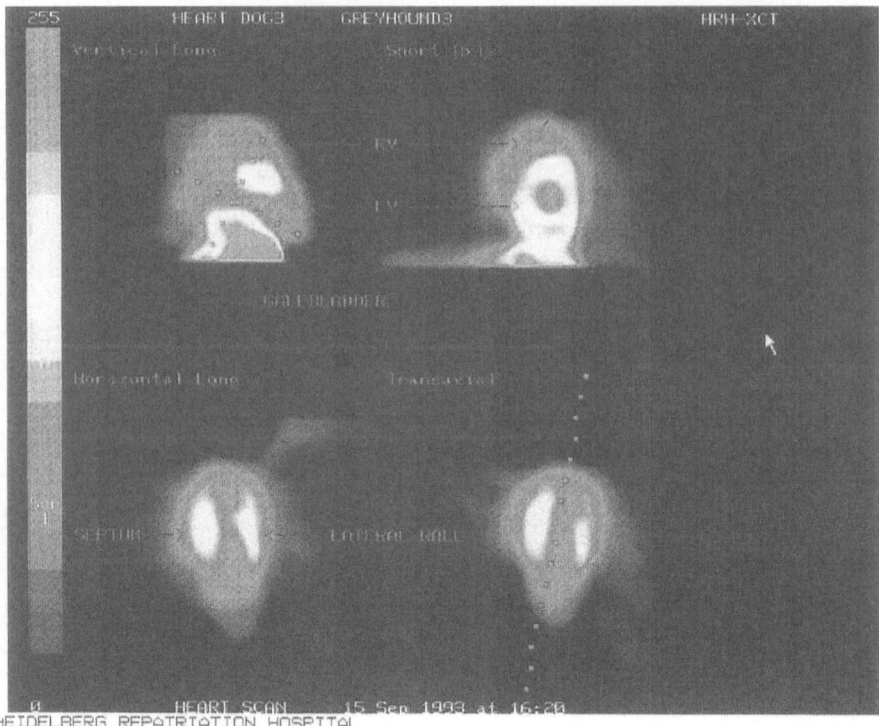

Figure 7. SPET imaging of [^{123}I]-N-methyl-4-iododexetimide revealed excellent cardiac definition in the greyhound with a myocardial to lung activity ratio of >10:1 at the mid-ventricular level. There was higher uptake of radiotracer in the inferior than in the anterior wall. (Reproduced by permission from Hicks et al., Eur J Nucl Med. 1995;22:343, Figure 4. © Springer Verlag)

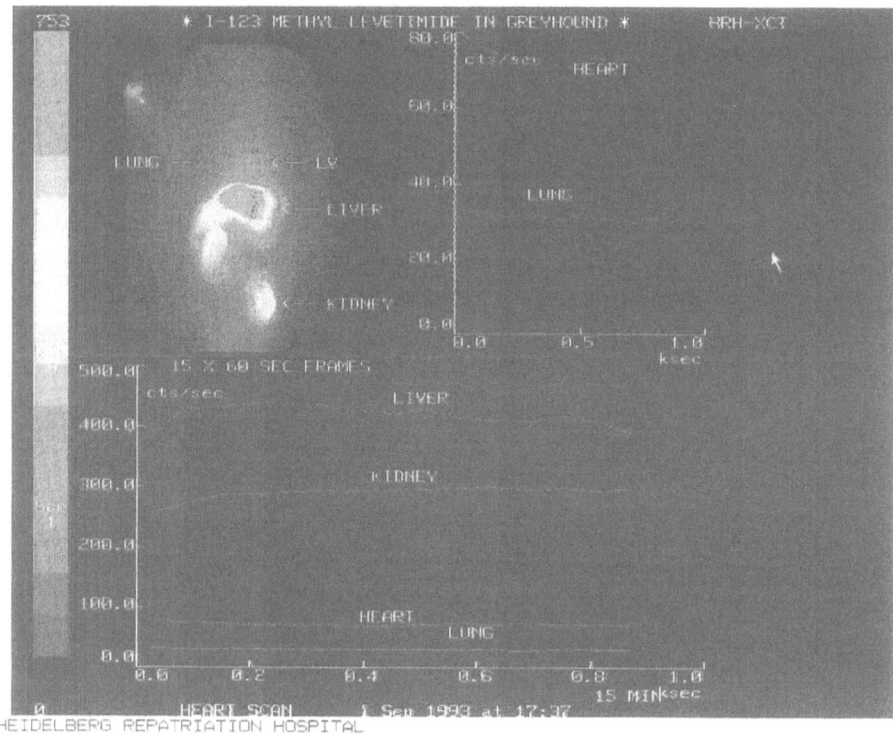

Figure 8. SPET functional imaging of [^{122}I]-N-methyl-4-iodolevetimide indicate there was no uptake of the pharmacologically inactive enantiomer in the heart of the greyhound. (Hicks, Lambrecht et al., unpublished data, 1994.)

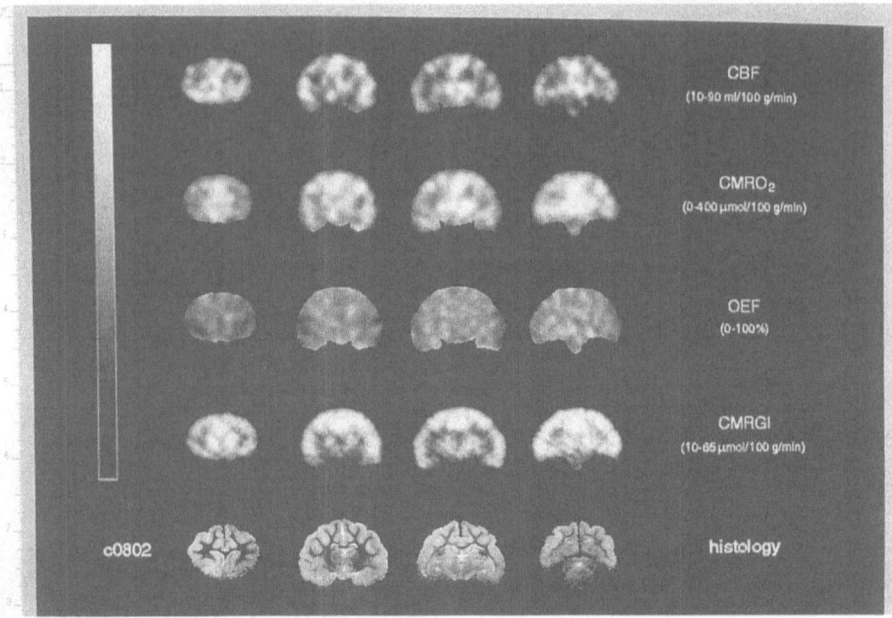

Figure 9. Matched transaxial tomographic brain sections at a 6-mm center-to-center slice distance show CBF, $CMRO_2$, OEF, CMR_{glc} (gray scale according to individual range) and histology of an anesthetized control cat administered $[^{15}O]$-O_2H_2O and $[^{18}F]$-FDG. Anatomical details are well represented particulary in CMR_{glc} and $CMRO_2$ images. (a) Anterior cortex, (b) posterior cortex, (c) caudato putamen, (d) thalamus, (e) cerebellum/brainstem and (f) white matter. (Reproduced with permission of the Society of Nuclear Medicine from Heiss et al., J Nucl Med. 1995;36:495. Figure 1)

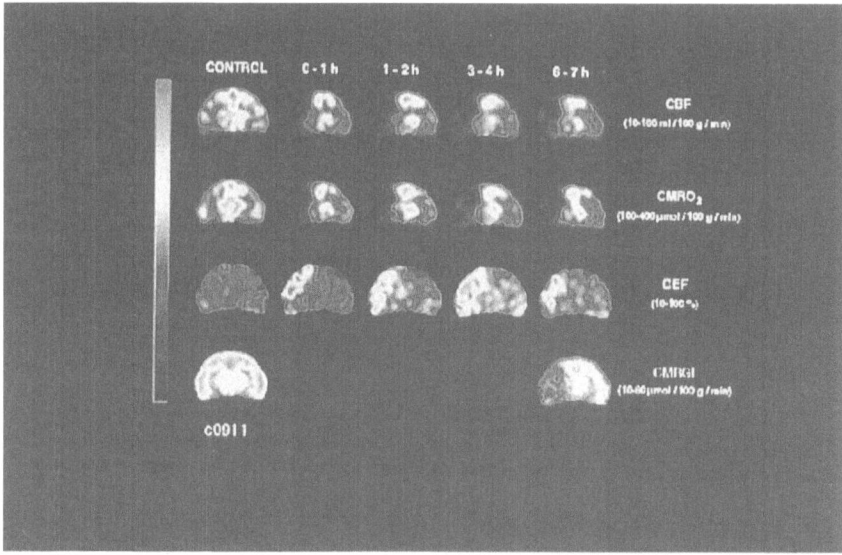

Figure 10. Matched transaxial slices in one plane at thalamic level before and at four time points after middle cerebral artery occlusion in a cat administered $[^{15}O]$-O_2 and H_2O. CBF is severely decreased immediately after MCA occlusion, while $CMRO_2$ is partially preserved because of increased OEF. Gray scale according to individual range of values. (Reproduced with permission of the Society of Nuclear Medicine from Heiss et al., J Nucl Med. 1995;36:496. Figure 2)

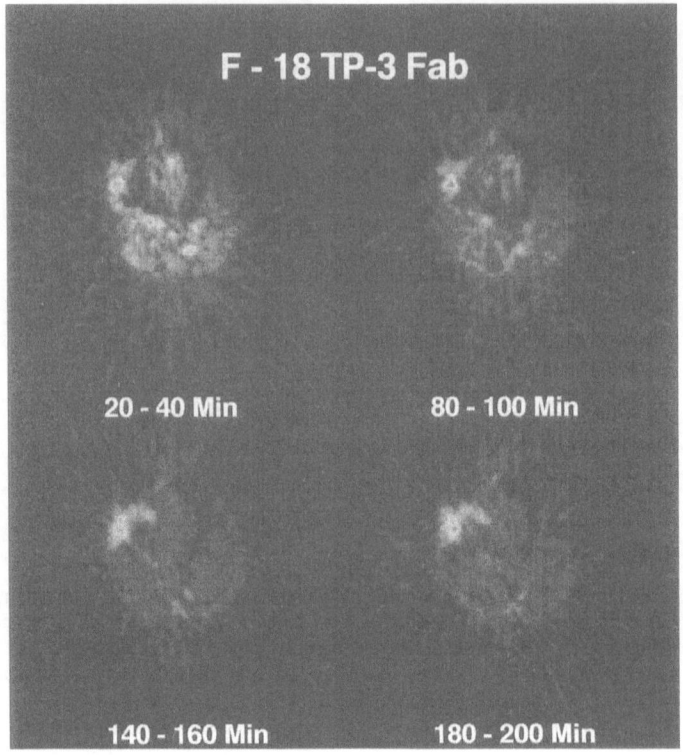

Figure 11. Selected transaxial PET images obtained [^{18}F]-TP-3 monoclonal antibody fragment during the study interval from a dog demonstrating accumulation of activity in a metastatic nodule associated with right anterior pleura. (Reproduced with permission of the Society of Nuclear Medicine from Page et al., J Nucl Med. 1995;36:1510. Figure 4)

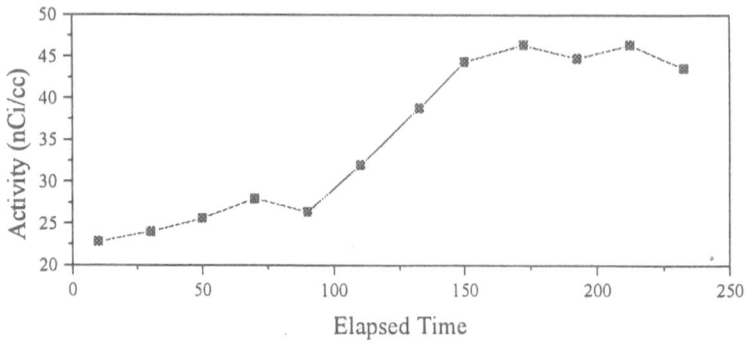

Figure 12. Activity as a function of time in the region of interest set over the center of the lesion depicted in Figure 6. (Reproduced with permission of the Society of Nuclear Medicine from Page et al., J Nucl Med. 1995;36:1510.)

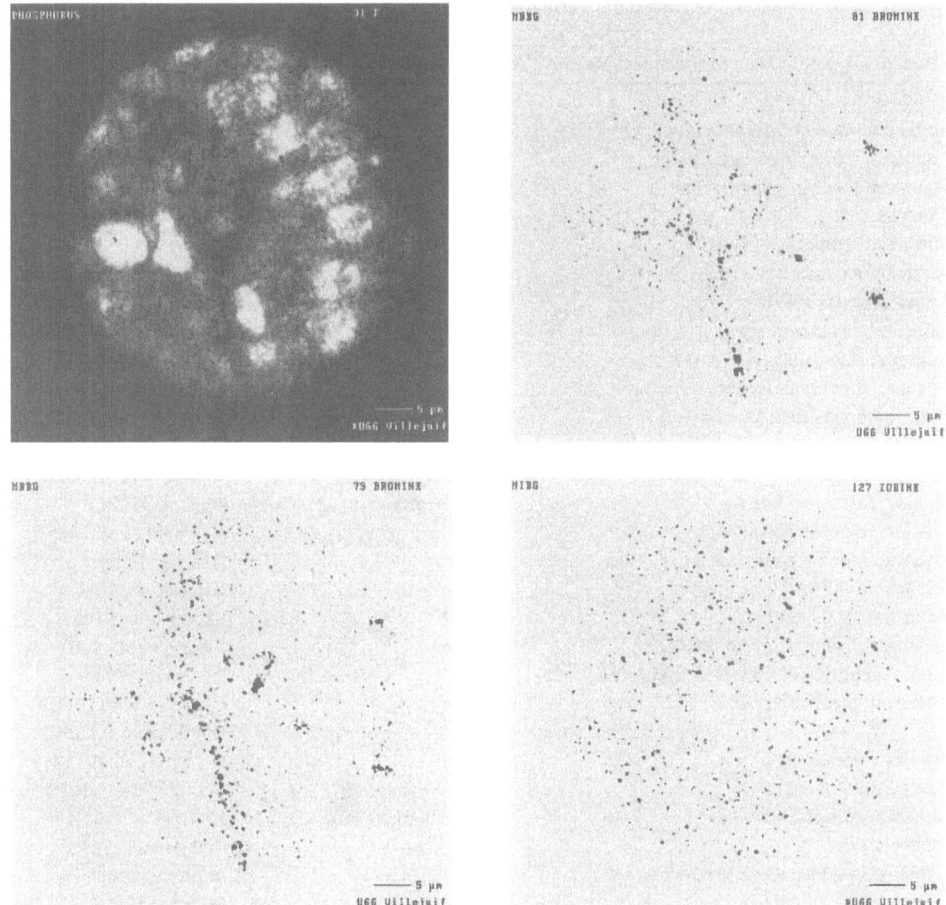

Figure 13. SIMS images of MBBG and MIBG within the PC12 xenograft after in vivo administration of 400 μg of the drugs and sample processing with cryotechniques. The phosphorus image indicates the tissue structure (A). The [^{127}I]MIBG is rather homogeneously distributed (B) compared to MBBG, which shows foci of accumulation (C and D). Since bromine has two stable isotopes of similar abundance, it is possible to map MBBG through the detection of [^{79}Br]MBBG (C) or [^{81}Br]MBBG (D). The two images are very similar and thus provide a powerful internal control for specificity detection. The minute differences observed between (C) and (D) are due to the fact that the two SIMS images are actually separated by approximately 50 nm. Image field: 60 μm. (Reproduced with permission of the Society of Nuclear Medicine from Clerc et al., J Nucl Med. 1995;36:864. Figure 6)

KEYWORD GUIDE TO SELECTION OF BIOLOGICAL MODELS

Table III. Keyword Guide to Biological Models Proposed for the Investigation of Human Diseases

Disease	Animal Model	Reference
Abdominal wall defects and cryptorchidism	Rat	Quinlan et al., 1988
Abnormal cyclic GMP metabolism	Models	Chader et al., 1987
Abnormal muscle mitochondria	Rat, in vitro	Lamperth et al., 1991
Abscess	Model	Mamedov et al., 1988
Abscess, intraabdominal	Rat	Casey et al., 1983
Abstinence syndrome	Rat	Kovalenko et al., 1984
Acanthamoeba keratitis	Wistar rat	Larkin & Easty, 1990
Accelerated senescence	SAM mice	Takeda et al., 1991
Acid aspiration	Dog	Griffith et al., 1988
Acquired immunodeficiency syndrome (AIDS)	Monkey	Letvin et al., 1983
Acquired subglottic stenosis	Dog	Supance, 1983
Acromegaly	Avian	Harvey, 1990
Action myoclonus	Model	Shohami et al., 1986
Acutely distressed fetus	Fetal sheep	Abitbol, 1993
Adenocarcinoma of rete testis	Mice	Newbold et al., 1986
Adenosine deaminase deficiency	Murine	Ratech, 1985
Adenosine receptor alterations	Pointer dog	Klein et al., 1987
Adhesion reduction	Rabbit	Linsky et al., 1987
Adrenergic nervous system function	Model	Sisson et al., 1987
Adult respiratory distress syndrome	Cat	St. John, 1991
African trypanosomiasis	Mice	Clarkson et al., 1983
	Sheep	Bouteille et al., 1988
Agammaglobulinemia	Horse	Perryman et al., 1983
Age related maculopathy	Rhesus macaque	Monaco et al., 1990
Age related mascular drusen	Rhesus monkey	Hope et al., 1992
Aged polyuria	IVCS mice	Ohba et al., 1985
Aggression and emotional stress	Model	Iumatov, 1988
Aging	Rodentia	Masoro, 1992
	WHHL-Hh rabbit	Esper et al., 1993
	Fischer 344 rat	Shimokawa et al., 1993
	Rat	Gallager & Nicolle, 1993
	Old animal	Hollander & Mos, 1986
	Models	Weindurch & Masoro, 19
Aging brain, search for drugs	Models	Pepeu et al., 1990
Aging of the isocortex	Dog	Braak et al., 1984
Aging penile vascular impotence	Chacma baboon	Bornman, 1985
Aging, body composition	Rat	Yasumura et al., 1993
AIDS	Macaca fasciaelanis	King, 1986
	Monkey	Letvin et al., 1985
	Chimpanzee	Alter et al., 1984
	Cat, chimpanzee troglodyte	Kindt, 1992
	Macaca nemestrina	Zuziak, 1992
	Macaca	Johnson & Hirsch, 1991
	Cat, goat, horse, monkey	Daristotle, 1992

Disease	Animal Model	Reference
AIDS	Cat	Shelton et al., 1990
	PBL-SCID mice	Mosier et al., 1991
	Macaque monkey	McClure et al., 1990
	Mice, human	Hersh et al., 1990
	African green monkey	Honjo, 1990
	SCID-hu mice	McCune et al., 1991
	Mice	Watson, 1989
	Rhesus macaque	Miller et al., 1989
	Models, human	Wohlhieter, 1992
	Naturally occuring models	Letvin & King, 1991
	Feline	Bendinelli et al., 1993
	Rhesus monkey	Gardner, 1989
	Mice	Mosier et al., 1988
	SCID-hu mice	Namikawa et al., 1988
	Chimpanzee	Nara et al., 1989
AIDS vaccine challenge	Primate	Warren et al., 1992
AIDS, changes due to morphine	Mice	Watson et al., 1988
AIDS, Friend leukemia complex	Mice	Soldaini et al., 1989
AIDS, leukemia and solid tumors	Mice	Shen, 1990
Air pouch inflammation	Rat	Tsurufuji et al., 1982
Airway disease	Monkey	Jackson & Eady, 1986
	Models	Wanner et al., 1982
Airway hyper-responsiveness	Models	Wanner et al., 1990
Albumin deficient + fatty strain	Rat	Shumiya & Nagase, 1984
Alcohol abuse	Mice, rat, genetic models	Crabbe et al., 1994
Alcohol consumption	Rat	Li et al., 1987
Alcohol dependence	Rat	Le Magnen et al., 1984
	Rat	Ruwe, 1986
Alcohol intake and preference	Rat	Li & Lumeng, 1984
Alcohol liver injury	Baboon	Lieber & De Carli, 1988
Alcohol research	Mice	McClearn, 1988
Alcohol tolerance development	Health rat	Tabakoff & Culp, 1984
Alcohol withdrawal	Model	Becker & Hale, 1993
Alcohol, chronic consumption	Rat	Rao et al., 1988
Alcohol, dose-specific effects	Mice	Schmidt et al., 1987
Alcohol-related cancer	Model	Mufti, 1990
Alcoholic cardiomyopathy	Rat	Hepp et al., 1984
Alcoholic liver disease	Models	Simpson & Peters, 1993
	Rodent	Goldin, 1994
Alcoholism	Rat	Burrov et al., 1983
	Mice	Dole & Gentry, 1984
	Pigtailed macaque	Clarren & Bowden, 1984
	Mice	Dole & Gentry, 1985
	Rat	Deitrich & Boher, 1984
	Models	Collins et al., 1987
	Rat	Abdrashitov et al., 1983
	Mice	Dole et al., 1988

Disease	Animal Model	Reference
Alcoholism	Rat	Vorob'eva & Geiko, 1990
	Rat	Lankford et al., 1991
	Albino rat	Vorob'eva, 1990
	Mini-pig	Osipov, 1988
	Models	Collins et al., 1993
	Rat	Vorob'eva, 1990
	Mice, rat	Tabakoff, 1983
Allergic alveolitis	Mice	Mantyjarvi et al., 1987
Allergic bronchoconstriction	Primate	Pritchard et al., 1983
	Guinea pig	Baumal et al., 1983
	Guinea pig	Montano et al., 1987
Allergic encephalomyelitis	Models	Satellite, 1984
Allergic orchitis	Murine	Kohno et al., 1983
	Guinea pig	Teuscher et al., 1983
Allergic reactions	Mice, rat, guinea pig	Nagai et al., 1990
	Guinea pig	Perpina et al., 1990
Allergy	Mice	Claman & Joffee, 1983
	Mice	Guschin et al., 1986
Alloimmune thrombocytopenia	Brown Norway rat	Mylvaganam et al., 1984
Alopecia	Rat	Holland, 1988
Alopecia aneata	DEBR rat	Michie et al., 1991
Alpha 1-antitrypsin deficiency	Pallid mice	Martorana et al., 1993
Alpha-L-iduronidase deficiency disease	Canine	Constantopoulos, 1985
Altered immunoregulation	Mice	Via et al., 1990
Altitude-induced pulmonary edema, acute	Rabbit	Ismailov, 1982
Alveolar hemorrhagic syndrome	Mice	Sakamoto, 1989
Alveolar hypoventilation	Dystrophic hamster	Schlenker et al., 1991
Alzheimer´s disease	Rat	Van den Bosch, 1984
	Rat	Pepeu et al., 1986
	Rodent	Sisodia & Price, 1992
	Transgenic models	Duff, 1994
	Transgenic mice	Price & Sisoda, 1994
	Monkey	Wenk, 1993
	Transgenic mice	Duff, 1994
	Transgenic mice	Lannfelt et al., 1993
	Model	Matsuda et al., 1990
Amitriptyline redistribution	Wistar rat	Hilberg et al., 1993
Amnesia	Rat	Lerer et al., 1986
	Monkey	Squire et al., 1988
	Models	Kameyama et al., 1986
Amniotic fluid embolism	Pregnant goat	Hankins et al., 1993
Amoebic liver abscess	Guinea pig	Gill et al., 1983
Amphetamine challenge	Rhesus monkey	Kraemer et al., 1983
Amphetamine psychosis	Rat	Lillrank et al., 1991
Amyloidosis	BALB/c mice	Ho & Fu, 1987
	Rat	Vargas & Stephens, 1983
	Transgenic mice	Araki et al., 1994

Disease	Animal Model	Reference
Amyloidosis	Mice, hamster	Gruys & Snel, 1994
	Model	Wagner et al., 1981
Amyloidotic polyneuropathy	Transgenic mice	Shimada et al., 1989
Amyotrophic lateral sclerosis	Guinea pig	Den Hartog Jager, 1985
	Mice	Appel et al., 1991
	Guinea pig	Sillevis et al., 1991
Amyotrophic leukospongiosis	Guinea pig	Votiakov et al., 1987
	Guinea pig	Kolomiets et al., 1987
	Models	Votiakov et al., 1986
	Squirrel monkey	Votiakov et al., 1985
Anaemia	Rat	Berger, 1982
Anaemia, aplastic	Rabbit	Den Ottolander, 1982
Anaerobic osteomyelitis	Rabbit	Johannson, 1991
Analgesic nephropathy	Rat	Henry et al., 1983
Anaphylactic shock	Mice	Ma, 1982
Anaphylaxis	Guinea pig	Verdier et al., 1994
Ancylostoma ceylanum infection	DSN hamster	Garside et al., 1989
Ancylostoma duodenale	Beagle, laboratory reared	Leiby et al., 1987
Andiogenetic alopecia	Macaque	Brigham et al., 1988
Androgen Insensitivity	Models	Bullock, 1986
Aneuploidy	Chinese hamster	Sheu et al., 1990
Aneurysm	Rat	Ammirati et al., 1986
	Dog	Yapor et al., 1991
Aneurysms, mural repair	Rat	Young et al., 1987
Angina coronary stenoses physiology	Dog	Momomura et al., 1984
Angiogenesis research	Mice	Gole et al., 1990
Angiotensin converting enzyme	Rat	Ibarra-Rubio et al., 1990
Anhedonia	Model	Papp et al., 1991
Aniridia-Wilms tumor deletion syndrome	Mice	Glaser, 1990
Anorexia	Mice	Maltais et al., 1984
Anoxic cardiopulmonary arrest	Pediatric model	Caputo et al., 1985
Anthelmintic model	Jird	Conder et al., 1990
Anti-anxiety drug action	Models	Treit, 1985
Anti-GMB glomerulonephritis	IgGza rat	Sado et al., 1992
Antiestrogen action	Models	Jordan, 1987
Antifilarial screening	Mice	Stables et al., 1988
Antifungal therapy	Mice	Herrera, 1982
Antigen-induced early and late reactions	Sheep	Abraham, 1988
Antiretroviral drug screening	Rat	Ohnota et al., 1990
Antitumor activity of natural products	Model	Marsh et al., 1985
Antral gastric ulcer	Rat	Uchida et al., 1991
Anxiety	Rat	Bodnoff et al., 1988
	Rat	File, 1983
	Rat	Emmet-Oglesby, 1983
	Dog	Gurguis et al., 1990
	Mice, monkey, Wistar rat	Borsini et al., 1993
	Mice	Costall et al., 1993

Disease	Animal Model	Reference
Anxiety	Wistar rat	Stefanski et al., 1992
	Mice, rat	Bill, 1992
	Rat, mice	Olivier et al., 1994
	Rat	Thiebot, 1983
	Wistar rat, Koletsky rat	Golda & Petr, 1990
	Dog	Griez, 1984
	Rhesus monkey	Skolnick et al., 1984
	Models	Lal et al., 1983
Anxiety and fearlessness	Rat	Marczynski et al., 1988
Anxiety disorders	Ethologically based mice	Lister, 1990
Anxiety neurosis	Rat	Eison, 1984
Anxiety, anticipatory	Mice	Lecci et al., 1990
Anxiety, receptor-mediated	Primate	Ninan et al., 1982
Anxiety, response to serotonergic drugs	Models	Handley et al., 1993
Anxiolytic action of GABA derivates	Model	Talalaenko et al., 1988
Anxiolytic drug action	Rat	Treit & Pesold, 1990
Aortic coartation	Puppy	Tarkka et al., 1982
Aortic regurgitation, chronic	Model	Magid et al., 1988
Aquaeductal lesions	Suckling mice	Aikawa et al., 1986
Arachnoiditis	Dog	Hoffman et al., 1983
Argentine hemorrhagic fever	Guinea pig	Oubina et al., 1984
Arrhythmia	Rabbit	Coker, 1989
	Guinea pig, etc.	Wascher et al., 1991
	Rat	Cheung et al., 1993
	Mice	Goa, 1981
Arrhythmia and infarction	Dog	Chezalviel-Guilbert, 1993
	Cat	Wetstein et al., 1985
Arrhythmia model for drug evaluation	Cat	Storozhuk, 1985
Arrhythmia, ouabain-induced	Guinea pig	Thomas & Varma, 1991
Arrhythmias in myocardial ischaemia and infarct	Rat	Curtis et al., 1987
Arrhythmias, hypoxia	Guinea pig	Dai, 1982
Arterial thrombosis	Dog	Pumphrey et al., 1983
	Rat	Cooley et al., 1992
Arteriosclerosis	Rat	Jellinek, 1982
	Macaca fasciculacis	Bush & Verlangieri, 1989
	Japanese quail	Jing, 1984
	Primate	Clarkson et al., 1985
	Golden Syrian hamster	Nikkari et al., 1991
	Rabbit	Esper et al., 1993
	Rabbit, guinea pig, rat	Wojcicki et al., 1985
	Cattle	Likar & Robertson, 1985
	Mice	Rubin & Smith, 1994
	Rabbit	Pearson, 1983
	Models	Vesselinovitch, 1988
	Japanese quail	Shih et al., 1983
Arteriosclerosis hypercholesterolemia	Rabbit	Watanabe, 1985
Arteriosclerosis obliterans	Rabbit	Murphy et al., 1992

Disease	Animal Model	Reference
Arteriosclerosis, diet-induced	Mice	Stewart-Phillips, 1988
	Gottingen miniature swine	Tanigawa et al., 1986
Arteriosclerosis, vascular	Yucatan microswine	Gal, 1990
Arteriosclerotic lumen	Dog	Spears et al., 1983
Arteritis	Mice	Nose, 1986
Artery occlusion, illiac	Dog	Kopchok et al., 1993
Arthritis	Rat	Zamma, 1983
	Rat	Coderre & Wall, 1987
	Athymic and euthymic rat	Kohashi et al., 1982
	Rat	Kerwar & Oronsky, 1986
	New Zealand white rabbit	Yamamoto et al., 1987
	Rat	Calvino et al., 1987
	MRL/LPR mice	Rordorf et al., 1987
	Mice	Wilhelmi & Maier, 1983
	Rat	Bendele et al., 1992
	Rat	Setnikar et al., 1991
	Lewis (LEW/N) rat	Wilder et al., 1991
	Rat	Mertz et al., 1991
	Rhesus monkey	Bakker et al., 1990
	Mice	Nabozny & David, 1994
	Mice	Yong et al., 1988
	Rat, rabbit	Mohr& Kirkpatrick, 1983
	Models	Trentham, 1989
	Guinea pig	Limb et al., 1989
	Rat	Hill & Yu, 1987
	Mice	Hunneyball et al., 1986
Arthritis (arthritic hip)	Sheep	Phillips & Gurr, 1989
Arthritis, antigen induced	Chediak-Higachi mice	Schalkwijk et al., 1990
Arthritis, chronic	Mice, rat	Breedveld et al., 1987
Arthritis, free oxygen cardial research	Rabbit	Linhart et al., 1990
Arthritis, type II collagen-induced	Rat	Probert et al., 1984
Arthropathy	Rhesus monkey, mice	Healy et al., 1989
Arthrosis	Models	Artlet & Gedeon, 1982
	Rabbit	Gluckert et al., 1983
Arthrosis by hyperpressure	Rabbit	Beju et al., 1986
Asbestosis	Mice	Bozekkla et al., 1983
Asphyxia	Beagle puppy	Ment et al., 1986
Aspiration pneumonia	Dog	Wynne, 1982
Asthma	Rat	Kuriyama et al., 1982
	Guinea pig	Vertes et al., 1987
	Guinea pig	Kallos & Kallos, 1984
	Models	Saetta et al., 1989
Ataxia telangiectasia	Mice	Nordeen, 1984
	Mice	Inoue, 1986
	Mice	Kaiserlian et al., 1986
Atherogenesis	Rabbit	Faggiotto, 1986
Atopy	Guinea pig	Engels et al., 1989

Disease	Animal Model	Reference
ATP-dependent hepatocanalicular transport	Wistar rat	Jansen et al., 1993
Atrioventricular block	Dog	Boucher et al., 1985
Atrophy and growth failure	Rat	Jaspers & Tischler, 1984
Atrophy of skeletal muscle	Model	Musacchia et al., 1988
Attention-deficit hyperactivity disorder	Hypertensive rat	Wultz et al., 1990
Attentional deficit	Rat	Feldon & Weiner, 1992
Atypical mycobacteria infection	Squirrel	Meissner, 1981
Autoallergic sialadenitis	C3H/He mice	Hayashi et al., 1989
Autoimmune diabetes	BB rat, NOD mice	Timsit et al., 1989
Autoimmune disease	Lewis rat	Broekhuyse et al., 1993
	SCID mice	Vladutiu, 1993
Autoimmune disease, picornavirus induced	Models	Craighead et al., 1990
Autoimmune disease, T-cell tolerance	Mice	Siegel, 1990
Autoimmune diseases	Models	Druet, 1992
Autoimmune endocrinopathy	Rat	Sternthal et al., 1981
Autoimmune liver affection	Mice	Briukhin & Grachev, 1990
Autoimmune motoneuron disease	Guinea pig	Engelhardt et al., 1989
Autoimmune myasthenia gravis	Mice	Jermy et al., 1989
Autoimmune orchitis	C3H/He mice	Itoh et al., 1991
Autoimmune renal disease	Mice	Neilson et al., 1984
Autoimmune thyroid disease	SCID mice	Volpe, 1993
Autoimmune thyroiditis	Buffalo strain rat	Cohen & Weetman, 1987
	Rat	Stott et al., 1988
	Chicken	Wick et al., 1982
	Chicken	Wick et al., 1989
Autoimmunity	RJH/Le rhino mutant	Roberts et al., 1989
	SCID mice	Hammerstrom, 1993
	DBA, C57 Bl mice	Via & Shearer, 1988
Autosomal dominant retinitis pigmentosa	Transgenic mice	Olsson et al., 1992
Axonal degeneration, central-peripheral	Rat	Ohnishi et al., 1985
Axonal transport	Rat	Medori et al., 1988
Bacertial prostatitis	Rat	Nickel et al., 1991
Bacteria-induced preterm pregnancy loss	Rabbit	Dombroski et al., 1990
Bacterial peritonitis	C57BL/6J mice	Goldman, 1991
Bacterial prostatitis, acute and chronic	Mastomys natalensis	Jantos et al., 1990
Bacterial sepsis	Rabbit	Trautmann et al., 1982
Balantidiasis	Rat	Karapetian et al., 1987
Bancroftian filariasis	Silvered leak monkey	Campbell et al., 1987
	Squirrel monkey	Campbell et al., 1987
Banti´s disease	Rabbit	Fukuda et al., 1985
Barbiturate dependence	Rat	Yutrzenka et al., 1985
Basal ganglia dysfunction	Rolling mice Nagoya	Yamaguchi et al., 1992
BB rat workshop	Bb wistar rat	Marliss, 1983
Behavioral and neurochemical change	Mice	Essnan & Essan, 1982
Behavioral changes	Rhesus monkey	Kato, 1985
Behavioral effects of interferon	Mice	Segall & Crnic, 1990
Benign prostatic hyperplasia	Transgenic mice	Tutrone et al., 1993

Disease	Animal Model	Reference
Berger´s disease (IgA nephropathy)	DdY mice	Tomino et al., 1993
Berry aneurysms of the aortic bifurcation	Rabbit	Stehbens, 1981
Beryllium-induced lung disease	Guinea pig	Barna et al., 1984
Beta-cell dysfunction	Dog	Tobin & Finegood, 1993
Beta-galactosidase-expressing melanoma	Nude mice	Dooley et al., 1993
Beta-hemolytic streptococcal infection	Horse	Powers et al., 1984
Beta-hexosaminidase	Cat	Rattazzi et al., 1982
Beta-thalessemia	Mice	Skow et al., 1983
Bile reflux	Ferret	Cabot & Fox, 1990
Biliary cirrhosis, primary	Model	Yamashiki et al., 1990
Bilirubin encephalophy	Models	Wennberg, 1993
Bilirubin glucuronidation	Gunn rat	Chowdhury et al., 1993
	Gunn rat	Chowdhury et al., 1993
Bilirubin metabolism	Sheep and rat	Nakamura et al., 1985
Biochemical research	Swine	Swindle et al., 1992
Biogenic amine defects	Dog	Mefford et al., 1983
Biological response modifiers	NCI	Talamadge et al., 1984
Biomedical research	Mice	Jonas, 1984
	Yucatan miniature pig	Panepinto & Phillips, 198
Biotindeficiency	Rat	Mock et al., 1988
Bismuth encephalopathy	Mice	Ross et al., 1988
Bladder carcinoma	Rat	Burkle et al., 1981
	Noble rat	Drago, 1984
	Noble rat	Drago & Nesbitt, 1987
	Nude mice	Keane et al., 1991
	Rodents, hamster, monkey,	Raghavan et al., 1986
	Model	Ahlering et al., 1987
Blastomycosis pneumonia	Mice	Sugar & Picard, 1988
Bleeding disorders	Models	Dodds, 1982
	Models	Dodds, 1983
Bleeding gastric ulcer	Dog	MacLeod et al., 1982
Bleeding time	Rat	Dejana et al., 1982
Blepharospasm	Cat	Klemm et al., 1993
Blood-brain barrier disruption, prolonged	Osborn mendel rat	Spigelman et al., 1983
Blood-brain barrier permeability	C57BL/6 mice	Wiranowska, 1988
	Mice	Wiranowska et al., 1988
Blood-to-tissue transport	Rat	Spence et al., 1987
Bone loss after cessation of ovarian function	Models	Rodgers et al., 1993
Bone marrow failure	W/Wr mice	Sharkis et al., 1984
Bone mass loss	Rat	Minne et al., 1984
Bone metabolism	Ovariectomized rat	Omi et al., 1992
	Rat	Seto et al., 1989
Bone physiology	Oroariectomized rat	Zallone & Teti, 1993
Bone repair	Rat femur	Barth et al., 1990
Bone resorption	Rat	Trechsel et al., 1987
Bone tumor	Dog	Pelfrene, 1985
	Mice	Shevrin et al., 1991

Disease	Animal Model	Reference
Borna disease virus	Mice	Kao et al., 1984
Bovine herpesvirus type 1 infection	Rabbit	Rock & Reed, 1982
Brain abscess	Rat	Matsuura et al., 1986
Brain ageing and dementia	Models	Sarter, 1987
Brain and pituitary gonadal disturbance	Mice	Charlton & Wood, 1992
Brain cannula tumor implantation	Wistar rat	Morreale et al., 1993
Brain development	Rat	Benesova & Pavlik, 1986
Brain dysfunction	Rat	Eisenberg et al., 1982
	Rat	Elsner, 1991
Brain edema	Rat	Takagi et al., 1983
Brain injury	Rat	Dixon et al., 1987
Brain ischaemia	Monkey	Gisvold et al., 1984
Brain lesions from acetaldehyde	Experimental animals	Phillips, 1987
Brain metastasis		Schackert & Fidler, 1988
Brain stem ischaemia	Rat	Shiroyama et al., 1991
Brainstem infarction	Model	Kuwabara et al., 1988
Brainstem, 5-HT receptor action	Guinea pig	Luscombe et al., 1986
Breast cancer	Mice, rat	Briand, 1983
	Rat	Escrich, 1987
	Cat	Prop et al., 1986
	Nude mice	Brunner et al., 1992
	Nude mice	Brunner et al., 1993
	Nude mice	Price & Zhang, 1990
Breast implant, soft tissue interaction	Rat	Picha et al., 1990
Breast tumor	Rat	Klamer et al., 1983
BRM screening	Mice	Dickneite et al., 1984
Bronchial asthma	Guinea pig	Misawa et al., 1989
	Model	Mue, 1981
Bronchial hyperactivity	Dunkin-Hartley guinea pig	Hayes et al., 1992
Bronchial infection, chronic	Mice	Tanaka et al., 1988
Bronchial injury, chronic	Dog	Fujita et al., 1986
Bronchiolitis obliterans	Dog	Mink et al., 1984
Bronze baby syndrome	Wistar rat	Jori et al., 1990
Brucella abortus infection	Pregnant goat	Meador & Deyoe, 1986
Brugia pahangi	Mongolian jird, hamster	Carraway et al., 1985
Bulimia nervosa	Rat	Hagan & Moss, 1991
Ca and P metabolism	Model	Ivic et al., 1988
Ca+ activation of cardiac contractile system	hamster	Herzig et al., 1987
Calcification of implanted vascular tissues	Rabbit, rat	Paule et al., 1992
Calcium cholelithiasis	Models	Hofmann, 1984
Calcium stone formation	Rat	Tur et al., 1991
Campylobacter coli	Suckling pigs	Kohler et al., 1988
Campylobacter diarrhea	Chicken	Ruiz-Palacios et al., 1981
Campylobacter enteritis	Rabbit	Caldwell & Walker, 1986
	Rabbit	Caldwell & Walker, 1983
Campylobacter jejuni diarrhea	Chicken	Sanyal et al., 1984
Campylobacter jejuni infection	Hamster	Humphrey et al., 1985

Disease	Animal Model	Reference
Campylobacter jejuni infections	Pig	Bossinger & Powe, 1988
Campylobacteriosis	Ferret	Fox et al., 1987
Cancer and nutrition	Panel on animal	Report, 1993
Cancer chemopreventative agent evaluation	Models	Boone et al., 1990
Cancer metastasis	Mice	Schirrmacher, 1984
Cancer research	Hamster	Mohr & Reznik, 1982
Cancer therapy	Mice	Martin et al., 1986
	C3H mice	Rak et al., 1988
Cancer therapy and radiation	Dog, ferret	Sagrada et al., 1991
Candida lesions skin and membranes	Models	Bykov & Karaev, 1986
Candide infection	Mice	Baklanova et al., 1987
Caractogenesis	Chick embryos	Doskocil et al., 1985
Carbon monoxide Intoxication, acute	Mice	Demaria Pesce, 1987
Carbonic anhydrase II deficiency syndrome	Mice	Lewis et al., 1988
Carcinogenesis	Mice, rat	Turusov, 1985
Carcinogenesis, bronchial	Syrian golden hamster	Hammond et al., 1993
Carcinogenesis, cheek	Syrian golden hamster	Gimenez-Conti, 1993
Cardiac arrhythmia	Rat	Burashnikov et al., 1991
	Rat	Cheung et al., 1993
	Rat	Carre et al., 1992
Cardiac arrhythmia, drug evaluation	Model	Schwartz & Vanoli, 1981
Cardiac failure	Sheep	Millner et al., 1991
Cardiac failure using adriamycin	Rabbit	Wanless et al., 1987
Cardiac hypertrophy	Rat	Mall et al., 1986
Cardiac retrograde conduction	Swine	Bowman & Hughes, 1984
Cardiomyopathy	Hamster	Franch et al., 1988
	Natural model	Dunningan, 1984
	Models, human	Davidoff et al., 1994
Cardiomyopathy - congestive heart failure	SHR/N-cp rat	Ruben et al., 1984
Cardiomyopathy sudden death	Rabbit	Rajs et al., 1982
Cardiomyopathy, congestive	Model	Noren et al., 1983
Cardiomyopathy, dilated	DBA mice	Matsumori et al., 1983
	Model	Matsumori, 1987
Cardiomyopathy, dilated type	Mice	Reyes et al., 1981
Cardiomyopathy, hypertrophic	Kangaroo	O'Rourke et al., 1986
Cardiopulmonary bypass and cardioplegia	Dog	Rosenblum et al., 1985
Cardiovascular disease + hyperlipidermia	Mice	Paigen et al., 1994
Cardiovascular research	Dog, human	Brugada et al., 1988
Carnitine deficiency	Sheep	Snowswell et al., 1989
Carotid artery aneurysms	Rat	Young & Yasargil, 1982
Carotid artery disease	Rat, rabbit	Holm & Hansson, 1990
Carotid artery occlusive disease	Mature pigmented rat	Slakter et al., 1984
Cartilage	Dog, guinea pig, macaca	Malemud, 1993
Cartilage matrix deficiency	Mice	Kimata, 1982
Cartilage-protective substance assay	Model	Weseloh et al., 1983
Castration-induced osteoporosis	Rat	Simmons et al., 1990
Catabolic rates of HDL-cholesterol + (APO) A-I	Control +transgenic mice	Hayek et al., 1993

Disease	Animal Model	Reference
Catecholamine uptake1 and uptake2	Models	Carr, 1983
Caudal dysgenesis	Models	Alles & Sulik, 1993
Caudate-putamen lesion	Primate	Hantraye et al., 1992
Caval syndrome	Dog	Buoro & Atwell, 1984
Celiac disease	Rat	Auricchio et al., 1984
	Rat	Kottgen et al., 1988
Cell-mediated immunity	Rat	Henningsen et al., 1984
Central distal oxonopathy	Mice	Mukoyama et al., 1989
Central nervous system	Cortisone-treated mice	Dixon, 1987
Cerebral aneurysms	Model	Hazama et al., 1987
Cerebral arachnoiditis	Model	Samosiuk, 1987
Cerebral arteriosclerose	Rhesus monkey	Bhardwaj et al., 1984
Cerebral arteriosclerosis	Rabbit	Masuda & Tanaka, 1984
Cerebral atherothromboembolism	NZW rabbit	Jeynes, 1988
Cerebral blood flow and metabolism	Cat	Heiss et al., 1995
	Baboon	Pappata et al., 1993
Cerebral embolization	Model	Phillips et al., 1988
Cerebral glioma	Syngeneic BD IX rat	Mella et al., 1990
Cerebral hemiatrophy	Pig, human	Pollak, 1989
Cerebral infarction	Rat	Kudo et al., 1982
	Rat	Laas & Igloffstein, 1983
	Rat	Kaneko et al., 1985
Cerebral infarction, focal	Rat	Tamura et al., 1986
Cerebral infarction, photochemical	Rat	Dietrich et al., 1987
Cerebral ischaemia	Rat	Busto & Ginsberg, 1985
	Cat	Kocsis et al., 1990
	Rat	Kawamura et al., 1991
	Rat	Rozvadovskii et al., 1985
	Models	Nakagawa, 1983
	Model	Labid, 1988
	Cat	Hossmann, 1991
	Rabbit	Yamamoto, 1983
Cerebral ischaemia and neurodegeneration	Fischer 344 rat	Benavides, 1990
Cerebral ischaemia brain edema	Rat	Todd et al., 1986
Cerebral ischaemia in hypertension	Rat	Delbarre et al., 1988
Cerebral ischaemia, 4 vessel occlusion	Rat	Todd, 1984
Cerebral ischaemia, complete	Dog	Mitro et al., 1983
Cerebral ischaemia, effects of Ginko biloba	Gerbil	Spinnewyn et al., 1986
Cerebral ischaemia, regional	Rat	Yan, 1988
Cerebral ischaemia, transient	Rabbit	Molnar et al., 1988
Cerebral ischaemia-induced behavioral changes	Mongolian gerbil	Chandler et al., 1985
Cerebral thrombosis	Dog	Hirschberg et al., 1988
Cerebral vasospasm	Monkey	Handa et al., 1991
	Squirrel monkey	Delgado-Zygmunt, 1992
Cerebral vasospasm, chronic	Primate	Frazee, 1982
Cerebral venous hypertension	Rat	Kurokawa et al., 1989
Cerebrovascular disease, stroke	Primate	Prusty et al., 1988

Disease	Animal Model	Reference
Ceroid-lipofuscinosis	Dog	Koppang, 1993
Chagas cardiomyopathy	Mice	Rowland et al., 1992
Chagas cardiopathy	Experimental models	Amorin, 1984
Chagas disease	Inbred III/J rabbit	Teixeira, 1986
	Dog	Lauricella et al., 1986
	Dog	Andrade et al., 1980
	Cebus apella monkey	Rosner et al., 1989
	Dog	Tafuri et al., 1988
Chagas heart disease	Experimental models	Amorin, 1985
Chancroid	Rabbit	Purcell et al., 1991
Chediak-Higashi syndrome	Models, human	Penner, 1987
	Cat	Kahraman & Prieur, 1990
	Mice	Roder, 1982
Chemoprevention	Model	Gould, 1993
Chemotherapy	Nude mice	Houchens et al., 1983
	Rabbit, mice, rat	De Carneri & Trane, 1983
Chemotherapy bronchial carcinoma	Mice	Fergusson et al., 1986
Chemotherapy of bladder cancer	Syngenic ACI/N rat	Yamashita & Ito, 1988
Chemotherapy, glioma	Rat	Kitahara et al., 1987
Chemotherapy, tumor	NMRI-mice	Fichtner et al., 1987
Chemotherapy-induced infertility	Rat	Gould et al., 1983
Childhood hyperactivity	Hypertensive rat	Sagvolden et al., 1992
Childhood rhabdomyosarcoma	CBA/CaJ mice	Houghton et al., 1982
Chlamydial genital disease	Model	Pasley et al., 1990
Chlamydial infection	Mice	Woodland et al., 1983
Chlamydiosis	Models	Rodolakis et al., 1987
Cholelithiasis	Hamster, rat	Cohen, 1987
	Guinea pig	Tadzhiev et al., 1991
Cholera	Suckling mice	Shimamura et al., 1981
Cholestasis	Wistar rat	Aller et al., 1993
Cholestatic liver disease	Rat	Deerns & Friedman, 1988
Cholestcystitis	Mongrel dog	Girglia & Danilenko, 1991
Cholesteatoma	Mongolian gerbil	Chole & Henry, 1981
Cholesteatoma induction	Cat, gerbil, hamster etc.	McGinn et al., 1981
Cholesteral storage disorder	BALB/c mice	Pentchev, 1986
Cholesterol cholelithiasis	Hamster	Cohen & Mosbach, 1993
Cholesterol gallstone disease	Hamster	Holzbach, 1984
Cholesterol-raising effect of coffee	Syrian hamster	Sanders et al., 1992
Cholestokinia receptor	Rat	Tani et al., 1990
Cholinergic denervation	Models	Smith, 1988
Cholinergic receptor sites	Dahl rat	McCaughran et al., 1984
Cholinergic supersensitivity	Genetic model	Golda & Petr, 1988
Cholinergic supersensitivity + affective disorders	Genetic models	Overstreet et al., 1988
Cholinergic systems	Models	Price et al., 1993
Choreoathetosis	Monkey	Jackson et al., 1984
Circulatory arrest	Rat	Garavilla et al., 1984
Circulatory shock	Long + short pig	Phillips, 1989

Disease	Animal Model	Reference
Cirrhosis	Rat	Kountouras et al., 1984
Cirrhosis, ascites and bacterial peritonitis	Rat	Runyon et al., 1991
Cirrhosis-like liver lesions	Rat	Muller et al., 1988
Cisplatin-induced emesis	Ferret	Florczyk et al., 1982
Clinical death	rat	Kapuscínski, 1987
Clinical significance	NMRI nu/nu tumor mice	Otto & Huland, 1982
Closed catheter drainage system	Rabbit	Nickel et al., 1991
Closed-chest myocardial ischaemia	Dog	Birkui et al., 1981
CNS infections		Tauber, 1986
CNS lymphoproliferative disease	SCID mice	Bashir et al., 1991
CNS phaeochyphomycosis	Mice	Dixon et al., 1982
CNS Syphillis	Rabbit	Marra et al., 1991
Cobalamin deficiency	Fruit bat	Metz, 1987
Cochlear hydrops	Cat	Eby, 1986
Cognitive decline	Aged mice	Gower & Lamberty, 1993
Cognitive dysfunction	Guinea pig	Fisher et al., 1991
Coliform mastitis	Mice	Anderson, 1983
Colitis	Hamster	Liu et al., 1985
	Rat	Ondrula et al., 1993
Colitis, chronic	Rat	Wallace, 1988
Collagen disease	Models	Hegreberg, 1982
Collateral circulation, 4-vessel occlusion	Rat	Pulsinelli et al., 1988
Colon cancer	Athymic nude mice	Lin et al., 1991
Colon carcinoma	Rodent	Rogers & Nauss, 1985
	Mice, rat	Rogers, 1985
Colon tumor	Nude mice	Bresalier et al., 1991
Colon tumor, antibody clearance	Nude mice	Pedey et al., 1989
Colonic cancer	WF rat	Takada et al., 1984
Colonic tumor metastases	Sprague Dawley rat	Rubio et al., 1987
Colorectal cancer	Rat	Gilbert, 1987
	Athymic nude mice	Schackert & Fidler, 1989
Colorectal cancer, receptor status	Rat	Summerton et al., 1985
Colorectal metastasis	Rat	Carter et al., 1992
Colorectal tumor expression of malignancy	Mice	Sordat & Wang, 1984
Complex anorectal malformations	SD-mice	Kluth et al., 1991
Conducting tissue	Dog	Andrade et al., 1984
Conflict situation	Monkey	Dzhalogoniia et al., 1983
Congenital coagulation defects	Models	Kase, 1981
Congenital contractures	Mice	Nonaka et al., 1986
Congenital hydrocephalus	Lamb	Di Tralani et al., 1990
	Rat	Kohn et al., 1988
Congenital hyperammonemia	Urease-infused rat	Batshaw et al., 1986
Congenital policystic kidney disease	C57BL/6J mice	Mandell et al., 1983
Congenital syphillis	Guinea pig	Wicher et al., 1992
Congestive heart failure	Rat	Desjaedins et al., 1988
	Rabbit	Chen et al., 1988
	Dog	Chong et al., 1985

Disease	Animal Model	Reference
Congestive heart failure	Rat	Bauer & Fung, 1990
	Dog	Wilson et al., 1987
Congestive heart failure and myocarditis	Rabbit	Edwards et al., 1992
Conjunctivitis	Rabbit	Langford et al., 1986
Connective tissue disease	Mice	Leader et al., 1983
	Autoimmune mice	Rosenberg, 1988
Contact eczema	Guinea pig	Boyera et al., 1992
Continous arteriovenous hemofiltration	Model	Werner et al., 1993
Controlled neuroimmunization	Rat	Zubova et al., 1991
Convergent strabismic amblyopia	Cat	Crewther et al., 1985
Convulsive liability of antibiotics	Model	Williams et al., 1988
Copper toxicosis	Dog, mice, rat, sheep	Schilsky et al., 1993
	Models	Schilsky et al., 1993
Corneal ulcer	Albino rat	Singh et al., 1990
Coronary angioplasty	Dog	Turi et al., 1990
Coronary artery embolization	Dog	Herr et al., 1988
Coronary artery ligation	Rat	Nadeau et al., 1987
Coronary artery spasm	Dog	Heupler et al., 1985
Coronary occlusion	Closed chest dog	Akizuki, 1984
	Pig	Alonso et al., 1991
Coronary stenosis, induced-vasoconstriction	Dog	Yokoyama et al., 1985
Coronary thrombosis	Pig	van der Giessen, 1983
Coronary thrombus formation	Dog	Benedict et al., 1986
Coronary vasospasm, variant angina	Rat	Vergona et al., 1984
Corpus callosum impingement	Sprague Dawley rat	Xiong et al., 1993
Cortical hypoplasia	Rat	Mercugliano et al., 1990
Cortical microcirculation	Model	Lindsberg et al., 1991
Cortical venous infarction, MR imaging	Rabbit	Secrist et al., 1989
Coxsackievirus B3 myocarditis	C3H/HeJ mice	Kiel et al., 1989
Craniosynostosis	Rabbit	Duncan et al., 1992
Creutzfeld–Jacob disease	Models	Tateishi, 1989
Creutzfeld–Jakob disease	Guinea pig	Dragansecu et al., 1981
Crohn´s disease	Pig	Nagel et al., 1988
Cryptococcus neoformans	Mice, human	Fromtling et al., 1988
Cryptorchidism	Wistar rat	Gracia et al., 1990
Cryptosporidiosis	Rat	Brasseur et al., 1988
	Guinea pig	Chrisp, 1990
Cryptosporidium infection	T-cell subset-depleted mice	Ungar et al., 1990
	Nude mice	Heine et al., 1984
Cushingoid degenerative changes	Obese/SHR	Wexler & McMurty, 1985
Cyanotic heart disease	Dog	Kohler et al., 1984
Cyclic hematopoiesis	Models	Jones & Lange, 1983
Cyclosporin A nephrotoxicity	Rat	McNally et al., 1990
	Rat	McNally et al., 1990
Cyclosporine nephrotoxicity	Laboratory animals	Sullivan et al., 1985
	Model	Faruco et al., 1991
Cyclosporine toxicity	Rat	Paller, 1985

Disease	Animal Model	Reference
Cyclosporine, toxicity, metabolism, drug interact	Models	Whiting et al., 1985
Cyclosporine-induced proximal tubular toxicity	Rat	Berty & Adler, 1991
Cystic disease development	Murine	Preminger et al., 1982
Cystic fibrosis	Rat	Martinez et al., 1983
	Rat	McCurdy et al., 1981
	Mice, rat	Sagstrom et al., 1990
	Rat	Park et al., 1987
	Reserpine-treated rat	Martinez et al., 1988
	Transgenic mice	Snouwaert et al., 1992
Cytochrome P-450 depleted	Model	Drummond et al., 1982
Cytomegaloviral infections	Guinea pig	Bia et al., 1983
Cytomegalovirus	Models	Kern, 1991
Cytomegalovirus infection	Model	Gonczol et al., 1985
Cytomegalovirus infection, acute	Brown Norway rat	Stals et al., 1990
D2 receptor supersensitivity	Macaca fasciculacis.	Graham et al., 1990
Debrisoquine metabolizer	DA rat	Ohta et al., 1990
Degeneration of dopamine system	Rat	Deutch, 1989
Degenerative diseases: Creutzfeld-Jakob	Guinea pig	Draganescu et al., 1985
Delayed aortic coarctation	Dog	Womble, 1982
	Dog	Womble et al., 1982
Delayed cerebral vasospasm	Dog	Varsos et al., 1983
Delirium	Wistar rat	Trzepacz et al., 1992
Dementia	Mice	Flood & Cherkin, 1986
	Model	Goudsmit, 1986
Dementia and memory dysfunction	Rat, human	Beatty, 1988
Demyelinating disease	Mice	Trotter et al., 1987
	Mice to human	Rose, 1992
	Models, in vitro - in vivo	Sorenson et al., 1981
	Models	Knobler et al., 1983
Demyelinating disease, acute and subacute	Rat	Wege et al., 1981
Demyelinating diseases	Quail, chicken	Le Douarin, 1987
Demyelination	Nude mice	Roos & Wollmann, 1984
	Guinea pig, mice	Raine & Traugatt, 1984
	Murine	Rodriguez et al., 1987
Demyelination of optic nerve	Mice	Illavia et al., 1982
	Cat	Caroll et al., 1985
Denervation-delymphatization kidneys	No reference	Shestakova et al., 1988
Dependence morphine	Rat	Suzuki et al., 1984
Dependence on tetrahydrocannabinol	Monkey	Beardsley et al., 1986
Depression	Rat	Gorka et al., 1985
	Rat	Downs et al., 1986
	Hamster	Crawley, 1984
	Rat	Hasey & Hanin, 1991
	Wistar rat	Golda & Petr, 1990
	Rat	Hartley et al., 1990
	Mice	Kostowski et al., 1990
	Rat	Muscat et al., 1990

Disease	Animal Model	Reference
Depression	Rat	Carlson & Glick, 1991
	Rat	Katz & Sibel, 1982
	Rat, mice	Renaud, 1988
	Rat	Simson & Weiss, 1988
	Model	Katz, 1982
Depression and chronic stress	Rat	Pignatiello et al., 1989
Depression with cholinergic supersensitivity	Rat	Schiller, 1991
Depression with muscarinic supersensitivity	Rat	Owens et al., 1991
Depression, 5 HT receptors	Rat	Edwards et al., 1991
	Rat	Edwards et al., 1991
Depression, central histaminergic	Mice	Nath et al., 1988
Depression, cholinergic supersensitivity	Rat	Overstreet et al., 1989
Depression, lack of tolerance to drugs	Rat	Wainstein et al., 1990
Depression, muscarinic supersensitivity	Flinders sensitive line rat	Daws et al., 1991
Depression, neurotransmitter release	Rabbit	Edwards et al., 1992
Depression, olfactory bulbectomized	Rat	Leonard, 1984
Depression, reversal	Rat	Sampson et al., 1991
Depression, separation-induced	Primate	Rosenblum et al., 1987
Depression, simulation	Models	Willner, 1991
Depression, swimming -induced head twitching	Mice	Naitoh et al., 1992
Depressive disorders	Models, human	Richardson, 1991
Dermatitis	Mice	Maguire et al., 1982
Dermatophytosis	Mice	Hay et al., 1983
	"hairless" guinea pig	Hanel et al., 1990
Detrusor instability	Pig	Sibley, 1985
Development of disease	Transgenic mice	Leonard et al., 1988
Developmental disorders	Models	Mailman, 1981
Deviant development	Primate	Sackett, 1984
Device-related infections	Models	Zimmerli, 1993
Diabetes	Guinea pig	Schlosser et al., 1984
	Juvenile pig	Gabel et al., 1985
	Rat	Cooper et al., 1990
Diabetes - obesity syndromes	Mice	Coleman, 1982
Diabetes and renal insufficiency	Animals, human	Bakris, 1991
Diabetes mellitus	Rabbit	Roth & Conaway, 1982
	Dog	Engerman et al., 1982
	Pig	Wilson et al., 1986
	BB ràt	Verheul et al., 1986
	Rodent	Coleman, 1982
	BB rat	Like et al., 1982
	Hamster	Gerritsen, 1982
	Aged Macaca mulatta	Kessler et al., 1985
	Mice	Jordan & Cohen, 1987
	Yucatan miniature swine	Phillips et al., 1982
	Primate, human	Howard, 1984
	Pregnant ewe	Dickinson et al., 1991
	Pregnant sheep	Lips et al., 1988

Disease	Animal Model	Reference
Diabetes mellitus	Pig	Stump et al., 1988
	Mystromys albicaudatus	Little, 1982
Diabetes obesity syndrome	CBA/CA mice	Connelly et al., 1989
Diabetes type 1 and 2	Streptozotocin-treated rat	Sullivan et al., 1990
Diabetes type I	Models	Bach & Boitard, 1986
Diabetes type II	KKA (y) mice	Castle et al., 1993
	SHR/N-cp rat	Voyles et al., 1988
Diabetes, genetic forms	Mice	Coleman, 1983
Diabetic cataract	Rat	Nakamoto et al., 1988
Diabetic glomerulopathy	Rat	Steffes & Mauer, 1984
Diabetic pregnancy	NOD-mice	Formby et al., 1987
Diabetic rat model	Sand rat	Kloting & Hahn, 1981
Diabetic retinopathy	BB Wistar rat	Sima, 1983
Diaphragmatic hernia	Sheep fetus	Rossotto et al., 1982
Diarrhoea	Rabbit	Spira & Sack, 1982
Diet-induced arteriosclerosis	Yacatan miniature swine	Reitman et al., 1982
Diffuse alopecia, acute	Sheep	Tonkin et al., 1982
Digeorge syndrome	Rat	Oster et al., 1983
Dipolar disorder	Rat	Cappeliez & Moore, 1990
Disc space infection, imaging	Rabbit	Szypryt et al., 1988
Discrimination conditioning	Rat	Gomita et al., 1985
Disease models	Transgenic mice	Brem, 1990
Disintegration of hormonal systems	Models	Ruzov, 1990
Disk displacement	New Zealand white rabbit	Tallents et al., 1990
Disorder-Vitiligo	Plymouth rock chicken	Boissy et al., 1988
Disseminated intravascular coagulation	Rat	Yoshikawa et al., 1983
DNA adduct measurements	Animal, human	Poirier & Beland, 1992
Domoate toxicosis	Swiss-Webster mice	Bose et al., 1990
Dopamine autoreceptor sensitivity	Rat	Muscat et al., 1988
Dopamine-mediated behavior	Rat	Hafner, 1991
Down´s syndrome	Mice	Cox et al., 1984
	Transgenic mice	Epstein et al., 1987
	Hamster	Ingalls, 1982
	Mice	Davisson et al., 1993
	Mice	Davisson et al., 1993
	Mice	Davisson et al., 1990
	Transgenic mice	Ceballos-Picot, 1991
Down´s syndrome (tongue pathology)	Transgenic mice	Yarom et al., 1988
Drug abuse	Mice, rat, genetic models	Crabbe et al., 1994
Drug action on arterial tissue	Turkey	Simpson & Boucek, 1983
Drug development, antimalarials	Chicks	Kinnamon et al., 1985
Drug effects	Models	Hutchings et al., 1991
Drug effects - cocaine	Albino rat	Ettenberg & Geist, 1991
Drug research, antibacterial	Mice, rabbit	Matti, 1984
Drug resistance	Golden hamster	Khanmirzoev et al., 1990
Drug studies	Cat	Wada et al., 1987
Drug testing	Models	Werner, 1984

Disease	Animal Model	Reference
Drug therapy	Rat	Humphrey et al., 1982
Duchenne muscular dystrophy	Dog	Valentine et al., 1992
	Dog	Valentine et al., 1988
Duet epithelial hyperplasia + nesidioblastosis	Hamster	Rosenberg et al., 1983
Duodenal Ulcer	Model	Eletskii et al., 1985
	Rat	Takeuchi et al., 1986
Dwarfism	Cat, dog	Sande, 1983
Dylipidermia and cardiovascular disease	Wistar rat	Storlien et al., 1993
Dysbacteriosis	Monkey	Dzhikidze et al., 1986
Dysentery	Model	Galikeyev et al., 1982
Dyskinesia	Primate	Clarke et al., 1987
	Primate	Crossman, 1987
Dyskinesia or nausea	Squirrel monkey	Rupniak et al., 1990
Dyslexia	Mice, rat	Galaburda, 1994
Dystrophy of the stomach	Rat	Voltenko et al., 1984
E. coli epidymitis	Rat	Tartaglione et al., 1991
Ear disease type II, collagen-induced	Guinea pig	Soliman, 1990
Ear inflammation	Chinchilla	Hamaguchi et al., 1988
Ear reattachment	Rat	Chiu et al., 1990
Early coronary artery dysrhythmia	Rat	Marshall et al., 1981
Eating disorders	Gorilla	Gould & Bres, 1986
Ebola infection	Rhesus monkey	Fisher-Hoch et al., 1983
Echinococcus multilocutaris	Golden hamster	Kovalenko et al., 1990
Edema of the lungs	Cat	Tel' et al., 1987
Edemas, permeability	Rabbit, sheep	Zelter & Dougvet, 1986
Eker renal tumor	Rat	Waynforth et al., 1981
Embolism in brain	Rat	Furlow, 1982
Embolism, massive pulmonary artery	Dog	Virganskii et al., 1990
Emotional postpartum disorders	Mice	Laviola, 1993
Emotional resonance	Rat	Meshcheriakova, 1988
Emotional stress	Monkey	Butovskaia et al., 1986
Emotional stress anxiogenic hyperalgesia	Rat	Vidal & Jacob, 1986
Emotional stress, chronic	Rabbit, cat	Vediaev, 1984
Emotionality	Model	Blizard, 1988
Emphysema	Rat	Yokoyama et al., 1987
	Rabbit	Gerovich et al., 1985
	Pig	Soskel et al., 1982
	Swine	Lucey, 1983
	Model	Reichart, 1986
Encephalitis	Squirrel monkey	Nagata, 1990
	Rabbit	Leib et al., 1988
Encephalitis, focal herpes simplex	Rabbit	Schlitt, 1986
Encephalitis, tick-borne	Clawed toad	Izotov & Chunikbin, 1982
Encephalomeningitis, chemotherapeutic model	Mice	Shipilova et al., 1982
Encephalopathy	Murine	Steinman et al., 1982
Endocarditis	Mice	Gutschik, 1983
	Rabbit, rat	Glauser & Francoili, 1987

Disease	Animal Model	Reference
Endocarditis	Rabbit	Sande, 1981
Endocarditis and meningitis	Models	Gerberding & Sande, 198
Endocarditis of mitral valve	Rabbit	Imataka et al., 1993
Endocarditis, aortic valve	Rat	Heraief et al., 1982
Endocarditis, streptococcal	Rabbit, human	Scheld, 1987
Endocrine parameters	Cynomolgus monkey	Udelsman et al., 1984
Endogenous depression	Rat	Vogel et al., 1990
Endolymphatic hydrops	Shark	Arenberg et al., 1981
	Models	Kimura, 1982
Endometrial adenocarcinoma	Nude mice	Zaino et al., 1985
Endometrial carcinoma	BD II/Han rat	Deeberg et al., 1987
Endometrial carinoma + steroid receptors	Nude mice	Satyaswaroop, 1987
Endometriosis	Rabbit	Dunselman et al., 1989
	Rat	Golan, 1984
	Rat	Golan et al., 1987
	Rabbit	Berthet et al., 1992
	Rat	Rajkumar et al., 1990
	Rat	Kadaba & Simpson, 1990
Endometriosis, cell culture model	Rat	Sharpe et al., 1992
Endometriosis-associated subfertility	Golden hamster	Steinleitner et al., 1991
Endotoxemia	Yucatan miniature swine	Fettman, 1986
	Sheep	Lubbesmeyer et al., 1989
Endotoxemia, chronic	Rat	Fish & Spitzer, 1984
Endotoxin-induced intravascular coagulation	Rat	Yoshikawa et al., 1981
Enteral and intranasal infection	Mice	Iakovleva et al., 1982
Enterocolitis	Rabbit	Miller et al., 1988
Enterocystoplasty	Long-Evans rat	Guan et al., 1990
Enteropathogenic E. Coli infection	Lamb	Gregory, 1983
Enterotoxin evaluation	Sealed adult mice	Richardson et al., 1984
Enzyme replacement therapy	Intestinal segment	Shelt et al., 1982
Epidemic hemorrhagic fever	Rabbit	Zhu et al., 1986
	Hamster	Yao, 1987
Epidermoid carcinoma	Chick eye	Gordon et al., 1986
Epididymitis	Rabbit	Hackett et al., 1988
Epididymitis, acute	Mice	Kuzan et al., 1989
Epidural compression of the spinal cord	Rat	Arbit et al., 1989
Epidymoepididymostomy	Sprague Dawley rat	McClatchey et al., 1991
Epilepsy	Rat	Beaumanoir, 1982
	Rat	Bo et al., 1986
	Cat	Kaijima et al., 1981
	Rat	Dailey & Jobe, 1985
	Rat	Zhao et al., 1985
	Rat	Buchhalter, 1993
	Wistar rat	Snead et al., 1992
	Epilepsy-prone rat	Reigel, 1986
	Rat, baboon	Jobe et al., 1991
	Rat	Serikawa, 1992

Disease	Animal Model	Reference
Epilepsy	Model, human	Fariello & Grant, 1992
	Primate	Engel, 1992
Epilepsy, chronic focal	Models	Louis et al., 1987
Epilepsy, drug development	Models	Loscher & Schmidt, 1988
Epilepsy, generalized	Genetic model	Olsen et al., 1986
Epilepsy, generalized non-convulsive	Rat	Vergnes et al., 1982
Epilepsy, spontaneous absence	WAG/Rij rat	Peeters et al., 1989
Epithelial cutaneous lesions	Dunkin-Hartley guinea pig	Gomez & Vicente, 1988
Epstein-Barr virus-induced lymphomagenesis	SCID mice	Purtillo et al., 1991
Erosive arthropathy	Guinea pig	Cashin, 1987
Esophageal motor disorder	Model	Keshavarzian et al., 1990
Esophageal tumor	Monkey	Beniashvilli et al., 1992
Esophageal varices	Dog	Jensen, 1983
	Rat	Tanoue et al., 1991
Essential hypertension	Dog	Bovee et al., 1986
Estrogen-induced diverticulosis	Mice	Newbold et al., 1984
Ethanol injury	Ferret	Roselle et al., 1986
Ethanol reinforcement	Rat	Samson, 1986
Ethanol self administration	Rat	Grant & Samson, 1985
Ethanol, behavioral changes	Rat	Shah & West, 1984
Excercise-induced muscle enlargement	Models	Timson, 1990
Excess weight gains in pregnancy	Rat	Bowen, 1989
Excessive eating: schedule-induced	Rat	Wilson & Cantor, 1987
Exencephaly	New Zealand white mice	Vogelweid et al., 1993
Eye disease	Subterranean mole rat	Cooper et al., 1993
Eye infection	New Zealand albino rabbit	Paschal et al., 1992
Facial nerve trauma	Pig	Barrs et al., 1991
Falciparum malaria	Wistar rat	Hershko et al., 1992
Familiar hypercholesterolemia	Rhesus monkey	Neven, 1990
Fanconi syndrome	Rat	Foreman et al., 1987
Fasciola hepatica	Rat, mice	Chapman et al., 1982
Fatty liver hemorrhagic syndrome	Chicken, cows, cats	Hansen & Walzem, 1993
Female behavioral endocrinology	Musk shrew	Rissman, 1990
Fetal alcohol effects	Pregnant rat	Hannigan et al., 1993
Fetal alcohol syndrome	Ferret	McLain & Roe, 1984
	Rat	West, 1989
Fetal brain development + iodine deficiency	Primate, Callithirix jacchus	Mano, 1987
Fetal death	Donkey-in-horse pregnancy	Allen et al., 1987
Fetal hydantoin syndrome	Rat	Lorente et al., 1981
	Rat	Parker, 1982
Fetal macrosomia	Rat	Kim & Kim, 1981
Fibrinolytic bleeding	Rabbit	Marder et al., 1992
Filaracidal activity	Rat	Denham et al., 1990
Filariacides	Leaf-monkey	Mak et al., 1990
Filariasis	Jird	Weil et al., 1990
	Model	Bastos et al., 1987
Focal cerebral ischaemia	Rabbit	Lyden et al., 1985

Disease	Animal Model	Reference
Focal cerebral ischaemia	Cat, rat	Bullock et al., 1990
Focal glomerulosclerosis	Hyperlipidemic lenai rat	Yoshikawa et al., 1991
Focal ischaemia	Cat	Traupe et al., 1982
Focal ischaemic stroke	Rat	Chen, 1986
Foetal wound healing	Sheep	Burd et al., 1990
Foeto-placental unit	BALB/c mice	Jensen & Hau, 1990
Forebrain ischaemia	Rat	Blomquist et al., 1984
Fracture repair	CD-1 mice	Bourque et al., 1992
Fraser syndrome	Mice	Darling & Gossler, 1994
	Mice	Darling & Gossler, 1994
Fulminant hepatitis	Long-Evans rat	Takeichi et al., 1988
Functional recovery, brain	Rat	Goldstein & Davis, 1990
G-6-pd deficient human erythrocytes	Sheep	Calabrese, 1984
Gallbladder inflammation, acute	Rabbit	Myers et al., 1990
Gallblader cancer	Syrian hamster	Gorin et al., 1988
Gastric and hepatic carcinomas	Transgenic mice	Ullrich et al., 1994
Gastric autral ulcer	Hamster	Kolbasa et al., 1988
Gastric carcinoma	Transgenic mice	Ullrich et al., 1994
Gastric heliobacter pylori infection	Nude and BALB/c mice	Karita et al., 1991
Gastric leiomyosarcoma	Rat	Cohen, 1984
Gastric ulcer	Rat	Kaminishi et al., 1987
	Rat	Ezer, 1989
	Sprague Dawley rat	Bui et al., 1991
Gastric ulceration, acute	Rat	MacLellan et al., 1986
Gastritis, chronic	Ferret	Tompkins et al., 1988
	Rhesus monkey	Baskerville et al., 1988
Gastro-duodenal ulcer	Models	Pillai et al., 1984
Gastroenteritis	Chicks	Welkos, 1984
Gastroesophageal reflux	Models	Beauchamp et al., 1986
Gastrointestinal bleeding	Sheep	Owunwanne et al., 1988
	Sheep	Owunwanne et al., 1987
Gastrointestinal carcinogenesis	Hamster, mice, rat	Mohn et al., 1992
Gastroschisis	Fetal rabbit	Phillips et al., 1991
Gaucher mouse	Gaucher mice	Kanfer et al., 1982
Gene targeting	Models	Melton, 1990
Gene therapy	Mice	Krauss et al., 1991
Genetic disease	Transgenic mice	Erickson, 1988
	Mice	Smithies, 1993
	Domestic animals	Patterson et al., 1982
Genetic diseases of connective tissues	Models	Minor, 1987
Genetic diseases with unknown etiology	Molecular, human	Yoshida & Wilson, 1992
Genetic significance	Primate	Stone et al., 1987
	Laboratory mice	Moriwaki, 1987
Genital herpes	Guinea pig	Stanberry, 1991
Genital herpes simplex virus infection	Guinea pig	Stanberry et al., 1985
Genital tract wound healing	Rat	Schlaff et al., 1987
Genital trichomoniasis	Squirrel monkey	Gardner et al., 1987

Disease	Animal Model	Reference
Gerontological research	Models	Hollander, 1984
Gestational diabetes	Rat	Hellerstrom et al., 1985
Giardia lamblia cysts	Mongolian gerbil, human	Visvesvara et al., 1988
Giardia lamblia infection	Gerbil	Lu, 1986
	Mice, rat	Kanwar et al., 1986
Gilbert's-like syndrome	Bolivian squirrel monkey	Cornelius, 1993
Glaucoma	Rabbit	Gherezghiher et al., 1986
	Rhesus monkey and rabbit	March et al., 1984
Glaucoma and buphthalmia	Rabbit	Bunt-Milam et al., 1987
Glioma disseminated via CSR	Rat	Rewers et al., 1990
Glioma line D45MG treatment profile	Athymic mice	Schold et al., 1987
Global cerebral ischaemia stroke	Cat	Todd et al., 1981
Globoid cell leukodystrophy	Twitcher mice	Takahashi et al., 1984
	Models	Suzuki, 1994
Glomerular basement membranes	Dog	Thorner et al., 1989
Glomerular metalloproteinase	Models	Le et al., 1992
Glomerular proteinases	Models	Teschner et al., 1992
Glomerulonephritis	Rat	Davin et al., 1989
	Mice, rat	Furness & Harris, 1994
Glomerulonephritis, antimyeloperoxidase-assoc.	Brown Norway rat	Brouwer et al., 1993
Glomerulonephritis, membranous	Rat	Brown et al., 1987
Glucose-6-phosphate dehydrogenase–deficiency	Sheep	Calabrese et al., 1983
Gluococorticoid resistance	Primate	Chrousos et al., 1986
Glutamatorgic denervation	Rat	Myhrer, 1993
Gluten sensitive enteropathy (coeliac disease)	BALB/c and BDF1 mice	Troncone et al., 1991
Glycogen storage disease	Models	Walvoort, 1983
Glycogen storage disease (Pompe's disease)	Dog	Walvoort et al., 1985
Glycolytic rates	Mice	Hawkins et al., 1993
Goldbatt hypertension	Model	Suzuki et al., 1987
Goodpasture disease	Mice	Wick, 1986
Goodpasture's syndrome	Mice	Fitzsimmons et al., 1991
Gout	Model	Hirai & Kumagai, 1982
Grafts in Parkinson's disease	Fetal models	Gagnon et al., 1994
Granulocytopenia, persistent	Rabbit	Walsh et al., 1984
Granuloma pouch	Rat	Dalhoff et al., 1983
Granulomatous bowel disease	Guinea pig	Mitchell & Turk, 1989
Granulomatous colitis, chronic	Lewis rat	Yamada et al., 1993
Granulomatous lung disease	Guinea pig	Fulmer et al., 1983
Growth	Premature rat	Glockner, 1986
Growth hormone-releasing and somatostation	Rat	Shakutsui et al., 1989
Growth of bowel segments	Dog	Weinberg et al., 1990
Growth of schwannomas	Nude mice	Lee et al., 1990
Growth sites for tumors	Tail vs flank	Moore, 1983
Guanethidine adrenergic neuropathy	Sprague Dawley rat	Zochone et al., 1988
Guillain-Barre syndrome	Rat	Hjorth et al., 1984
H2-receptor gastric pathology	Rat	del Soldato, 1982
Haemochromatosis, primary	Wistar rat	Ward et al., 1991

Disease	Animal Model	Reference
Haemolytic-uraemic syndrome in shigellosis	Rabbit	Butler et al., 1985
Haemonchus contortus infection	Guinea pig	Wagland et al., 1989
Haemophilus influenzae type b infection	Mice	Marks et al., 1982
Haemorrhagic and haemolytic anaemias	Rabbit	Benestad et al., 1983
Hair patches	Mice	Shultz et al., 1991
Hallucinogenic activity	Rat	Adams et al., 1985
Halothane hepatitis	F344 rat	Knights et al., 1987
Halothane hepatotoxicity	Rat	Strunin et al., 1983
HBV and HDV infections	Duck, marmota	Cova et al., 1993
Head and neck squamous cell carcinoma	Rnu/Rnu athymic rat	Moses et al., 1993
Heart circumflex artery occlusion	Dog, pig	McDonough et al., 1984
Heart damage using oxygen	Rat	Ravingeroka et al., 1989
Heart disease	Mice	Gauntt et al., 1993
Heart failure	Dog	Unverferth et al., 1983
	Wistar rat	Oka et al., 1993
	Dog	Lucas et al., 1992
	Mini-pig	Nutall et al., 1985
	Model	Moe et al., 1988
Heart failure, autonomic innervation	Hamster, dog, guinea pig	Lund et al., 1983
Heart failure, congestive	Dog	Riegger & Liebau, 1982
Heart failure, muscarinic receptor	Dog	Vatner et al., 1988
Heart ischaemic	Rat	Hultman, 1982
Heart transplantation	Rat	Miller et al., 1985
Heliobacter pylori active chronic gastritis	Mice	Lee et al., 1990
Heliobacter pylori gastritis	Rat	Fox et al., 1991
	Ferret	Fox et al., 1990
	Mice	Dick-Hegedus, 1991
Hematogenous osteomyelitis, acute	Chicken	Emslie & Nade, 1986
Hematoma formation after bone biopsy	Dog	Robertson et al., 1983
Hematopoetic disease	Mice	Dick, 1991
Hematopoiesis	Nude mice	Lapidot et al., 1993
Hematopoietic and endocrine systems	Dog	Lothrop et al., 1987
Hematopoietic stem cells	Model	Mueller-Sieburg, 1992
Hemi-Parkinson syndrome, D1 and D2 receptor	Monkey	Przedborski et al., 1991
Hemochromatosis	Rat	Iancu & Shiloh, 1988
	Rat	Bonkovski et al., 1987
Hemoglobin regulation	Mice	Alter et al., 1982
Hemolytic disease of the newborn	Rabbit fetus	Moise, 1992
Hemophilia therapies	Models	Giles, 1994
Hemophilic model	Dog	Kingdon et al., 1981
Hemophilus somnus infection	Chicken embryos	Nivard et al., 1982
Hemorrhage and thrombosis in the neonate	Models	Kisker, 1987
Hemorrhagic pancreatitis, acute	Rat	Redha et al., 1990
Hemorrhagic shock	Rat	Sato et al., 1985
	Dog	Vivaldi et al., 1983
	Monkey	Bar-Joseph et al., 1991
	Model	Fleisher et al., 1987

Disease	Animal Model	Reference
Hemorrhagic shock-induced lesions	Rat	Teribble Wiel, 1982
Hepatectomy, hepatic ischaemia	Rat	Omokawa et al., 1991
Hepatectomy, subtotal	Rat	Edmond et al., 1988
Hepatic carcinoma	Transgenic mice	Ullrich et al., 1994
Hepatic collagen cirrhosis	Rat	Tanner et al., 1981
Hepatic coma	Model	Ignatovski & Borcic, 1981
Hepatic encephalopathy	Rabbit	Basile et al. et al., 1988
	Rat	Morony et al., 1983
	Rat	Basile et al., 1990
	Rat	Gammal et al., 1990
Hepatic encephalopathy, acute	Rabbit	Rossle et al., 1989
Hepatic encephalopathy, benzodiazepine	Sprague Dawley rat	Yurdaydin et al., 1993
Hepatic failure	Rabbit	Ferenci et al., 1983
Hepatic failure, acute	Rat	Minato et al., 1982
	Pig	De Groot et al., 1987
	Dog	Karrer et al., 1984
	Pig	Henne-Bruns et al., 1988
Hepatic fibrosis	Rat	Sun et al., 1990
	Pig	Peterson, 1993
Hepatic fibrosis and cirrhosis	Rat	Trivedi & Mowat, 1983
Hepatic insufficiency, acute	Rat	Marni et al., 1983
Hepatic iron overload	Baboon	Brissot et al., 1983
Hepatic ischemia-anoxia and reperfusion injury	Sprague Dawley rat	Pretto, 1991
Hepatic lipase deficiency	Rabbit	Clay et al., 1989
Hepatic Metastases	Murine	Lafreniere et al., 1986
Hepatic metastasis	Sheep	Dilley et al., 1993
	Nude rat	Graf et al., 1992
Hepatic periportal fibrosis	Mice	Andrade et al., 1993
Hepatic phospholipidosis	Guinea pig	Pirovino et al., 1988
Hepatic release of vitamin A in liver disease	Rat	Scholmerich et al., 1991
Hepatic schistosoma mansoni egg granulomas	Mice	Botros et al., 1986
Hepatic tumor, solitary	Rat	Tamura et al., 1990
Hepatitis A	Green monkey	Ugriumov, 1982
	Old World monkey	Lapin, 1988
Hepatitis A and Hepatitis non-A, non-B	Ssanguinus mystax tamarin	Poleshchuk et al., 1990
Hepatitis A virus	New World owl monkey	LeDuc et al., 1983
Hepatitis A, hepatitis B, non-A, non-B hepatitis	Primate	Tabor et al., 1983
Hepatitis B	Woodchuck	Gerin, 1983
	Mice	Chisari et al., 1985
	Nude mice	Feitelson et al., 1988
	Duck	Long et al., 1993
	Tree shrews	Su, 1987
	Indian palmtree squirrel	Mehrota et al., 1990
Hepatitis B virus infection, chronic	Duck	Bishop et al., 1990
Hepatitis delta infection	Woodchuck	Ponzetto et al., 1987
Hepatitis E	Pregnant Macaca mulatta	Arankalle et al., 1993
	Rhesus monkey	Li, 1992

Disease	Animal Model	Reference
Hepatitis hepatocellular carcinoma	Marmola	Snyder et al., 1982
Hepatitis research	Chimpanzee	Muchmore, 1983
Hepatitis, chronic active	Models	Ramos-Martinez, 1988
Hepatitis, D-galactosamine-induced	Rat	Sugrobova et al., 1992
Hepatitis, delta virus	Chimpanzee	Purcell et al., 1987
Hepatitis, hepatocellular carcinoma	Mutant rat	Thorgeirsson, 1992
Hepatobiliary tracers	Models	Fritzberg et al., 1983
Hepatocarcinogenesis	Rat	Dragan et al., 1991
Hepatocarcinoma for MAb serotherapy	Guinea pig	Key et al., 1983
Hepatocyte transplantation	Clinical model	Henne-Bruns et al., 1987
Hepatogenic encephalopathy	Model	Mossakowski, 1981
Heptic alveolar echinococcocis	Rat	Ohnishi, 1984
Heptic amoebiasis	Mice	Bhol et al., 1989
Hereditary brain disease	Mice	Inoue, 1986
Hereditary nephritis	Samoyed dog	Jansen et al., 1986
Herpes simplex encephalitis	Pig	Boogerd & Peters, 1986
	Rat	Clator et al., 1987
	Rat	Cleator et al., 1988
	SJL mice	Hudson et al., 1991
Herpes simplex eye disease	NIH mice	Claoue, 1986
Herpes simplex retinitis	Mice	Cousins et al., 1989
Herpes simplex virus genital infection	Guinea pig	Stephanopoulos, 1989
Herpes simplex virus in trigeminal ganglia	Rabbit	Green et al., 1982
Herpes simplex virus infection	Guinea pig	Stanberry, 1989
Herpes virus infection	Patas monkey	Achili et al., 1984
Herpes virus sylvilagus infection	Cottontail rabbit	Hesselton et al., 1988
Herpetic infection	Cotton rat	Marennikova et al., 1986
	Guinea pig	Vales et al., 1991
Herpetic keratitis	Inbred mice	Metcalf & Michaelis, 1984
Hindlimb wound	Rat	O'Connor et al., 1982
Hip dislocation, in vivo + in vitro	Newborn rabbit	Asplund et al., 1983
Hip dysplasia	Dog	Schoenecker et al., 1984
Hip implant evaluation	Arthritic sheep	Phillips et al., 1990
Hipoxaemia, chronic fetal	Sheep	Daniel et al., 1989
Hippocampal lesions	Models	Schmajuk, 1987
Hirschsprung's disease	Mice	Wood et al., 1986
HIV-1	Mice, rabbit, rat, primate	Agy & Katze, 1993
HIV-1 in utero infection	Chimpanzee	Eichberg et al., 1988
HIV-1 infection	Cat	Siebelink et al., 1990
	SCID-hu mice	Aldrovandi et al., 1993
	Macaque monkey	Voss & Hunsmann, 1993
	Macaque	Voss & Hunsmann, 1993
HIV-1 vaccines	Macaca	Schultz & Hu, 1993
HLA-B27-associated disorder	Transgenic rat	Hammer et al., 1990
Hodgkin's disease	Mice	Kapp et al., 1992
Homocysteinemia	Pig, human	Reddy & Wilcken, 1982
Hookworm infections	Mice	Carroll et al., 1983

Disease	Animal Model	Reference
HSV-1 infection, oral	Mice	Park et al., 1982
HSV-induced retinitis	Von Sizily model	Zierhut, 1994
HTLV-1 (human T-cell leukemia virus type I)	Rat	Suga et al., 1991
Human filarial parasitic Loaloa	Macaca fasciaelanis	Pinder et al., 1990
Humoral hypercalcemia of malignancy	CD 1 mice	Gkonos et al., 1984
	Rat	Ikeda et al., 1988
Huntington's disease	Rodent	Rieke et al., 1984
	Rat	Schwartz & Block, 1993
	Rat	Sanberg et al., 1989
Hyaline membrane disease	Rabbit	Nilsson, 1982
Hydrocephalus	Wistar-Imamichi rat	Koto et al., 1987
	Rat, rabbit	Brent & Beckman, 1986
	C57 black mice	Kanno et al., 1987
Hydronephrosis	DDD inbred mice	Nakajima & Goto, 1983
Hydroxyapatite bone graft	Dog	Sartoris, 1986
Hyperactivity but without hypertension	Rat	Hendley et al., 1986
Hyperactivity following postnatal anoxia	Rat	Speiser et al., 1983
Hyperammonemia	Rat	Azorin et al., 1989
Hyperbilirubinemia	Rat	Leyten et al., 1986
	Bolivian squirrel monkey	Cornelius, 1993
Hypercalcemia nephrolithiasis	Rabbit	Eddy et al., 1986
Hypercalcemia of malignancy	Murine	Burtis et al., 1986
	Athymic mice	Shipley et al., 1988
	Nude mice	Mehdizadeh et al., 1989
Hypercholesterolemia	WHHL rabbit	Havel et al., 1982
	WHHL rabbit	Phelan et al., 1985
	Watanabe rabbit	Kita et al., 1987
	Watanabe rabbit	Buja et al., 1990
	WHHL rabbit	Tilton et al., 1985
	Rabbit	Ishii et al., 1988
	Rabbit	Saku et al., 1990
Hypercholesterolemia and arteriosclerosis	Pig	Rapacz et al., 1986
Hyperdynamic sepsis, chronic	Rat	Mela-Riker et al., 1988
Hyperkinesis	Mice	Sackler & Weltman, 1985
Hypermagnesemia	Pregnant goat	Wians et al., 1990
Hypermetabolic sepsis	Rat	Lang et al., 1983
Hyperoxaluria type 2	Cat	Danpure et al., 1989
Hyperparathyroidism	Rat	Jaeger et al., 1987
	Long-Evans rat	Demeter et al., 1991
Hyperparathyroidism, primary	Athymic nude mice	Schachter et al., 1989
Hyperphenylalaninemia and hyperthyrosinemia	Rat	Lewis et al., 1985
Hyperplasia in vein grafts	Dog	Landymore et al., 1985
	Model	Murday et al., 1983
Hyperprolactinemia, chronic	Buffalo rat	Adler et al., 1991
Hyperprolactinemic hypogonadism	Rat	Park & Selmanoff, 1991
Hypersensitivity pneumonia	Rat	Quezada et al., 1983
Hypersensitivity pneumonitis	Rabbit	Butler et al., 1983

Disease	Animal Model	Reference
Hypersensitivity pneumonitis	Nude mice	Takizawa et al., 1992
Hypersensitivity, allergic asthma	Dog	Lewis et al., 1982
Hypersplenism	Rat	Roncoroni, 1982
Hypertension	Hypertensive rat	Williams et al., 1982
	Rat	Bianchi et al., 1986
	Wistar rat	Benediktsson et al., 1993
	Rat	Yamori et al., 1984
	Rat	Hatton & McCarron, 1994
	African green monkey	Martin et al., 1990
	Transgenic mice	Lang et al., 1994
	Dahl rat	Friedman, 1988
	Munich + Kyoto Wistar rat	Gamerman et al., 1985
Hypertension and diabetes	Rat	Fein et al., 1984
	Hypertensive diabetic rat	Sato et al., 1987
Hypertension research	Wooly monkey	Muller et al., 1989
	Rat	Lovenberg, 1987
Hypertension with diabetes	Rat	Cooper et al., 1990
Hypertension, aldosterone-binding	Rat	Nowaczynski, 1983
Hypertension, arterial	Broad-brested white turkey	Scannapieco et al., 1983
	Rat	Ribeiro et al., 1981
Hypertension, chronic alimentary imbalance	Wistar rat	Strekalova et al., 1991
Hypertension, chronic salt loading	Wistar rat	Strekalova et al., 1989
Hypertension, Deoxycorticosterone acetate	Sheep	Mitchell, 1984
Hypertension, DOCA and aldosterone	Yucatan miniature swine	Terris & Simmonds, 1982
Hypertension, environmentally induced	Rat	Lawler et al., 1988
Hypertension, essential arterial	Rat	Grana et al., 1989
Hypertension, pregnancy-induced	Pregnant sheep	Thatcher & Keith, 1986
Hypertension, progressive	Rat	Martin et al., 1984
Hypertension, severe	Rat	Heidemann et al., 1985
Hypertension, spontaneous	Rat	Pravenec, 1986
Hypertension, stroke	Rat	Yamori, 1991
Hypertensive, genetic markers	Rat	Yamori et al., 1981
Hyperthermia	Mice	De Feo et al., 1989
	Pig	Mayzner-Zawadzka, 1983
Hyperthyroid tissue	Nude mice, human	Vignaud et al., 1984
Hypertrophic neuropathy	Tibetian Mastiff dog	Sponenberg et al., 1981
Hyperventilation	Guinea pig	Hosenpud et al., 1983
Hypocholinergic syndrome	Model	Jenden et al., 1987
Hypophosphaetamia and phosphate depletion	Rat	Knochel, 1982
Hypothyroidism	Albino mice	Gonzalez Reimers, 1988
Hypoxanthine phosphoribosyl transferase	Mice	Monk et al., 1987
Hypoxia	Mice	Grau & Balasch, 1985
	Murine	Dunn, 1980
	Perfused rat heart	Korneev et al., 1991
	Model	Hlinak & Krejci, 1990
	Cardiomyocyte culture	Stvolinska et al., 1988
Hypoxia - post infarction	Rat	Manukhina et al., 1991

Disease	Animal Model	Reference
Hypoxia and ischaemia, cerebral	Rabbit	Fekete et al., 1988
Hypoxia, fetus in utero	Cat, rat, guinea pig	Sohmer et al., 1991
Hypoxia, heart	Rat	Ivanov & Khitrov, 1983
Hypoxia, muscle	Rat	Schroder et al., 1990
Hypoxial, cerebral	Rat	Ivanova & Bobkov, 1984
Hypoxic brain damage, perinatal	Rat	Lun et al., 1990
Hypoxic neuropathy	Rat	Low et al., 1986
Hypoxic-ischaemic brain injury	Rodent	Silverstein et al., 1984
Ichthyosis	Nude mice	Elias et al., 1983
Idiopathic dystonia	Syrian gold hamster	Richter et al., 1993
Idiophatic torticollis	White Pekin duck	Gopalakrishnakone, 1985
IGA nephropathy	Mice	Lamm et al., 1984
	C3H/HeJ mice	Genin et al., 1986
	Models	Scivittaro et al., 1993
Immotile cilia syndrome	Mice, human	Bryan, 1983
	WIC-Hyd rat	Torikata et al., 1991
Immune complex glomerulonephritis	Rat	Oite et al., 1983
Immune complex glomerulopathy	Mice	Sawtell et al., 1987
Immune reproductive failure	DBA mice	Strassburger et al., 1992
Immune-complex-induced inflammatory reaction	Hamster	Bjork et al., 1984
Immune-mediated motor neuron disease	Guinea pig	Smith et al., 1993
Immunity & pasteurellosis	Rabbit	Corbeil et al., 1983
Immunocytoma	LOU/M/WSL X CF Y/F1 rat	Puskas et al., 1984
Immunodeficiency	Guinea pig	Antonenko et al., 1989
Immunodeficiency syndrome	Chimpanzee	Fultz et al., 1987
	Chimpanzee	Fultz, 1989
Immunodeficiency virus type I	Chimpanzee	Lusso et al., 1990
Immunologic asthma	Guinea pig	Obata et al., 1992
Immunosuppressants	Models + clinic	Tufveson et al., 1993
Implanted onchocerca volvulus	Mice, rat	Rajan et al., 1992
In vitro fertilization	Mice	Santalo et al., 1992
In-situ immune complex disease	Model	Boyce et al., 1988
Inborn error of metabolism of urea cycle	Mice	Spector et al., 1983
Inborn errors, cancer and evolution	Cat	O'Brien et al., 1982
Incomplete circle of willis	Gerbil	Delbarre et al., 1987
Induction of cholesteral gallstones	Ground squirrel	Pemsingh et al., 1987
Infant respiratory failure	Sheep, goat	Tsuno et al., 1987
Infantile amnesia	Rat	Campbell et al., 1984
Infantile polycystic kidney disease	Mice	Fry et al., 1985
Infants-at-risk	Models	Resnick et al., 1983
Infarcted myocardium	Rat	Bogers et al., 1983
Infection	Mice	Blaser et al., 1983
	Beige mice	Bertram et al., 1986
	Mice, rat	Berti, 1982
	SCID and SCID/beige mice	Percy & Barta, 1993
Infection immunodeficiency	Rabbit	Filice et al., 1988
Infection model	Gnotobiotic piglet	Tzipori et al., 1985

Disease	Animal Model	Reference
Infection model	Primate	Kodama et al., 1990
Infection, Brugia malayi	Ferret	Crandall, 1984
Infection, Brugia spp.	Nude rat	Cruiekshank, 1983
Infection, Giardia lamblia	Rat	Craft, 1982
Infection, intestinal helminth	Trichuris muris mice	Grencies, 1993
Infection, Ostertagia circumcinta	Gerbil	Court et al., 1988
Infection, Pixuna	White mice	Chizhow et al., 1985
Infection, plasmodium knowlessi	Presbytis entellus	Dutta et al. et al., 1981
Infection, salmonella typhi	Newborn guinea pig	Dima et al., 1989
Infection, schistosoma mansoni	Monkey	Del Portillo et al., 1986
Infection, strongyloides stercoral	Ferret	Davidson, 1988
Infection, Yersinia enterocolitica	Mice	Chiesa et al., 1987
Infections	Monkey	Dzhikidze, 1986
Infections bovine keratoconjunctivitis	Model	Chandler et al., 1982
Infections hookworm infection	Dog	Caroll, 1984
Infections, chronic urinary tract	Rat	Davis, 1987
Infections, pseudomonas aeruginoas	Leukopenic mice	Cryz et al., 1983
Infectious mononucleosis-like response	Marmoset	Wedderburn, 1984
Inflamatory pain + endogenous opid system	Mice	Shibata et al., 1986
Inflamatory pain, effect of opiods	Rat	Shippenberg et al., 1988
Inflammation	Rat	Carbonell et al., 1989
	Rat	Johnson et al., 1986
	Sprague Dawley rat	Zuccato et al., 1992
	Mice	Henriques et al., 1987
	Model	Pawlowski, 1983
	Horse	Higgins et al., 1987
	Rat	Isaji et al., 1989
Inflammation of bladder	Rat	McMahon & Abel, 1987
Inflammation, acute	Horse	Lees et al., 1987
Inflammation, air pouch	Rat	Yoshino et al., 1985
	Rat	Yoshino et al., 1984
Inflammatory bowel disease	Sprague Dawley rat	Moyana & Lalonde, 1990
	Wistar rat	Matsumoto et al., 1993
	Sprague Dawley rat	Selve, 1992
	Models	Warren & Watkins, 1994
	Rat	Wallace et al., 1989
	Models	Warren & Watkins, 1994
Inflammatory demyelinating polyneuropathy	Mice	Dib et al., 1987
Inflammatory myopathies	Models	Rosenberg, 1993
Inflammatory pain, chronic	Mice, rat	Okuyama & Aihara, 1984
Inflammatory polyneuropathy	Monkey	Heininger et al., 1984
Inflammatory-resorptive bone destruction	Hamster, rat	Seichter, 1983
Influence of x-chromosome on immunity	CBA/N mice	Scher, 1982
Influenza	Ferret	Smith & Sweet, 1988
Influenza C virus infection	Rat	Takiguchi et al., 1990
Influenza illness	Ferret	Reuman et al., 1989
Information file	WHHL rabbit	Kawamata, 1984

Disease	Animal Model	Reference
Informational neuroses	Model	Chkhikvishvili, 1984
Infrahepatic bile duct proliferation	Rat	Bourdelat et al., 1983
Inhalant abuse	Rat	Gause et al., 1985
Inhalation injury	Goat	Walker et al., 1981
Inherited hematologic disease	Models	Kaneko et al., 1987
Inhibition of Na+/K+ pump	Models	Pamnani et al., 1981
Inhibition of S-alpha-reductase	Rat	Imperato-McGinley, 1985
Insulin-dependent diabetes mellitus	Mice	Blay et al., 1985
Interstitial lung disease	Motheaten mice	Rossi et al., 1985
Intestinal infarction or obstruction, acute	Rat	Kazmierczak et al., 1988
Intestinal ischaemia	Dog	Parks et al., 1982
Intestinal ischaemia, MRI imaging	Lewis rat	Temes, 1991
Intestinal mucosal hyperplasia	Rat	Senior et al., 1985
Intraabdominal abscess	Rat	Fry et al., 1982
	Rat	Bartlett et al., 1990
Intraabdominal infection	Rat	Muhvich et al., 1988
Intracerebral hematoma	Rabbit	Kaufman et al., 1985
Intracerebral hematomas	Rat	Romanova, 1989
Intracerebral hemorrhage	Dog	Lillehei et al., 1984
Intracerebral infection	Monkey	Carballal et al., 1987
Intracerebral toxoplasmosis	Murine	Hofflin et al., 1987
Intracutaneous melanoma	DBA/ 2J mice	Levine et al., 1982
Intrahepatic infection	Murine	Liance et al., 1984
Intraperitoneal infection	Mice	Petrovskaia et al., 1983
Intraperitoneal sepsis	Sprague Dawley rat	Short, 1983
Intrapulmonary implantation	Rat	Kal et al., 1986
Intrauterine exposure to phenylalanine	Rhesus monkey	Pueschel, 1985
Intrauterine growth retardation	Models	Evans et al., 1983
	Rat	Hayashi & Dorko, 1988
	Model	Zhang, 1989
Intrauterine infection	Guinea pig	Griffith et al., 1986
Intraventricular blood clot	Dog	Pang et al., 1986
Intraventricular hemorrhage	Premature rabbit	Kasik et al., 1985
	Premature rabbit and pup	Coulter et al., 1984
	Beagle puppy	Ment et al., 1984
	Beagle puppy	Ment et al., 1983
	Beagle puppy	Ment et al., 1982
Intraventricular hemorrhage in the fetus	Pregnant Sprague Dawley	Howe & Webster, 1990
Intraventricular hemorrhage in the premature	Beagle puppy	Johnson et al., 1987
Invalidation of neuroleptic response	Models, human	Wetzel et al., 1991
Invasive aspergillosis	New Zealand white rabbit	Spreadbury et al., 1989
Iodine deficiency + fetal brain development	Cotton eared marmoset	Mano, 1985
Iron deficiency	Syrian hamster	Rennie et al., 1982
	Syrian hamster	Ranasinghe et al., 1983
Ischaemia	Baboon	Opie et al., 1983
Ischaemia of extremities	Rat	Kosnikova, 1987
Ischaemia, acute	Skeletal muscle	Kuzon et al., 1986

Disease	Animal Model	Reference
Ischaemia, bilateral hemispheric	Rat	Sugio et al., 1988
Ischaemia, chorodial	Monkey	Sterkers & Larsen, 1985
Ischaemia, forebrain	Rat	Smith et al., 1984
Ischaemia, global forebrain	Rat	Dirnagl et al., 1993
Ischaemia, regional	Dog	Sunagawa et al., 1983
Ischaemia, reversible	Model	Vas et al., 1981
Ischaemia, spinal cord	Dog	Zhan et al., 1989
Ischaemic attacks	Gerbil	Tomida et al., 1987
Ischaemic bowel necrosis	Rat	Goonzales-Crussi, 1983
Ischaemic cortical lesions	Rat	Rubino & Young, 1988
Ischaemic heart	Pig	Klein, 1986
Ischaemic injury of spinal cord	Dog	Sulla et al., 1989
Ischaemic left ventricular failure, acute	Dog	Smiseth & Mjos, 1982
Ischaemic liver failure	Rat	Asakawa et al., 1989
Ischaemic myocardium, transient	Ischemic swine heart	Mousa et al., 1992
Ischaemic renal failure	Rat	Zager, 1987
Isolating intact retinal vascular beds	Models, human	Laver et al., 1993
Jaundice	Wistar rat	Ker & Wu, 1992
Jaundice, obstructive	Rat	Diamond et al., 1991
Jejunal injury	Rat	Warren et al., 1982
Juvenile diabetes	BB rat	Workshop, 1982
Kallmann syndrome - neuronal targeting	Adult chicken	Rugarli et al., 1993
Kaposi's sarcoma	Murine	Sato et al., 1986
Kashin-Beck disease	Mice	Yang et al., 1993
	Rhesus monkey	Yang, 1992
	Macaque monkey	Zhang & Liu, 1989
Kawasaki disease	Mice, human	Miyamoto et al., 1987
	Mice	Tomita et al., 1993
	Mice	Lehman et al., 1988
	Dog	Burns et al., 1991
	Mice	Murata, 1983
Keralitis	Nu/nu mice	Paniagua-Crespo, 1989
Keratoacanthoma	Dog	Rudolph, 1983
Kidney allograft	Rat	Lander et al., 1986
Kidney concentrating ability	Rabbit	Kekomaki et al., 1985
Kidney disease + chemical exposure, chronic	Mice, rat, human	Kluwe et al., 1984
Kidney lesions	NZB-NZW F1 mice	Prause et al., 1986
Kidney stone disease	Rat	Khan & Hackett, 1985
Labyrinth diseases	Mice	Nakai, 1982
Lagionella pneumophila	Models	Tartakovskii, 1984
Large bowel tumor promotion	Rat	Kusche et al., 1988
Larval multilocular echinococcosis liver + lungs	Rat	Kovalenko et al., 1986
Laryngeal carcinoma	Nude mice	Zhang, 1990
Lassa virus infection	Guinea pig	Jahrling et al., 1982
Learned helplessness	Rat	Maier, 1984
	Model	Telner & Singhal, 1984
Learning ability	Mice	Hunter et al., 1986

Disease	Animal Model	Reference
Left-to-right shunts in the newborn	Pig	Mavroudis et al., 1984
Left-ventricular bypass	Donkey	Chilaia & Khodeli, 1990
Legionella pneumofila infection	Guinea pig	Fitzgeorge et al., 1983
Legionnaire´s pneumonia	Guinea pig	Winn, 1982
	Guinea pig, rat	Winn et al., 1982
Leishmania aethiopica	Laboratory models	Huber et al., 1989
Leishmania mexicana	Inbred balb/c mice	Anderson, 1983
Leishmaniasis	Hamster	Ghosh & Ghosh, 1987
	East African primate	Githure et al., 1987
	Laboratory animals	Pleskanovskaia, 1986
Leprosy	Hairless mice	Packchanian et al., 1982
	African green monkey	Baskin et al., 1987
	Primate	Martin et al., 1984
	Monkeys - 3 species	Wolf et al., 1985
	Mice	Lovik, 1987
	Mangabey monkey	Modlin et al., 1986
	Mexican armadillo	Quesada-Pascul, 1987
Leprous infections	Mice	Vishnevetskii et al., 1988
Leptomeningeal heterotopias	Rat fetal tissue	Tamagawa et al., 1989
Leptomeningeal neoplasia	Guinea pig	Zovivkian & Youle, 1988
Leptospirosis	Mice	Hathaway et al., 1983
Lesch-Nyhan syndrome	Rat	Minana et al., 1984
	Monkey	Goldstein et al., 1986
	Mice	Kuehn et al., 1987
	HPRT-deficient mice	Jinnah, 1990
Lesions in the tracheal wall	Syrian hamster	Reuzel et al., 1984
Leukaemia	Nude mice	Potter et al., 1984
	Wild mice	Gardner, 1987
Leukaemia infection	Sheep	Burkhardt et al., 1989
Leukaemia transplant model	Fischer rat	Dieter et al., 1990
Leukaemia, comparative	Mice, human	Pasqualini, 1981
Leukemia-related disorders	F344 rat	Stromberg, 1990
Leukemias	Models	Daley, 1993
Leukemias, induced	Transgenic mice	Daley, 1993
Leukemias, pH-positive	Transgenic mice	Groffen et al., 1993
Leukemogenesis	Chicken	Graf, 1984
	Murine	Van Etten, 1993
Leukocyte adhesion deficiency	Mice	Krauss et al., 1991
Leukodystrophy (Krabbe´s disease)	Mice	Suzuki & Suzuki, 1983
Leutivirus disease	Cow	Gonda et al., 1990
Limbic epilepsy	Rat	Robertson, 1983
Lipid keratopathy	Rabbit	Stock et al., 1985
Lipid metabolism	Models	Suckling et al., 1993
Lipid peroxidation	Sprague Dawley rat	Morrow et al., 1992
Listeriosis	Mice	Hof & Kuhn, 1984
Listeriosis, T-cell deficiency	BALB/c mice	Schaffner, 1983
Lithiasis	Rat	Sakly et al., 1991

Disease	Animal Model	Reference
Liver abscess	New Zealand white rabbit	McDonald et al., 1984
	Rabbit	Kryshen et al., 1984
Liver allograft rejection	Lewis rat	Nakamura et al., 1993
Liver cells, injury, death, changes	Models	Taoka, 1985
Liver cirrhosis	Rat	Toth et al., 1991
	Model	Nadkarni et al., 1991
	Model	Shiga & Mori, 1985
Liver evaluating hepatoprotective drugs	Model	Trcka & Siblikova, 1985
Liver failure 90% hepatectomy, acute	Rabbit	Mullen, 1987
Liver failure, acute	Rat	Bates et al., 1989
Liver injury and disease, Kupffer cells	Models, human	Winwood & Arthur, 1993
Liver ischemia	Sprague Dawley rat	Portugal et al., 1993
Liver lesions, focal and nodular	Rodent	Vesselinovitch, 1988
Liver metastases	Rabbit	Toda, 1992
Liver metastasis from gastric VX2 cancer	Model	Tada et al., 1992
Liver oval cells, effect of treatment	Rat	Tatematsu et al., 1984
Liver transplantation	Pig	Cywes et al., 1992
Liver transport system	Rat	Dixit & Chang, 1990
Liver tumor	Rat	Hamm & Jaupitz, 1993
Liver tumors, extrapolation to man	Rodent	Roe, 1987
Lung cancer	Dog	Benfield et al., 1981
	Rat	Byhardt et al., 1984
	Hamster	Hammond et al., 1991
	Model	Tran et al., 1981
Lung cancer, responsiveness to drugs	Nude mice	Tashiro et al., 1989
Lung carcinogenicity of cell	Rat	Maximilien et al., 1992
Lung confusion	Rat	Fricke, 1982
Lung disease	Rat	Chang et al., 1986
	Equine	Breeze et al., 1984
Lung disease, chronic	Swine	Donham et al., 1984
Lung fibrosis, subchronic	Hamster	Zia et al., 1992
Lung hyperactivity to bronchial hyperreactivity	Guinea pig	Pretolani et al., 1993
Lung infection, chronic	Wild rodent	Maciver et al., 1991
Lung injury	Sheep	Begin et al., 1983
	Models	Chang et al., 1991
Lung injury, acute	Sheep	Simpson et al., 1991
Lung radiogenic pneumopathy	Piglet	Herrmann et al., 1986
Lung response to elastase	Sheep	Susskind et al., 1984
Lung surfactant	Fetal monkey	Rooney et al., 1983
Lung transplantation	Rat	Corris et al., 1987
Lupus syndrome	Models	Meyer, 1981
Lupus syndrome, drug related	Rapid + slow acetylator rat	Weber & Tannen, 1981
Lyme arthritis	LEW/N rat	Barthold et al., 1988
Lyme disease	Rhesus monkey	Philipp et al., 1993
	Gerbil	Preac et al., 1990
Lymph node metastasis	Murine	Vandendris et al., 1985
Lymphadenophy-associated virus	Chimpanzee	Francis et al., 1984

Disease	Animal Model	Reference
Lymphatic filarial infection	Dog	Snowden et al., 1989
Lymphoblastic leukemia, acute	Sprague Dawley rat	Mullenix, 1990
	Sprague Dawley rat	Schunior et al., 1990
Lymphocytic leukaemia	Murine	Slavin et al., 1981
Lymphocytic leukemia, chronic	Mice	Schrek, 1990
Lymphocytic thyreoditis	Rat	Penhale et al., 1982
Lympholeukemia	Cattle	Kukain et al., 1983
Lymphoma	Rabbit	Iakovleva et al., 1987
	Athymic mice	Baird et al., 1982
Lysocomal storage disease	Feline	Baker et al., 1982
Malabsorption	Rat	Wild & Murray, 1992
Malaria	Mice	Bastien et al., 1987
	Japanese monkey	Kawai et al., 1993
	Transgenic models	Shear, 1993
	Rat, primate	Langhorn, 1994
Malaria, cerebral	Mice	Rest, 1982
	Squirrel monkey	Gysin, 1992
Malaria, plasmodium bergei	White rat	Desowitz et al., 1989
Male -pattern baldness	Androchronogetic mice	Matias, 1989
Male infertility	Mice	Chubb & Nolan, 1985
	Wistar rat	Engel et al., 1988
	Inbred mice	Anderson et al., 1983
	Black mink	Tung, 1981
	Mice	Chubb & Nolan, 1985
Male reproductivity toxicology	Animal, human	Working, 1988
Malignancy-associated humoral hypercalcemia	Athymic mice	Kukla et al., 1984
Malignant fibrous histiocytoma	Rat	Konishi et al., 1984
Malignant hematologic disorders	BALB/c mice	Ackerstein et al., 1981
Malignant melanoma	Swine	Tissot et al., 1987
Malignant mesothelioma	Nude mice	Chahinian et al., 1991
Mammary sarcoma tumor	BALB/cKa mice	Lord & Burkhardt, 1984
Mammary tumor model	Sprague Dawley rat	Kort et al., 1987
Mannosidosis	Guinea pig	Huxtable & Darling, 1982
	Cattle	Jones & Abbitt, 1993
Mannosidosis: ocular lesions eye	Bovine	Jolly et al., 1987
Marfan syndrome	Calf	Besser et al., 1990
Masseter muscle	Cow, dog, cat, rabbit, rat	Tuxen & Kirkeby, 1990
	Pig	Tuxen, 1993
Mastectomy	Rat	Lindsey et al., 1990
Medullary thyroid carcinoma	Mice	Horiuchi et al., 1991
Megacaryocytopoiesis	CH3 mice, human	Jackson et al., 1990
Melanocyte dysfunction	Chicken	Buissy et al., 1986
Melanoma	Swine	Hook et al., 1982
	Dog, guinea pig, hamster	Epstein, 1992
Melanoma LOX	Nude mice	Fodstad et al., 1988
Melanoma metastasis	Nude mice	Kerbel et al., 1984
Membranous nephropathy	Rat	Couser et al., 1982

Disease	Animal Model	Reference
Membranous nephropathy	Rat	Gabbai, 1987
Memory disorders	Rabbit	Solomon et al., 1988
Menetrier's disease	Cattle	Snider et al., 1983
Mengo virus infection	Mice	Guthke et al., 1987
Meningeal gliomatosis	Mice	Yoshida et al., 1986
	Wistar, F344 rat	Yoshida et al., 1984
Meningeal leukemia	Model	Varakis et al., 1981
Meningeal neoplasia	Rat	Kooistra et al., 1986
Meningo-encephalitis	Murine	Hay et al., 1985
Meningocele + meningoencephalocele	Rhesus monkey	Hendrickx & Tarara, 1990
Meningococcal infection	Mice	Mironova et al., 1984
Meningoencephalitis	Rabbit	Smego & Durack, 1984
Menke's disease	Brindled mottled mice	Martin et al., 1991
Menkes' kinky-hair disease	Cu-induced toxicity in mice	Shiraishi et al., 1991
Menkes' kinky-hair syndrome	Mutant mice	Shiraishi et al., 1988
Mental disease	Rhesus monkey	Goosen, 1981
Mental retardation	Rat	Hendrich et al., 1984
	Rat	Anderson, 1994
	Rat	Strupp et al., 1984
Metastatic brain tumor	Mice	Conley, 1984
Metastatic colon carcinoma	Rat	Dunnington et al., 1987
Metastatic liver involvement	Model	Udintsev et al., 1992
Microvascular dysfunction	Rabbit	Tilton et al., 1983
Migastenia gravis	SCID mice	Martino et al., 1993
Mineralocorticoid resistance	Models	Meyer, 1986
Mite infection	Guinea pig	Rothwell et al., 1991
Mitochondrial myopathy	Rat	Cooper et al., 1988
Moebius syndrome	Rat	Lipson et al., 1989
Monoamine receptors, affective disorder	Rat	Martin et al., 1990
Mononucleosis-like syndrome	Marmoset	Emini et al., 1986
Morphine dependence	Mice	Suzuki et al., 1984
Motion sickness	Models	Ossenkopp, 1985
	Rat	Puko & Orozd, 1990
	Rat	Morita, 1989
Motion sickness syndrome	Monkey	Wilpizeski & Lowry, 1987
Motor neuron degeneration	Mice	Messer, 1987
Mozambique virus infection	Rhesus monkey	Walker et al., 1982
Mucocutaneous disease	Mice	Barral et al., 1983
Mucopolysaccharidosis	Dog	Shull et al., 1982
	Mice	Biekenmeir et al., 1989
Mucosa cancer	Nude mice, hamster	von Glass et al., 1992
Mucositis induced by chemotherapy	Golden Syrian hamster	Sonis et al., 1990
Multiple acyl-CoA dehydrogenase deficiency	Raboflavin-deficient rat	Montgomery et al., 1991
Multiple myeloma	SCID mice	Huang et al., 1993
	Mice	Radl et al., 1988
Multiple osteochrondrial lesions	Mice	Hosoda et al., 1981
Multiple sclerosis	Mice	Lindsley et al., 1992

Disease	Animal Model	Reference
Multiple sclerosis		Tsukada et al., 1987
	Model	Lassman, 1983
	Models	Fleming, 1985
Muscarinic receptor function	Dog	Vatner et al., 1988
Muscarinic receptor, hypersensitivity	Rat	Carrier & Aronstam, 1987
Muscle degeneration and regeneration	Rat	Narukami, 1991
Muscle type 2B fibres damage	Rat	Brumback, 1983
Muscular dystrophy	White Pekin duck	Gopalakrishnakone, 1986
Myasthenia gravis	Dog	Garlepp et al., 1984
Myasthenia gravis, acetylcholine receptor	Rabbit, electric ray	Tu, 1988
Myasthenia, acetylcholine receptor	Rat	Gomez et al., 1984
Mycobacterium avium complex infection	Beije mice	Bermudez et al., 1992
Mycobacterium bovis infection	Badgers (Meles meles)	Pritchard et al., 1987
Mycobacterium intracellular disease	Beige mice	Gangadharan, 1983
Mycobacterium leprae	Hibernating ground squirrel	Galleti et al., 1982
Mycobacterium ulcerans research	Mastomys natalenis	Singh et al., 1984
Mycoplasma chronic infection	Monkey	Marantidi et al., 1991
Myelin deficiency	Syrian hamster	Nunoya, 1985
Myelin formation deficiency	Models	Tsuji, 1981
Myelocytic leukemia	Mice	Zhao, 1985
Myelocytic leukemia, acute	Rat	Hagenbeck et al., 1990
	Brown Norway rat	Martens, 1990
Myelodysplastic syndrome	Cat	Testa et al., 1988
Myelogenous leukemia	RF mice	Wolman et al., 1982
Myeloma	ST2 mice	Croese et al., 1987
Myocardial anti-infarct research	Rat	Somora et al., 1987
Myocardial dysfunction, transient	Dog	Raberger, 1986
Myocardial hypertrophy	Rat	Batra et al., 1991
Myocardial infarction	Dog	Browne et al., 1983
	Dog, baboon	Flameng et al., 1986
	Rat	Erlebacher, 1985
	Rat	Cammileri et al., 1981
	Dog	Sakai et al., 1982
Myocardial infarction, occlusion-reperfusion	Rabbit	Shvilkin et al., 1991
Myocardial ischaemia	Pig	White et al., 1986
	Pig	Verdouw et al., 1983
	Dog	Shi, Sinvas et al., 1995
	Rabbit	Dwived et al., 1987
Myocardial ischaemia / Salvage	Ferret	Gomoll & Lekich, 1990
Myocardial ischaemia, focal	Dog	Obelinius et al., 1981
Myocardial necrosis	Mice	Khatib et al., 1982
Myocardial occlusion-reperfusion	Pig	Naslund et al., 1986
Myocardial perfusion	Dog	Mousa, 1991
Myocardial reperfusion	Pig	Garcia-Dorado, 1987
Myocardial stunning	Dog, rabbit, rat	Abd-Elfattah, 1993
Myocardial stunning and preconditioning	Rabbit, rat	Abd-Elfattah et al., 1993
Myocarditis	BALB/c mice	Sun et al., 1988

Disease	Animal Model	Reference
Myocarditis, gaint cell	Lewis rat	Kodama et al., 1990
Myocardium protection from ischaemic damage	Models	Hale & Kloner, 1994
Myoclonic encephalopathy, acute	Hamster	Sugita et al., 1984
Myoclonus	Rat	Angel, 1986
Myofibrillar disarray	Rat	Olsen, 1985
Myoglobinuric acute renal failure	Rat	Abul-Ezz et al., 1991
Myohypotransferrinemia with hemosiderosis	Murine	Bernstein, 1987
Myosin isoform expression	Sprague Dawley rat	Caiozzo et al., 1992
Narcolepsy-cataplexy	Mutant rat (taiep)	Prieto et al., 1991
Nasal allergy	Guinea pig	Tanaka et al., 1988
Nasal polyposis	Chimpanzee	Jacobs et al., 1984
Necrotizing enterocolitis	Models	Toplian & Ziegler, 1984
Negative schizophrenic symptomatology	Rat	Carnoy et al., 1986
Neisseria meningitidis	Mice	Brodeur et al., 1986
Nematode infection chronic trichuriasis	Mice	Lee et al., 1983
Nematovirus spathiger infection	Rabbit	Hoste & Fort, 1992
Neonatal biliary atresia	Macaca mulatta	Cornelius et al., 1985
Neonatal hyperbilirubinemia	Rat carrybunn mutation	Stobie et al., 1991
Neonatal intraventricular hemorrhage	Beagle puppy	Pasternak et al., 1983
Neonatal lung disease, acute and chronic	Preterm rat	Tanswell et al., 1989
Neoplasia	Transgenic mice	Fowlis & Balmain, 1993
Neoplastic disease	SCID mice	Williams et al., 1993
Neoplastic invasion of arterial wall	Rabbit	Moshakis & Carter, 1984
Nephritis	Mice	Assmann et al., 1985
Nephrolithiasis	Rat	Kumar et al., 1991
Nephropathy	Rat	Lorentz et al., 1987
Nephrotic syndrome	Rat	Abramowsky et al., 1984
	Rat	Jiang, 1989
	Mutant mice (ICGN)	Ogura et al., 1989
	Rat	Wang et al., 1990
Nephrotoxic acute renal failure	Rabbit, rat	Stein & Fried, 1985
Nephrotoxicity of hemoglobin tetamer	Model	Moss et al., 1986
Nerve compression, chronic	Rat	MacKinnon et al., 1984
Nerve growth factor	Mice	Scott et al., 1983
	Rat	Williams, 1989
Nerve sensory function	Rat	De Koning et al., 1986
Neural basis of behavior	Models	Sanberg, 1990
Neural tube defects	Mice	Elmazar et al., 1988
	Genetic mammalian model	Copp, 1994
	Rhesus monkey	Michejda et al., 1987
	Manx cat	Green & Green, 1987
Neuroaxonal dystrophy	Scrapie	Liberski et al., 1989
Neurobehavioral teratology	Ferret	Rabe et al., 1985
Neuroblastoma	Mice	Della Penta, 1982
Neuroblastoma metastasis	Mice	Gilbert, 1988
Neuroendocrine lung cancer	Hamster	Schuller et al., 1988
Neurofibromatosis	Bicolor damselfish	Schmale et al., 1983

Disease	Animal Model	Reference
Neurofibromatosis	Rat	Cardesa et al., 1989
	Natural models	Riccardi et al., 1994
Neurogenic stress gastric ulcer	Rat	Ohashi et al., 1983
Neurogenic vesical dysfunction	Manx cat	Woodside et al., 1982
Neuroleptic anxiety syndrome	Rat	Russell et al., 1987
Neurologic deficit, glucose exacerbation	Rat	Le May et al., 1987
Neurologic diseases	Dog, cat	Tokuriki et al., 1981
Neurological deficit amd cerebral infarction	Cat	Weinstein, 1986
Neuromuscular disease	Guinea pig	McVicker et al., 1982
Neuron tube defect	Curly-tail mice	Seller et al., 1981
Neuronal degeneration	Models	Price et al., 1992
Neuronal responses to aging and injury	Models	Price et al., 1990
Neuropathy	Rabbit	Chiba et al., 1985
	Chicken	Padilla & Veronesi, 1988
Neuropsychiatric disorders	Primate	Howard & Pollard, 1983
Neuropsychiatric disorders Tourette syndrome	Models	Shaywitz, 1982
Neurosis	Developing rat	Krybus, 1984
	Dog	Airapetiants et al., 1986
Neurotoxicity	Model	Kobat et al., 1985
Neurovascular compression syndrome	Model	Segal et al., 1982
Neurovisceral toxic syndrome	Mice	Glavin et al., 1990
Nicotine addiction	White rat	Khodzagel'diev, 1984
Niemann-Pick disease	Mice	Miyawaki et al., 1982
	Mice	Sakiyama et al., 1982
Non-A and non-B viral hepatitis	Macaca mulatta	Uchida et al., 1988
Non-A, non-B Hepatitis	Monkey	Andzhaparidze, 1986
	Model	Karasawa et al., 1981
Non-Hodgkin's lymphoma	Baboon	Bukaeva et al., 1984
	Mice	Pattengale et al., 1983
Non-human models	Primate	McClure, 1984
Non-immunologic contact urticaria	Hartley guinea pig	Lahti & Maibach, 1987
Non-insulin-dependent diabetes	Rat	Portha et al., 1988
Non-insulin-dependent diabetes mellitus	Sand rat	Marquie et al., 1991
	Wistar fatty rat	Jiao et al., 1991
	Hypertensive rat	Iwase, 1991
Non-obese diabetic (NOD) mouse	Mice	Leiter et al., 1987
Non-obstructive bladder instability	Minipig	Sethia et al., 1990
NON-Thyroidal disease	Model	Tibaldi & Surks, 1985
Nutritional factors in carcinogenesis	Rat	Kroes et al., 1986
Nystagmus	Guinea pig	Miyamura et al., 1987
Obese-hypertensive model	Rat	Chanh et al., 1988
Obesity	Rat	Fisler et al., 1987
	C57B1/6, T/O mice	Webb et al., 1982
	Models	Guy-Grand, 1988
Obesity - theories of aetiology	Models	Proietto et al., 1994
Obesity research	Models	Mrosovsky & Melnk, 1986
Obstructive jaundice, reversible	Fischer 344 rat	Posner et al., 1990

Disease	Animal Model	Reference
Obstructive uropathy	Cat	Radzinski et al., 1991
Occlusive arterial disease	Rat	Angerbach et al., 1988
Occult filariasis	Ferret	Thompson et al., 1985
Ocular autoimmunity	Mice	Caspi et al., 1990
Ocular disease	Models	Tabbara & Cello, 1984
Ocular herpes, keratitis, retinitis and cataract	Mice	Anderson & Field, 1984
Ocular inflamation	Rabbit	Gherezghiher et al., 1989
Ocular lesions, herpes simplex virus	Newborn rabbit	Brick et al., 1981
Ocular toxocariasis	Mice	Ghafoor et al., 1984
Ocular toxoplasmosis	Murine	Dutton, 1986
	Rabbit	Friedrich & Muller, 1988
Ocular vasculaturis	Beagle puppy	Flower, 1990
Onchocerca gutturosa	Rodent	El Sinnary et al., 1987
Onchocercosis	Primate	Greene, 1987
	Rodent	Bain et al., 1985
	Mangabey monkey, chimp	Eberhard et al., 1991
Oncological models for radiotracer evaluation	Models	Wiebe, 1983
	Models	Wiebe, 1991
Ontogenesis	Mice	Hilbig et al., 1986
Opiate abstinence head-shaking	Infant rat	Perez-Saad, 1984
Opiate induced euphoria + analgesia	Model	Kornetsky et al., 1982
Opiate self-administration	Macaque monkey	Mello et al., 1983
Opiate-dependency	Macaca mulatta	Donahoe et al., 1993
Opistorchis infection	Cotton rat, white rat	Gitsu & Kovalenko, 1983
Opportunistic infection	Mice	Imai et al., 1984
Oral cancer	Hamster	Meng et al., 1981
Oral candidiasis	Hamster, macaca, mice, rat	Allen, 1994
Oral carcinomas	Mice	Feinberg, 1983
Oral mucosa cancer	Nude mice	Frohlich et al., 1986
Oral pulse granuloma	Rat	Talacko & Radden, 1988
Osmoregulatory disturbances	Prattleboro rat	Van Leeuwen, 1992
Ossicular and otic capsular	PL/J mice	Chole & Henry, 1985
Ossifying enthesopathy	Rat	Gillet et al., 1989
Osteoarthritis	Rabbit	Butler et al., 1983
	Rabbit	Malemud et al., 1986
	Mice	Van der Kraan, 1990
	Rhesus macaque	Chateauvert et al., 1990
	Rabbit	Coulais et al., 1983
	Adult merino sheep	Ghosh et al., 1993
	Guinea pig	Schwartz et al., 1981
	Rabbit	Colombo et al., 1983
	Guinea pig	Bendele et al., 1987
	Guinea pig	Meacock, 1990
	Dog	Tenenbaum, 1984
	Dog	Brandt, 1994
	Models	Pritzker, 1994
	Models	Carney, 1991

Disease	Animal Model	Reference
Osteoarthritis	Pond-Nuki dog	Pelletier et al., 1983
Osteoarthritis - process, problems, prospects	Models	Pritzker, 1994
Osteoarthrosis	Guinea pig	Kopp et al., 1983
	Models	Rohozkova et al., 1990
Osteoarthrotic changes after transarticular load	Dog	Thompson et al., 1991
Osteogenesis imperfecta	Mice	Sillence, 1993
Osteomyelitis	Model	Madel, 1985
Osteomyelitis, chronic	Rat	Rissing et al., 1985
Osteopenia	Castrated rat	Grynpas et al., 1987
Osteopetro-rickets	Model	Milhaud et al., 1981
Osteoporosis	Rat	Pazzaglia et al., 1990
	Models	Aufdemorte et al., 1993
	Sprague Dawley rat	Giardino et al., 1993
	Dog	Brandt, 1994
Osteoporosis, postmenopausal	Rat	Matsumoto et al., 1985
Otitis media	Chinchilla, Mongolian gerbil	Fulghum et al., 1982
	Guinea pig	Kohubu & Amatsu, 1985
	Mongolian gerbil	Fulghum et al., 1985
	Guinea pig	Hozawa, 1985
	Chinchilla	Giebink, 1989
Otitis media with effusion	Wistar rat	Hamada et al., 1993
Otitis media, acute	Cat	Brenna & Clarke, 1985
Otosclerosis-like condition	LP/J mice	Henry & Chole, 1987
Otosclerosis-like lesions	LP/J mice	Cramer & Chole, 1986
Ovarian cancer	Rabbit	Tu, 1993
Ovarian carcinoma	Nude mice, human	Fu & Hoffman, 1993
Ovarian epithelial adenocarcinoma	Nude mice	Li & Qian, 1993
Ovarian tumors	Rat	Burenin et al., 1987
Ovariectomy	Dog	Martin et al., 1987
Pain, arthritis, chronic	Rat	Chudler & Dong, 1981
	Rat	de Castro Costa, 1982
	Rat	Colpaert, 1987
Pain, chronic	Rat	Calvino et al., 1991
	Models	Sweet, 1981
Pancreas carcinoma	Rat	Longnecker, 1981
	Rat	Longnecker et al., 1984
Pancreas regulations	Rat	Goke, 1990
Pancreas spontaneous tumor formation	Rat	Stace et al., 1987
Pancreas, partially diabetic	Rabbit	Meehan et al., 1987
Pancreatic cancer	Syrian hamster	Chester et al., 1989
	Transgenic animals	Working group, 1987
Pancreatic cancer transplantation	Nude mice, human	Vezeridis et al., 1989
Pancreatic cancer transplants	BALB/c -nu/nu nude mice	Liu, 1992
Pancreatic carcinogenesis	Hamster, rat	Birt & Roebuck, 1986
Pancreatic carcinomas	Wistar/Lewis rat	Redding, 1984
Pancreatic closed duodenal loop	Cat	Goulbourne et al., 1986
Pancreatic diseases	Mice	Kubota et al., 1989

Disease	Animal Model	Reference
Pancreatic duct adenocarcinoma	Syrian gold hamster	Townsend et al., 1982
Pancreatic ductal ligation + excision	Hamster	Pour et al., 1983
Pancreatic insufficiency, chronic	Rat	Kataoka et al., 1988
Pancreatic pseudocysts	Dog	Salinas et al., 1985
Pancreatic transplantation	Baboon	Du Toit et al., 1987
Pancreatic tumor, induction	Rat	Taylor et al., 1989
Pancreatitis, acute	Dog	Estourgie et al., 1983
	Sprague Dawley rat	Schmidt et al., 1992
	Rat	Rueda et al., 1991
	Rat	Tani, 1990
Pancreatitis, chronic	Dog	Strombeck et al., 1984
	Wistar Bonn/Kobori rat	Ohashi et al., 1990
Pancreatitis, infectious	Rat, dog	Kenmochi et al., 1989
Papillomavirus infection	Athymic mice	Howett et al., 1990
Papovavirusi	Golden hamster	Borodina et al., 1984
Parainfluenza virus type 1 and 3	Marmoset	Hawthorne et al., 1982
Parainfluenza virus type 3 disease	Cotton rat	Murphy et al., 1981
Parasitic disease	Models	Poleshchuk et al., 1983
Parasitic diseases	SCID mice	McKerrow et al., 1993
Parathyroid function	Chicken	Cole et al., 1989
Parkinson syndrome	Monkey Macaca rhesus	Burov et al., 1992
Parkinson-like symptoms	Sheep	Hammock et al., 1989
Parkinson-like syndrome	Primate	Barsoum et al., 1986
Parkinson's disease	Rat	Bjorklund et al., 1982
	Rat	Curran & Becker, 1991
	Macaca fasciculacis	Graham et al., 1990
	MPTP-induced mice	Sershen et al., 1987
	Rat	Dymecki et al., 1985
	Primate	Doudet et al., 1985
	Rhesus monkey	Chen et al., 1988
	Mice	Heikkila & Sonsalla, 1987
	Model	Renkawek, 1986
	Monkey	Bankiewicz et al., 1990
	Rat	Horellou et al., 1990
	Rat	Perese et al., 1989
	C57 BL/6 mice	Sundstrom et al., 1990
	Mice	Bankiewicz et al., 1993
	MTP-usioned mice	Nakashima, 1991
	Genetic cell lines	Freed et al., 1990
	Models	Hansen et al., 1989
	Models	Gagon et al., 1994
	Rabbit	Zigmond et al., 1984
Parkinsonian syndrome	Rat	Kryzhanovskii et al., 1987
	Primate	Hantraye et al., 1993
Parkinsonism	C57 black mice	Arai et al., 1990
	Rhesus monkey, C57 mice	Chen, 1990
	Rhesus monkey, C57 mice	Chen, 1990

Disease	Animal Model	Reference
Parkinsonism using selective neurotoxins	Rat	Zigmond & Stricker, 1989
Partial liver graft	Dog	Terpstra et al., 1983
Partial nephrectomy	Rat	Gretz et al., 1988
Passive lung anaphylaxis	Rat	Wu et al., 1985
Pasteurella haemolytica infection	Mice	Chengappa et al., 1983
Pelvic inflammatory disease	Cat	Kane et al., 1985
Penale bloodflow	Baboon	DeBruin et al., 1991
Penicillin-induced epileptic activity	Wistar rat	Kryzhanovskii et al., 1992
Peptic ulcer	Model	Malov et al., 1982
Peptic ulceration	Model	Hinder, 1986
Periductal fibrosis and fat-storing cells	Lamprey	Yamamoto, 1986
Perilymphatic fistulas	Chinchilla	Wall & Casselbrant, 1992
Perinatal asphyxia	Models	Raju, 1992
Perinatal carcinogenesis	Opossum	Jurgelski, 1983
Perinatal human megalovirus infection	BALB/c, H2d mice	Fitzgerald et al., 1990
Perinatal transmission of pathogenic viruses	Models	Ruprecht et al., 1993
Periodontal disease	Rat	Klausen, 1991
	Cat	Boyce, 1992
	Sheep	Ismaiel et al., 1989
Periotoneal metastasis	BALB/c mice	Hirayama et al., 1987
Peripheral nerves in malnutrition	Rhesus monkey	Rana et al., 1984
Peritonitis	Dog	Ashurmetov et al., 1992
Persistent infection	Mice	Goriumova et al., 1987
Perthes´ disease	Hypertensive rat	Hirano et al., 1988
Petit mal epilepsy	Rat	Serikawa, 1987
	Rat	Scherkl & Voits, 1991
	Wistar rat	Snead et al., 1990
Petit mal-like seizures	Rat	Marescaux et al., 1984
Phenylketonuria	Rat	Lacey, 1984
	Rat	Loo et al., 1984
	Model	Roux et al., 1991
Phlebovirus-induced disease	C57 BL/6J mice	Pifat & Smith, 1987
Phospholipid metabolism	Rat	Hosokawa, 1991
Photoaging	Miniature pig	Fourtanier et al., 1989
Photoallergenicity	Guinea pig	Maurer, 1984
Photoallergic contact dermatitis	Guinea pig	Jordan, 1982
Photochemotherapy	Wistar rat	van Iperen et al., 1992
Photodermatology	Hairless guinea pig	Horio et al., 1991
	Pig	Sambuco, 1985
Photodynamic therapy	Mice	Hill et al., 1986
Photoporphyric hepatopathy	Sprague Dawley rat	Berenson et al., 1992
Photothrombic occlusion of cerebral artery	Sprague Dawley, Wistar rat	Markgraf et al., 1993
Pigment gallstones	Model	Rege et al., 1993
Pituitary miniaturism	Miniature rat Ishikawa	Serizawa, 1993
Pituitary tumor	Rat	Trouillas & Girod, 1988
Plasmodium Brasilianum	Marmoset	Wedderburn et al., 1985
Plasmodium falciparum, malaria	Monkey	Collins et al., 1985

Disease	Animal Model	Reference
Plasmodium falciparum, malaria	Monkey	Collins et al., 1986
	Monkey	Rossan et al., 1985
	Aotus monkey	Espinal et al., 1984
	Mice	Clark et al., 1992
	Bolivian squirrel monkey	Whiteley et al., 1987
	Squirrel monkey	Fajfar-Whesotne, 1987
	Squirrel monkey	Campbell et al., 1986
	Saimiri saureus	Gysin et al., 1983
	Saimiri + Aotus monkey	Kakoma et al., 1992
Plasmodium species infection	Thamnonys rutilans	Landau & Chabaud, 1994
Plasmodium vivax	Squirrel monkey	Campbell et al., 1983
	Monkey	Collins et al., 1987
Plasmodium Yoelli yoelli	Vertebrate hosts	Amanmuradov, 1990
Platelet storage pool deficiency	Sandy mutant mice	Swank, 1991
	Mice	Novak et al., 1988
Pleurisy	Guinea pig	Satoh, 1982
Pleuropneumonia	Pig	Sebunya et al., 1983
Pneumociniosis	Mice, rat	Hatch et al., 1984
Pneumococcal bacteremia	Tamarin	Chudwin et al., 1987
Pneumococcal infection	Splenectomized rat	Alwmark, 1981
Pneumococcal otitis media	Chinchilla	Supance, 1982
Pneumoconiosis	Models	Elovskaia et al., 1986
Pneumocystis carinii	Rat	Bartlett et al., 1987
	Rabbit	Soulez et al., 1988
Pneumocystis carinii infection	Rat	Bartlett et al., 1988
Pneumocystis carinii pneumonia	Mice	Walzer et al., 1983
	Ferret	Stokes et al., 1987
	Rat	Bartlett, 1987
	Rat	Bartlett et al., 1989
	Lewis rat	Walzer, 1984
Pneumocystis pneumonia	Rat	Bartlett et al., 1990
Pneumonia	Mice	Kohno et al., 1986
	Large animal	Patterson & Todd, 1982
Pneumonia: interstitial lung disease	Swine	Edwards et al., 1983
Pneumonitis	Rabbit	Konishi et al., 1984
Polio virus - sensitive	Transgenic mice	Koike et al., 1993
Polioarthritis, chronic	Rabbit	Aoki et al., 1985
Poliomyelitis	TgPVR mice	Racaniello et al., 1993
Polyarthritis	Mice	Boissier et al., 1987
	Rat	Wozniczko-Orlows, 1983
	MRL 1pr/1pr mice	Pataki et al., 1985
Polycystic kidney and liver disease	Springbok	Iverson et al., 1982
Polycystic kidney disease	SPRD rat	Kaspareit-Ritting., 1990
Polycystic ovarian disease	Model	Mahajan, 1988
Polycystic ovarian syndrome	Guinea pig	Quandt & Hutz, 1993
Polycystic ovaries	Rat	Shanbhag et al., 1984
Polyhydramnios	Fetal lamb	Anderson & Faber, 1989

Disease	Animal Model	Reference
Pompe's disease	Calf	Reichmann, 1989
	Cattle	Reichmann et al., 1989
Porphyria	Rat	Enriquez de Sala., 1982
Portacaval transposition	Rat	Benjamin et al., 1984
Portal hypertension	Japanese white rabbit	Komeichi et al., 1990
Portal hypertension, chronic	Model	Landa Garcia et al., 1988
Post partum infection	Rabbit	Bawdon et al., 1989
Post-irridation reaction	Model	Trott & Huczkowski, 1991
Post-ischaemia immunosuppression	Yucatan miniature swine	Miller & Lim, 1986
Post-ischaemic neuronal damage, menadione	Rat	White & Clark, 1988
Post-radiation motor disorders	Albino mice	Bokk et al., 1990
Post-traumatic osteomyelitis	Rabbit	Worlock et al., 1988
Post-traumatic stress disorder	Model	Foa et al., 1992
Postmenopausal osteoporosis	Macaca fasciaelanis	Bowles et al., 1985
Postnatal hypoxia, chronic	Rat	Lun, 1989
Postprandial hyperinsulinemia	Miniature swine	Weingand, 1989
Posttraumatic stress disorder	Models	Yehuda et al., 1993
Pregnancy failure	Mice	Chaonat et al., 1989
Pregnancy-induced hypertension	Pregnant baboon	Cavanagh et al., 1985
Preleukemia myelopoietic dysplasias	Rat	Fohlmeister et al., 1981
Premature birth	Rabbit	Lorenzo, 1985
Premature ovarian failure	Mice	Miyake et al., 1988
Prenatal alcohol exposure	Models, human	Driscoll et al., 1990
Preneoplastic hepatocyte nodules	Rat	Roomi et al., 1985
Presbyopia	Rhesus monkey	Bito, 1984
	Macaca mulatta	Kaufman et al., 1982
Presbyopia: ocular ageing	Macaca mulatta	Bito et al., 1987
Primary reaction to radiation	Rabbit	Arlaschenko et al., 1984
Proctitis	Cynomolgus monkey	Quinn et al., 1986
Progressive cytomegalovirus glomerulonephritis	MA/ICR mice	Wehner & Smith, 1983
Progressive glomerular sclerosis + renal failure	Nephrectomized rat	Makino, 1990
Progressive hydronephrosis	Mice	Horton et al., 1988
Prolactinoma	Wistar/Furth rat	Trouillas et al., 1990
Proliferative glomerulonephritis	BALB/c mice	Cavallo et al., 1984
Proliferative vitreoretinopathy	Rabbit	Araiz, 1993
Prophylactic irradiation	Model	Mildenberger et al., 1990
Prostate	Monkey	Habenicht et al., 1987
Prostate adenocarcinomas	Lobund-Wistar rat	Pollard & Luckert, 1987
Prostate cancer	Dunning 3327 rat	Carter et al., 1989
	Nude mice	Passaniti et al., 1992
	Transgenic mice	Thompson et al., 1993
	Rat	Juniewicz et al., 1991
Prostate cancer model	Lobund-Wistar rat	Pollard, 1992
Prostate carcinogenesis	Rat	Bosland, 1992
Prostate carcinoma	Nb rat	Noble, 1982
Prostatic cancer	Rat	Isaacs, 1987
Prostatic hyperplasia	Mice	Chung et al., 1984

Disease	Animal Model	Reference
Prostatic hyperplasia	Mice	Chung & Auble, 1985
Prostatitis	Monkey	Dilworth et al., 1990
Prostatitis, acute	Monkey	Neal, 1990
Prostatitis, chronic	Dog	Barsanti, 1982
Prostrate adenocarcinoma	Rat, human	Dahlberg et al., 1980
Prostrate androgen-sensitive tumor	Rat	Drago, 1983
Protein induced enteropathy	Mice	Malo & Morin, 1986
Proteinase regulation	Mice	Hart, 1989
Proteinuria	Mice, rat	Howie, 1989
Prurigo	Dog	Rudzki et al., 1982
Pseudomonas pneumonia, chronic	Rat	Graham et al., 1990
Pseudotuberculosis	Models	Timchenko et al., 1983
Pseudotuberculosis infection	Mice	Polotskii et al., 1983
Psoriasis	Mice	Huang, 1984
Psychiatric disorders	Models	McGuire et al., 1989
Psychosis	Rat	Krendal & Kudrin, 1982
	Cat	Kryzhanovskii et al., 1987
	Macaca	Schlemmer et al., 1983
Psychotic disease	Rat	Kline & Reid, 1985
Psychotropic	Monkey	Startsev et al., 1986
Pulmonary edema	Sheep	Coggeshall et al., 1987
	Sprague Dawley rat	Ahn et al., 1993
	Sheep	Garnett et al., 1987
	Cat, dog, rabbit, rat, etc.	Tel'l et al., 1985
Pulmonary edema, acute	Wistar rat, dog	Manenti et al., 1992
Pulmonary edema, high altitude	Pig, rat	Schoene et al., 1992
Pulmonary edema, unilateral	Model	Tel', 1991
Pulmonary embolism	Dog	Kornacewicz-Jach, 1985
Pulmonary eosinophilia	BALB/c mice	Egwang & Kazura, 1990
Pulmonary fibrosis	Models	Homma, 1981
Pulmonary granulomata	Rat	Votto et al., 1987
Pulmonary granulomatous vasculitis	Rat	Johnson et al., 1984
Pulmonary hypersensitivity	Guinea pig	Griffiths-Johnson, 1991
Pulmonary hypertension	Dog	Shelub et al., 1984
Pulmonary hypertension, persistent	Lamb	Soifer et al., 1987
Pulmonary hypoplasia	Rat	Moessinger, 1983
	Rabbit	Nakayama et al., 1983
Pulmonary inflammation	Mice	Sunderrajan et al., 1986
Pulmonary injury, pneumonitis, fibrosis	Rabbit	McCall et al., 1983
Pulmonary interstitial fibrosis	Hamster	Stein-Streilein, 1987
Pulmonary interstitial inflammation	Guinea pig	Schuyler et al., 1987
Pulmonary ischaemia	Chacma baboon	Reichart et al., 1987
Pulmonary lesions	Mice	Kono, 1986
Pulmonary mucormycosis	Mice	Waldorf et al., 1982
Pulmonary paracoccidioidomycosis	Hamster	Tani, 1987
Pulmonary radiation fibrosis	Mice	Karvonen et al., 1987
Pulmonary response	Rabbit in vivo / in vitro	Marshall et al., 1988

Disease	Animal Model	Reference
Pulmonary vascular resistance	Sheep	Pearl et al., 1992
Purine nucleoside phosphorylase deficiency	Rat, dog	Osborne et al., 1986
Q fever	Inbred mice	Scott et al., 1987
	Mice	Mourya et al., 1983
Q-fever	Sheep	Perry et al., 1994
Radiation injury	Rodent	Hurn et al., 1983
Radiation injury of intestine	Rat	Hauer-Jensen, 1988
Radiation myelitis	Stem cell depletion	Yaes & Kalend, 1988
Radiation oncology brain metastases model	Nude mice	Bamberg et al., 1988
Radiation therapy	Mice	Loor et al., 1988
Radiation-induced leukemia	Rat	Wright, 1991
Radioimmunotherapy, monoclonal antibodies	Models	Shah & Sands, 1990
Radiolabeled monoclonal antibody evaluation	Models	Gallagher, 1983
Radiorenography dehydrated and rehydrated	Primate	Dormehl et al., 1983
Radiotherapy and bone growth	Rat	Wechsler-Jentzsch, 1993
Ras activation in tumor	Rabbit, mice	Corominas et al., 1991
Reactive arthritis	Mice	Toivanen et al., 1986
Receptor deficiencies	Mice, rat	Tsuji & Matsumoto, 1982
Rectal mucoid adenocarcinoma	Nude mice, human	Xu, 1989
Recurrent herpetic eye disease	Mice	Shimeld et al., 1990
Reduced renal mass	Os/+mice	Zalups, 1993
Reflex epilepsy	Mongolian gerbil	Bartoszyk et al., 1987
Reflux pancreatitis, acute	Rat	Infantino, 1992
Refractory diseases	Mice, rat	Kyogoku, 1982
Regional chemotherapy	Rabbit	Davidson et al., 1986
Renal ablation	Rat	Moskowitz et al., 1992
Renal arachidonic aced metabolism	Rabbit	Schwartz et al., 1984
Renal autoimmunity	MAXX rat	Henry, 1988
Renal cell carcinoma	Models	Rangel, 1989
	Nude mice	Fidler et al., 1990
Renal cell carcinoma cholesterol acquisition	Wistar-Lewis rat	Clayman et al., 1986
Renal cystic disease	Sprague Dawley rat	Gardner et al., 1987
	Models	Resnick, 1981
Renal disease	Rat	Baylis, 1987
Renal failure	Dog	Ash et al., 1982
Renal failure utero-placental circulatory	Chinchilla	Klimenko et al., 1986
Renal failure, acute	Rat	Burdman et al., 1993
	Rat	Gretz et al., 1988
Renal failure, chronic	Models	Friedman, 1986
	Rat	Christensen et al., 1983
	Mice	Gagnon & Duguid, 1983
	Dog	Vaneerdeweg et al., 1992
	Rat	Acott et al., 1987
	Daunomycin rat	Shimizu et al., 1990
	Rat	Kumano et al., 1986
Renal hypertensive, chronic	Rabbit	Kurz et al., 1981
Renal papillary necrosis	Syrian hamster	Carlton et al., 1989

Disease	Animal Model	Reference
Renal papillary necrosis	Models	Bach & Hardy, 1985
Renal syndrome	Rat	Roth et al., 1991
Renal tuberculosis	Rabbit	Bispen et al., 1992
Renal tumor	Murine	Vandendris et al., 1983
Renititis pigmentosa	Miniature poodle dog	Acland et al., 1990
Reperfusion injury	Model	Hardy & Gough, 1991
Reproduction and growth	Mice	Erdman et al., 1987
Reproductive failure, autoimmune	Mice	Gleicher, 1987
Respiratory distress syndrome	Pig	Modig & Berg, 1986
	Pig	Mustard et al., 1989
	Sprague Dawley rat	Simons et al., 1991
	Models	Lachman, 1989
	Rabbit	Sandhar et al., 1988
Respiratory failure	Pig	Olson et al., 1985
	Porcine	Dehring et al., 1983
Respiratory failure syndrome, acute	Model	Rogatskii, 1984
Respiratory failure, acute	Porcine	Dehring et al., 1983
	Pig	Kesecioglu et al., 1992
Respiratory lung distress syndrome	Rat	Takeda, 1989
Respiratory mycoplasmosis	Rat	Tsinzerling et al., 1981
Respiratory syncytical infection	Mice	Taylor et al., 1984
Respiratory tract disease	Cotton rat	Pacini et al., 1984
	Models	Wanner, 1990
Respiratory tract infection	Beagle puppy	Quan et al., 1991
	Cotton rat	Sadowski et al., 1987
Respiratory tract infections	Cotton rat	Sadowski et al., 1987
Response of myocardium to injury	Rat	Vracko & Thorning, 1985
Resuscitation research, criteria	Primate, swine, canine	Yearly, 1993
Retina diseases	Models	Khodtsev, 1986
Retinal degeneration	Mice	Smith & Yielding, 1986
Retinopathy of prematurity	Rat	Penn & Thun, 1989
Retrolental fibroplasia	Beagle puppy	Flower & Blake, 1981
Reversible left ventricular volume overload	Dog	Swindle et al., 1991
Reye's syndrome	Chicken	Awrich & Wolf, 1983
	Ferret	Deshmukh et al., 1985
	Mice	Davis & Kornfeld, 1986
	Mice	Davis et al., 1983
	Ferret	Kilpatrick-Smith, 1989
	Rat	Kilpatrick et al., 1989
	Rat, margosa oil	Sinniah et al., 1985
Rheumatism	Model	Koizumi, 1980
Rheumatoid arthritis	Rabbit	Puschel et al., 1982
	Chicken	Marquardt et al., 1983
Rickets	Arctic fox	Ogden et al., 1981
Rift valley fever virus	Rhesus monkey	Cosgriff et al., 1989
Right ventricular function	Dog	Wackers et al., 1981
Saccular aneurysms	Rat	Van Alphen, 1990

Disease	Animal Model	Reference
Saccular aneurysms	Rat	Gao & Kamphorst, 1990
Salpingitis	Rabbit	Patton et al., 1982
	Mice	Swenson et al., 1983
Salpingitis and resitual tubal infertility	Mice	Zana et al., 1990
Salpingitis, chronic	Rabbit	Slaveikova et al., 1986
Sandhoff's disease	Cat	Neuwelt et al., 1985
Sandimmun metabolites	Models, human	Fahr et al., 1990
Sarcomas	Model	Mankin, 1990
Schedule-induced self injection of drugs	Model	Singer & Wallace, 1984
Schistosoma mansoni infection	Verve monkey	Sturrock et al., 1984
Schistosome immunity	Mice	Smithers et al., 1987
Schistosomiasis	Mice	Campos et al., 1984
	In vitro models	Warren, 1982
Schistosomiasis mansoni	Guinea pig	Pearce, 1983
Schistosomiasis mansoni infection	Albino mice	Machado et al., 1991
Schizophrenia	Rat	Port et al., 1991
	Models	Kaufmann et al., 1988
Schizophrenia, infection, temperature	Rat	Rubinstein, 1993
Schizophrenia, Sigma receptor	Sprague Dawley rat	Ruckert & Schmidt, 1993
Schizophrenic symptomatology	Macaca fasciaelanis	Dubach & Bowlen, 1983
SCID mouse	SCID mice	Kaneshima et al., 1990
Scleroderma	Tight-skin mice	Russell, 1983
	Models	Claman, 1990
Sclerosis panencephalitis	Ferret	Thormar et al., 1985
Scoliosis	Rabbit	Barrios et al., 1987
	Primate	Pincott & Taffa, 1982
	Chicken	Rucker et al., 1986
	Monkey	Thomas & Dave, 1985
	Rat	Salzman et al., 1988
Screening anti-inflammatory drugs	BUF rats	Ishizuki et al., 1984
Scrub typhus	Models	Ridgway et al., 1986
Secondary antiphospholipid syndrome	MRL-1 pr/pr1 mice	Smith et al., 1990
Secondary hemochromatosis	Wistar rat	Figueiredo et al., 1993
Secretory diarrhoea	Rat	Rolston et al., 1987
	Rat	Elliott et al., 1991
Sedlarik's pulmonary embolism	Miniature swine (minipig)	Lesser et al., 1989
Seizure, infusion model	Rat	Pollack & Shen, 1985
Seizures	Gerbil	Frey, 1987
Selective lenticulostriate occlusion	Primate	Yonas et al., 1981
Selective loss of cholinergic neurons	Rat	Kudo et al., 1989
Selective retardation	Trysomy 16 mice	Kiss, 1989
Semichronic diarrhea	Rat	Mir & Alioto, 1982
Senile idiopathic osteoporosis	Rat	Simon, 1984
Senile osteoporosis	Mice	Matsushita et al., 1986
Sensitization mechanisms	Guinea pig	Scheper et al., 1990
Sensorimotor gating and schizophrenia	Model, human	Braff & Geyer, 1990
Sensorimotor gating defects	Sprague Dawley rat	Swerdlow & Geyer, 1993

Disease	Animal Model	Reference
Sensorimotor gating deficiency	Mice, schizophrenic human	Swerdlow et al., 1994
Sensory neuropathy	Dog	Cummings et al., 1983
Sepsis	Models	Cross et al., 1993
	BALB/c mice	Dunn, 1988
	Piglet	Schimmel, 1988
	Bacteria	Cross et al., 1993
	Dog	Shaw & Wolfe, 1984
Sepsis and endotoxic shock	Rat	Wise, 1989
Sepsis and endotoxic shock	Rat	Wise et al., 1989
Sepsis in chronic biliary obstruction	Rat	Tanaka et al., 1985
Sepsis, "hyperdynamic state"	Baboon	Hinshaw et al., 1983
Septic arthritis	CD 1 mice	Tissi et al., 1990
	Rat	Gordon et al., 1986
Septic lung disease	Rabbit	Miyata et al., 1993
Septic shock	Dog	Natanson, 1986
	Dog	Yuan et al., 1984
	Dog	Hinshaw, 1989
	Dog	Chung et al., 1991
	Baboon (Papio ursinus)	Dormehl et al., 1991
	Pony	Sembrat et al., 1979
Serotonin models of myoclonus	Guinea pig	Wolfson et al., 1986
Sexually transmitted disease	Feline	Miller, 1994
	Models	Miller, 1994
Shigellosis	Guinea pig	Hartman et al., 1991
Shock	Swine	Traverso et al., 1984
Shock and starvation	Rat	Barillo et al., 1985
Shock, anaphylactic	Rabbit	Orlowaski, 1986
SHT sensitive action myoclonus	Rat	Pratt et al., 1986
Sickle cell disease	Transgenic models	Fabry, 1993
Silicosis	Rat	Struhar et al., 1989
Sinusitis	Rabbit	Brugmann et al., 1993
Sinusoidal liver cell damage	Murine	Kirn et al., 1983
SIV encephalopathy	Rhesus macaque	Hurtrel et al., 1991
Sjogren's syndrome	MRL/MP mice	Alexander, 1986
	Models	Fox, 1994
	Mice	Cutler et al., 1987
	Mice	Jabs et al., 1994
	Transgenic mice	Mountz & Gause, 1993
	Models	Tarkowski et al., 1986
Skeletal muscle dysfunction	Mice	Hettleman et al., 1983
Skeletal muscle ischaemia	Gracilis	Lindsay, 1994
Skin and hair abnormalities	Mice	Sundberg, 1993
Skin atopic reactivity	Monkey	Winkenmann, 1986
Skin carcinogenesis	Athymic nude mice	Das et al., 1986
Skin disease	Hairless guinea pig	Moon et al., 1990
Skin infection	Mice	Lloyd & Nobel, 1982
Skin penetration	Guinea pig, rat, human	Priborsky et al., 1990

Disease	Animal Model	Reference
Skin tumor (keratoacanthomas)	Rabbit, human	Leon, 1988
Skin-flap survival	Rat, procine	Smith et al., 1992
Sleep-disordered breathing	English bulldog	Hendricks et al., 1987
Slow viral infections	Models	Gudnodottir, 1981
Sly syndrome	Dog	Haskins et al., 1991
Small Bowel ischemia	Dog	Cohen et al., 1987
Smoke inhalation injury	Sheep	Hubbard et al., 1988
Spasticity	Wistar rat	Ossowska et al., 1992
	Mice	Wright & Rang, 1990
Spinal cord injury	Rat	Black et al., 1986
	Cat	Ford, 1983
Spinal cord injury, chemically induced	Rat	Wehling et al., 1990
Spinal cord injury, photochemical induced	Rat	Watson et al., 1986
Spinal cord Krabbe disease	Mice	Kodama et al., 1982
Spinal epidural abscess	Rabbit	Feldenzer et al., 1987
Splenic dysfunction	Models	Dumont, 1983
Splenic injuries, severe	Beagle dog, human	Rogers et al., 1991
Spondylarthrophy	Mice	Mahowald et al., 1988
Spondyloarthropathy	Mice	Krug et al., 1989
	Models	Taurog, 1990
Spontaneous diabetes mellitus	BB rat	Chappel et al., 1983
Spontaneous diabetic kidney disease	Models	Velasquez et al., 1990
Spontaneous recurrent seizures	Rat	Cavalheiro et al., 1982
Squamous cell carcinoma	Sheep	Ladds & Daniels, 1982
Staphylococcal blepharitis	Rabbit	Mondino et al., 1987
Staphylococcal osteomyelitis	Dog	Varshney et al., 1989
Staphylococcus aureus chronic osteomyelitis	Rat	Power et al., 1990
Staphylococcus aureus infection	Rabbit, pig, baboon	Kohrman et al., 1989
Stasis thrombosis	Rabbit	Thomas et al., 1989
State of clinical death from acute blood loss	Rat	Stepanov et al., 1983
Stationary night blindness	Briard dog	Narfstrom et al., 1989
Stimulus deprivation amblyopia	Chicken	Marg, 1982
Stomach ulcer	Model	Vertelkin et al., 1987
Streptococcal pneumonia	Wistar rat	Rhodes et al., 1989
Streptococcus pneumoniae pneumonia	Dog	Moser et al., 1982
Streptococcus type III	Murine, human neonate	Gotoff et al., 1986
Streptococcus zooepidemicus	Horse	Varma et al., 1984
Stress	Hypertensive rat	Cox et al., 1991
	Rat	Drugan et al., 1989
	Rat	Kuznetsov, 1991
Stress and mental illness	Rat	Ottenweller et al., 1989
Stress, weightlessness	Rat	Durnova et al., 1987
Stroke	Dog	Brenowitz & Yonas, 1990
	Gerbil	Holaday et al., 1982
	Stroke-prone rat	Yamori et al., 1982
	Models	Zivin & Grotta, 1990
	Rat	Kotwica et al., 1989

Disease	Animal Model	Reference
Stroke	Primate	Nehis, 1986
Stroke index	Gerbil	Ohno et al., 1984
Stroke, focal ischaemic	Rat	Chen et al., 1986
Strongyloidiasis	Erythrocebus patas	Genta et al., 1984
Strongyloidiasis venezuelensis infection	Mice	Sato et al., 1990
Sub-glottic stenosis	Dog	Koufman et al., 1988
Subarachnoid hemorrhage	Baboon	Zawirski et al., 1985
	Rat	Solomon et al., 1985
	Baboon	Sahlin et al., 1987
	Models	Logothetis et al., 1983
Subdural hematoma, acute	Rat	Miller et al., 1990
Subluxation, chronic	Rabbit	De Boer McKnight, 1988
Sudden coronary death	Dog, rat, human	Patterson, 1983
	Dog	Chi & Lucchesi, 1991
	Model	Spear et al., 1982
Sudden death and malarian lung syndromes	Mice	Weiss & Kubat, 1983
Sudden infant death syndrome	Rabbit pup	Gingras et al., 1990
Supersensitivity	Rat	Chalon et al., 1990
Suppression of reproductive function	NZB/W mice	Keisler & Walker, 1987
Syndrome of inappropriate antidiuretic hormone	Rat	Verbalis, 1984
Synovitis in air pouch	Rat	Sedgwick et al., 1985
Syphillis	Guinea pig	Pierce et al., 1983
Sysmorphogenesis	Chicken embryos	Fineman et al., 1987
Systemic amyloidosis	Transgenic mice	Araki et al., 1994
Systemic candidiasis	Mice	Papadimitriou, 1986
Systemic candidiasis and systemic aspergillosis	DBA/ 2N mice	Hector et al., 1990
Systemic lupus erythematosus	Naive mice	Shoenfeld & Mozes, 1990
	Mice	Appleby et al., 1989
	BALB/c mice	Kalush et al., 1992
	Models	Shoenfeld et al., 1989
	NZW mice	Tron, 1990
	Mice	Mendlovic et al., 1988
	Model	Hirose & Shirai, 1985
	Mice	Theofilopoulus, 1985
Systemic scleroderma	Chicken, mice	Serakovski et al., 1989
Systemic sclerosis	Chicken, mice, rat	Jimenez et al., 1994
T-cell lymphocyte leukaemia	Rat	Stromberg, 1985
T-cell malignancy expressing IL-2 receptor	BALB/c mice	Lugasi, 1990
Tachycardia	Dog	Iesaka et al., 1983
Tardative diskinesia	Models	Casey, 1984
Tardative diskinesia, effect of neuroleptics	Rat	See & Ellison, 1990
Tardative dyskinesia	Macaca	Beddard et al., 1988
	Cebrus apella monkey	Barany et al., 1983
	Rat	Goetz et al., 1983
Targeted radiotherapy	Mice	Chiou, 1991
Temporomandibular articular complex	Pig	Bermejo et al., 1993
Tendon adhesions	Primate	Pruzansky, 1987

Disease	Animal Model	Reference
Testicular cancer, heterograft	Nude mice	Osieka et al., 1985
Tetanus, automic over-activity	Model	Shibuya et al., 1987
Thalassemia	Mice	Whitney & Popp, 1984
	Mice	Martinell et al., 1981
	Mice	Anderson et al., 1982
Therapeutic efficiency of immunomodulators	Rat with tumor	Talmadge et al., 1984
Therapeutic screening	Rat	Nakamura et al., 1982
Thoracic empyema	Guinea pig	Mavroudis et al., 1987
Thrombogenicity	Rabbit	Herring et al., 1993
Thrombogenicity, arterial graft	Sheep	Lundell et al., 1991
Thrombosis	Baboon	Dormehl et al., 1987
	Rat, mice	Bekemeier et al., 1985
	New Zealand white rabbit	Kersh et al., 1989
	Rat	Vogel et al., 1989
	Model	Valji & Bookstein, 1987
Thrombosis and bleeding	Rat	Meuleman et al., 1982
Thrombosis and bleeding time	Rat, rabbit	Just et al., 1991
Thrombosis, arterial	Dog	Mestre et al., 1985
	Syrian hamster	McMartin & Dodds, 1982
	Rabbit, rat	Ubatuba, 1989
Thrombosis, deep vein	Baboon	Wakefield et al., 1991
Thrombosis, laser-induced	Wistar rat	Vesvres et al., 1993
Thrombosis, middle cerebral artery	rat	Umemura et al., 1993
Thrombosis, venous	Dog, rabbit	el Kouri, 1992
Thrombotic thrombocytopenia	Rat	Sanders et al., 1988
Thyroid disease	SCID and nude mice	Volpe et al., 1993
	Cattle, goat, mice	Ledent et al., 1994
Thyroidectomy	Rat	Hananeur, 1989
Tibia fracture	Rabbit	Ashhurst, 1982
Tinnitus	Guinea pig	Jastreboff & Sasaki, 1994
	Rat	Jastreboff et al., 1988
	Rat	Kellerhals & Zogg, 1991
Tissue calcium and vascular function	Sprague Dawley rat	Cannon & Williams, 1990
Tissue shizontocide test	Monkey	Zhang, 1982
Tobacco-inhalation studies	Model	Homburger et al., 1985
Toluene-induced neurotoxicity	Model	Pryor, 1990
Tongue carcinogenesis	Hamster	Eveson, 1981
Tongue squamous cell carcinogenesis	Nude mice	Wang, 1988
Topical photoallergy	Mice	Gerberick & Ryan, 1990
Total cerebral ischaemia	Dog	Arai et al., 1986
Tourette syndrome	Rat	Diamond et al., 1982
Tourniquet-induced limb ischaemia	Rat	Chabel et al., 1990
Toxemia	Pregnant guinea pig	Golden et al., 1980
	Rat	Abitbol, 1982
Toxic shock syndrome	Mice	Tierno et al., 1987
Toxicant-induced epithelial transformations	Rat	Harkemia et al., 1993
Toxicological evaluation	Rat	Oser, 1981

Disease	Animal Model	Reference
Toxin production in gut	Rabbit	Kesel & Ellis, 1988
Toxin-induced neurobiological disorders	Models	Woodruff et al., 1994
Toxoplasmic retinochoroiditis	Mice	Hay et al., 1984
Toxoplasmosis	Aotus monkey	Escajadillo et al., 1991
Transplacental congenital cytomegaloviral infect	Guinea pig	Strauss & Griffith, 1991
Transplant arteriosclerosis	Rat	Mennander et al., 1991
Transplantable stomach cancer	Rat	Shimizu, 1986
Transplantation Dirofilaria immitis	Lewis rat	Grieve et al., 1985
Transplantation of bladder and renal carcinoma	NMRI nu/nu mice	Otto et al., 1987
Transport of phosphate by plasma membranes	Hypophosphatemic mice	Nakagawa et al., 1993
Trauma disease	Rabbit	Dedushkin et al., 1990
Trauma-sepsis	Rat	Pedersen et al., 1984
Traumatic coma	Primate	Gennarelli et al., 1982
Traumatic tatoo	Guinea pig, human	Sunde et al., 1990
Treponema hyodysenteriae infection	Mice	Suenaga et al., 1984
Treponema pallidum infection	Mice	Folds et al., 1983
Trichinella spiralis infection	Ferret	Campbell et al., 1982
Trichocephaliasis	Mice	Rashid, 1991
Trichomoniasis	Squirrel monkey	Hollander et al., 1985
Trisomy 16 model	Mice	Kornguth et al., 1986
Trombosis in the inner ear, microcirculation	Rat	Umemura et al., 1990
Tru anosoma (Nannomonas) congolense	Microtus montanus	Bafort & Schmidt, 1984
Trypano tolerance	West african dog	Horchner et al., 1985
Trypanosoma brucei infection	Deer, mice	Anosa & Kaneko, 1983
Tuberculosis	Deer (Cervus elaphus)	Buchan & Griffin, 1990
	Guinea pig	Khomenko, 1981
	Models	Smith et al., 1989
	Mice	Someya, 1984
Tuberculosis, infection	T-cell deficient mice	Orme, 1987
Tuberculosis, intracerebral	Guinea pig	Grashchenkova, 1985
Tuberculosis, uterine tube	Rabbit	Rekel'lul, 1982
Tumor growth	Mice	Volk & Ershler, 1991
Tumor induced hypercalcemia	Rat	Berger et al., 1982
Tumor invasion, V2 carcinoma	Rabbit	Strauli et al., 1984
Tumor progression	Models	Leibovici et al., 1984
Tumor response	Nude mice, human	Fiebig, 1984
Tumor-associated granulocytosis	New Zealand rabbit	Hough et al., 1983
Tumors + evaluation of antitumor drug	Mice	Shirai et al., 1991
Tumors of model	Djungarian hamster	Pogosianz, 1982
Tympanic membrane perforations	Rat	Spandow et al., 1993
Tympanosclerosis	Guinea pig	Yazawa et al., 1985
Tyramine-induced toxicity	Mongrel dog	Faraj, 1983
Ulceration, chronic	Guinea pig	Manna et al., 1982
Ulcerative colitis	Marmoset	Clapp et al., 1985
Ulcerative colitis, acute and chronic	Mice	Okayasu et al., 1990
Unilateral 6-OHFA model	Rat	Carey, 1990
	Rat	Carey, 1991

Disease	Animal Model	Reference
Unilateral cartoid artery ligation	Mongolian gerbil	Costello et al., 1990
Unilateral cryptorchidism	Model	Stewart & Brown, 1990
Update on model	Flinders sensitive line rat	Overstreet, 1993
Ureal melanoma	Chicken embryos	Luyten et al., 1993
Ureaplasmas	Cattle	Ball et al., 1987
Urethral obstruction, gradual	Guinea pig	Mostwin, 1991
Urinary bladder tumor	Rabbit	Nemoto et al., 1981
Urinary retention	Rat	Tita et al., 1988
Urinary tract chronic infection	Rat	Miller, 1987
Urinary tract infection	Mice	Ketyi, 1981
Urogenital infections	Monkey	Moller & Freundt, 1983
Urogenital tract infection	Monkey	Marantnidi et al., 1987
Urolithiasis	Rat	Mel'nishkov et al., 1984
Urolithiasis, chemically induced	Weanling rat	Wolkowski-Tyl, 1982
Urologic malignant tumors	SCID mice	Shibayama et al., 1991
Uveitis	Rabbit	Rosenbaum et al., 1988
Uveoretinitis	Monkey	Faure et al., 1981
Vaginitis	Grivet monkey	Mardh et al., 1984
Vagus-cardiac pacemaker interactions	Model	Somsen et al., 1991
Validation criterias of mental disorders	Models	Willner, 1986
Validation of models	Depression models	Willner, 1984
Varicella-Zaster virus	Marmoset	Provost et al., 1987
Vascular disorders, radiotracer evaluation	Models	Mathias & Welch, 1983
Vascular graft infection	Sheep	Fletcher et al., 1990
Vascular responsiveness during pregnancy	Rabbit	Lee et al., 1982
Vasculitis	Mice	Lehman et al., 1988
Vasculitis in common tissue	MRL/Mp autoimmune mice	Alexander et al., 1985
Vasculogenic impotence	Model	Floth et al., 1991
	Dog	Breza et al., 1990
	Dog	Aboserf, 1990
Vasectomy	Mice, human	Schwartz, 1991
Vasospasm	Rat femoral artery	Okada et al., 1990
Veneral and congenital syphilis	Hamster	Kajdacsy-Balla, 1987
Veno-venous extracorpal lung assist	Small dog	Otsu, 1985
Venous incompetence in erectile function	Dog	Aboseif et al., 1990
Ventricular dysrhythmias	Dog	Garson, 1984
Ventricular fibrillation	Cat	Vol'pert et al., 1984
Ventricular hypertrophy	Pig	Guerreiro, 1988
Ventricular repolarization and refractory period	New Zealand white rabbit	Manley et al., 1989
Ventricular septal defect	Dog	Nakai et al., 1983
Ventricular tachyarrhythmia	Dog	Michelson, 1981
Ventricular tachycardia	Rat, guinea pig	Tripathi, 1986
	Dog	Gessman et al., 1983
Vesicoureteral reflux	Monkey	Roberts, 1983
Vibrio cholerae infection	Rabbit	Guinee et al., 1985
Viral disease	Primate	Soike et al., 1984
Viral hepatitis	Monkey	Balaian, 1986

Disease	Animal Model	Reference
Viral-induced astrocytomas	New World primate	Houff et al., 1983
Virology models	Inbred mice	Maiboroda, 1983
Virus infection, herpes simplex	Mice	Dix et al., 1983
Virus susceptibility	Murine	Brinton et al., 1981
Visceral leishmaniasis	German shepherd dog	Keenan et al., 1984
	Owl monkey	Broderson et al., 1986
	Squirrel monkey	Chapman & Hanson, 198
	Opossum, armadillo, ferret	White et al., 1989
	Opossum	White et al., 1989
Viscosity of fluids in epilidymis	Rat	Wen & Wong, 1988
Vitamin A and Newcastle disease	Chicken	Sijtsma et al., 1989
Vitamin D-dependent rickets type II	Marmoset	Suda et al., 1986
Vitamin K deficiency	Mice	Komai et al., 1988
Vitiligo	Mice	Lerner et al., 1986
Von Recklinghausen's neurofibromatosis	Syrian gold hamster	Nakamura et al., 1989
Von Willebrand factor	Models	Brinkhaus et al., 1991
Waardenburg syndromes	Mice and hamster mutants	Asher & Friedman, 1990
Water balance	Brattleboro rat	Edwards, 1982
Wheat-sensitive enteropathy	Dog	Batt et al., 1987
Wilson's disease	Dog	Owen & Ludwig, 1982
	Long-Evans cinnamon rat	Li et al., 1991
Wound healing	Diabetic mice	Tsuboi et al., 1992
Wucheria bancrofti infection	Silvered leaf monkey	Palmieri et al., 1983
	Silvered leaf monkey	Palmieri et al., 1982
Wucheria bancrofti, transmission of	Leaf monkey	Sucharit et al., 1982
Xenogenic neoplasms	Gray opossum	Fadem & Hill, 1985
Yersiniosis	Mice, rabbit, rat	Heesemann et al., 1993
Yolk sac tumor	Rat	Vandeputte et al., 1988
Zinc deficiency	Rat	Van Herck et al., 1989

REFERENCES

AAAS Board (1990). Resolution on the use of animals in research, treating and education. American Association Advancement of Science. Science 244:611.

Aas M., Fjeld J.G. (1993). Animal models for radiolabeled monoclonal antibodies in cancer research. Acta Oncol. 32(7-8):819-24.

Abd-Elfattah A.S., Ding M., Wechsler A.S. (1993). Myocardial stunning and preconditioning: age, species, and model related differences: role of AMP-5'-nucleotidase in myocardial injury and protection. J Card Surg. 8(2 Suppl):257-61.

Abdrashitov Akh., Listvina V.P., Nuzhnyi V.P., Uspenskii A.E. (1983). Comparative characteristics of methods for forced alcoholization of rats. Farmakol Toksikol. 46:94-8. (Russian).

Abitbol M.M. (1982). Simplified technique to produce toxemia in the rat: considerations on cause of toxemia. Clin Exp Hypertens [B]. 1:93-103.

Aboseif S., Wetterauer U., Breza J., Benard F., Bosch R., Stief CG., Lue T., Tanagho E. (1990). The effect of venous incompetence and arterial insufficiency on erectile function: an animal model. J Urol 144(3):790-3.

Abraham W.M. (1988): The role of leukotrienes in allergen-induced late responses in allergic sheep. Ann N Y Acad Sci. 524:260-70.

Abramowsky C.R., Aikawa M., Swinehart G.L., Snajdar R.M. (1984). Spontaneous nephrotic syndrome in a genetic rat model. Am J Pathol. 117:400-8.

Abul-Ezz, S., Walker, P., & Shah, S. (1991). Role of glutathione in an animal model of myoglobinuric acute renal failure. Proc Natl Acad Sci U S A, 88 (21):9833-7.

Achilli G., Sarasini A., Gerna G., Iltis J.P., Madden D.L. (1984). Antibody response of patas monkeys to experimental infection with Delta herpesvirus. Eur J Clin Microbiol. 3:158-9.

Achiron A. (1986). New aspects in myopia development-models in experimental animals--a literature review. Harefuah. 110:152-4.

Ackerstein A., Kedar E., Slavin, S. (1991). Use of recombinant human interleukin-2 in conjunction with syngeneic bone marrow transplantation in mice as a model for control of minimal residual disease in malignant hematologic disorders. Blood 78(5):1212-5.

Acland G., Halloran-Blanton S., Boughman J., Aguirre, G. (1990). Segregation distortion in inheritance of progressive rod cone degeneration (prcd) in miniature poodle dogs. Am J Med Genet 35(3):354-9.

Acott P.D., Ogborn M.R., Crocker J.F. (1987). Chronic renal failure in the rat. A surgical model for long-term toxicological studies. J Pharmacol Methods. 18:81-8.

Adams L.M., Geyer M.A. (1985). Effects of DOM and DMT in a proposed animal model of hallucinogenic activity. Prog Neuropsychopharmacol Biol Psychiatry. 9:121-32.

Adams M.E., Billingham M.E. (1982). Animal models of degenerative joint disease. Curr Top Pathol. 71:265-97.

Adams, J., Cory, S. (1991). Transgenic models for haemopoietic malignancies. Biochim Biophys Acta, 1072 (1):9-31.

Adler, R., Krieg, R., Farrell, M., Deiss, W., & MacLeod, R. (1991). Characterization of a new animal model of chronic hyperprolactinemia. Metabolism, 40 (3):286-91.

Aguzzi A., Brandner S., Sure U., Ruedi D., Isenmann S. (1994). Transgenic and knock-out mice: models of neurological disease. Brain Pathol. 4(1):3-20.

Agy M.B., Katze M.G. (1993). HIV-1 infection of animals: the search for a pathogenesis model continues. AIDS 7(Suppl 1):S37-42.

Ahlering T.E., Dubeau L., Jones P.A. (1987). A new in vivo model to study invasion and metastasis of human bladder carcinoma. Cancer Res. 47 (24 Pt 1):6660-5.

Ahn C., Sandler H., Glass M., Saldeen, T. (1993). Effect of a synthetic leukocyte elastase inhibitor on thrombin-induced pulmonary edema in the rat. Exp Lung Res 19(2):125-35.

Aikawa H., Kobayashi S., Suzuki K. (1986). Aqueductal lesions in 6-aminonicotinamide-treated suckling mice. Acta Neuropathol (Ber). 71:243-50.

Airapetiants M.G., Mekhedova A. Ia., Kozlovskaia M.M., Neznamov G.G. (1986). Modeling neurosis in the dog and a study of the effects of antidepressants. Zh Vyssh nerv Deiatl. 36:1131-8. (English Abstract) (Russian).

Akizuki S. (1984). Simple technique for coronary occlusion in a closed-chest dog. Kokyu To Junkan. 32:921-4(Japanese).

Aldrovandi G., Feuer G., Gao L., Jamieson B., Kristeva M., Chen I., Zack, J. (1993). The SCID-hu mouse as a model for HIV-1 infection. Nature 363(6431):732-6.

Alexander E.L. (1986). Immunopathologic mechanisms of inflammatory vascular disease in primary Sjogren's syndrome- a model. Scand J Rheumatol [Suppl]. 61:280-5.

Alexander G.E., Delong M.E., Strick P.L. (1985). Two histopathologic types of inflammatory vascular disease in MRL/Mp autoimmune mice. Model for human vasculitis in connective tissue disease. Arthritis Rheum. 28:1146-44.

Allen C.M. (1994). Animal models of oral candidiasis. A review. Oral Surg Oral Med Oral Pathol. 78(2):216-21.

Allen W.R., Kydd J.H., Boyle M.S., Antczak D.F. (1987). Extraspecific donkey-in-horse pregnancy as a model for early fetal death. J Reprod Fertil [Suppl]. 35:197-209.

Aller M., Lorente L., Alonso S., Arias J. (1993). A model of cholestasis in the rat, using a microsurgical technique. Scand J Gastroenterol 28(1):10-4.

Alles A.J., Sulik K.K. (1993). A review of caudal dysgenesis and its pathogenesis as illustrated in an animal model. Birth Defects 29(1):83-102.

Alonso M. J., Garcia-Dorado D., Soriano T. J., Botas R., Fernandez A. F., Munoz A. R., Duran H. JM., Elizaga C. J., Esteban P. E., Theroux P. (1991). [The intracoronary infusion of superoxide dismutase during the initial liberation of oxygen free radicals induced by reperfusion. The effect on the infarct size after 60 minutes of coronary occlusion in the pig model] Infusion intracoronaria de superoxido dismutasa durante la liberacion inicial de radicales libres del oxigeno inducida por la reperfusion. Efecto sobre el tamano del infarto tras 60 minutos de oclusion coronaria en el modelo porcino. Rev Esp Cardiol 44(7):462-72.

Alroy J., Warren C., Raghavan S., Kolodny E. (1989). Animal models for lysosomal storage diseases: their past and future contribution. Hum Pathol 20(9):823-6.

Alter B.P., Campbell A.S., Holland J.G., Friend C. (1982). Increased mouse minor hemoglobin during erythroid stress: a model for hemoglobin regulation. Exp Hematol. 10:754-60.

Alter H.J., Eichberg J.W., Masur H., Saxinger W.C., Gallo R., Macher A.M., Lane H.C., Fauci A.S. (1984). Transmission of HTVL-III infection from human plasma to chimpanzees: an animal model for AIDS. Science. 226:549-52.

Altshuler H.L. (1981). Animal models for alcohol research. Curr Alcohol. 8:343-57.

Alwmark A., Bengmark S., Gullstrand P., Schalen C. (1981). Improvement of the splenectomized rat model for overwhelming pneumococcal infection. Standardization of the bacterial inocula. Eur Surg Res. 13:339-43.

AMA (1992). Engaging physicians in the campaign against animal activists. J Nucl Med. 33:24N.

Amanmuradov A. (1990). [The modelling of the development of Plasmodium yoelli yoelli in different vertebrate hosts] Modelirovanie razvitiia Plasmodium yoelii yoelii v raznykh pozvonochnykh khoziaev. Med Parazitol (Mosk) (6):20-2.

Ammirati M., Cozzens J., Eller T., Ciric I., Tarkington J., Rabin E. (1986). Technique of experimental aneurysm formation in the rat common carotid artery using the milliwatt carbon dioxide laser and the adventitial patch model. Neurosurgery. 19:732-4.

Amorim D.S. (1984). Chagas' cardiopathy. Experimental models. Arq Bras Cardiol. 42:243-7.

Amorim D.S. (1985). Chagas' heart disease: Experimental models. Heart Vessels. [Supl]. 1:236-9.

Amsel A. (1992). Frustration theory: an analysis of dispositional learning and memory. Cambridge; New York, NY, USA: Cambridge University Press. 278 P.

Anderson B. (1994). Role for animal research in the investigation of human mental retardation. Am J Ment Retard. 99(1):50-9.

Anderson C.J., Schwarz S.W., Connett J.M., Cutler P.D., Guo L.W., Germain C.J., Philpott G.W., Zinn K.R., Greiner D.P., Meares C.F., Welch M.J. (1995). Preparation, biodistribution and dosimetry of copper-64-labeled anti-colorectal carcinoma monoclonal antibody fragments 1A3-F(ab')$_2$. J Nucl Med. 36:850-8.

Anderson D., Faber J. (1989). Animal model for polyhydramnios. Am J Obstet Gynecol. 160(2):389-90.

Anderson D.E., Kearns W.D., Worden T.J. (1983). Progressive hypertension in dogs by avoiding conditioning and saline infusion. Hypertension 5:286-91.

Anderson J.R., Field H.J. (1984). An animal model of ocular herpes, keratitis, retinitis and cataract in the mouse. Br J Exp Pathol. 65:283-97.

Anderson R.A. Jr., Willis B.R., Oswald C., Zaneveld L.J. (1983). Ethanol-induced male infertility: impairment spermatozoa. J Pharmacol Exp. Ther. 225:479-86.

Anderson W.F., Maritnell J., Whitney J.B. 3d, Popp R.A. (1982). Mouse models of human thalassemia. Prog Clin Biol Res. 94:11-26.

Andrade Z.A., Andrade S.G. (1980). Pathology of experimental Chagas disease in dogs. Mem Inst Oswaldo Cruz. 75:77-95. (English Abstract) (Portugese).

Andrade Z.A., Andrade S.Q., Sadiqursky M. (1984). Damage and healing in the conducting tissue of the heart (experimental study in dogs infected with Trypanosoma cruzi). J Pathol. 143:93-101.

Andrade, Z., Cheever, A. (1993). Characterization of the murine model of schistosomal hepatic periportal fibrosis ('pipestem' fibrosis). Int J Exp Pathol, 74 (2):195-202.

Andzhaparidze A.G., Balaian M.S., Savinov A.P., Braginskii D.M., Paleshchuk V.F. (1986). Reproduction in monkeys of non-A, non-B hepatitis transmitted via the fecal and oral routes. Vopr Virusol. 31:73-81. (English Abstract) (Russian)

Angel A. (1986). Animal models of myoclonus using 1,2-dihydroxybenzene (catechol) and chloralose. Adv Neurol. 43:589-609.

Angerbach D., Nicholson C. (1988). Enhancement of muscle blood cell flux and pO_2 by cromakalim (BRL 34915) and other compounds enhancing membrane K+ conductance, but not by Ca2+ antagonists or hydralazine, in an animal model of occlusive arterial disease. Naunyn Schmiedebergs Arch Pharmacol 337(3):341-6.

Anosa V.O., Kaneko J.J. (1983). Pathogenesis of Trypanosoma brucei infection in deer mice (Peromyscus maniculatus): hematologic, erythrocyte biochemical, and iron metabolic aspects. Am J Vet Res. 44:639-44.

Antal A., Bodis-Wollner I. (1993). Animal models of Alzheimer's Parkinson's and Huntington's disease. A minireview. Neurobiology 1(2):101-22.

Antonenko V., Kovrikova N., Korulia V., Shalimov V., Iashchenko O. (1989). [Modelling of a combined immunodeficiency state by splenectomy and alloimmunization with lymph node antigens] Modelirovanie kombinirovannogo immunodefitsitnogo sostoianiia splenektomiei i alloimmunizatsiei antigenami limfaticheskikh uzlov. Vrach Delo, (9):99-101.

Aoki S., Ikuta K., Nonogaki T., Ito Y. (1985). Induction of chronic polyarthritis in rabbits by hyperimmunization with Escherichia coli. I. Pathologic and serologic features in two breeds of rabbits. Arthritis Rheum. 28:522-8.

Appel S., Engelhardt J., Garcia J., Stefani E. (1991). Autoimmunity and ALS: a comparison of animal models of immune-mediated motor neuron destruction and human ALS. Adv Neurol 56:405-12.

Appel S., Engelhardt J., Garcia J., Stefani E. (1991). Immunoglobulins from animal models of motor neuron disease and from human amyotrophic lateral sclerosis patients passively transfer physiological abnormalities to the neuromuscular junction. Proc Natl Acad Sci. 88(2):647-51.

Appleby P., Webber DG., Bowen J. (1989). Murine chronic graft-versus-host disease as a model of systemic lupus erythematosus: effect of immunosuppressive drugs on disease development. Clin Exp Immunol 78(3):449-53.

Arai N., Misugi K., Goshima Y., Misu Y. (1990). Evaluation of a 1-methyl-4-phenyl-1,2,3,6-tetrahydropyridine (MPTP)-treated C57 black mouse model for parkinsonism. Brain Res 515:57-63.

Arai T., Tsukahara I., Imon H., Dote K., Kuzume K. (1986). A new model for total cerebral ischemia in dogs. Masui. 35:1107-13. (English Abstract). (Japanese)

Araiz J., Refojo M., Arroyo M., Leong F., Albert D., Tolentino F. (1993). Antiproliferative effect of retinoic acid in intravitreous silicone oil in an animal model of proliferative vitreoretinopathy. Invest Ophthalmol Vis Sci 34(3):522-30.

Araki S., Yi S., Murakami T., Watanabe S., Ikegawa S., Takahashi K., Yamamura K. (1994). Systemic amyloidosis in transgenic mice carrying the human mutant transthyretin (Met 30) gene. Pathological and immunohistochemical similarity to human familial amyloidotic polyneuropathy, type I. Mol Neurobiol. 8(1):15-23.

Arankalle V., Chadha M., Banerjee K., Srinivasan M., Chobe L. (1993). Hepatitis E virus infection in pregnant rhesus monkeys. Indian J Med Res 97:4-8.

Arbit E., Galicich W., Galicich J., Lau N. (1989). An animal model of epidural compression of the spinal cord. Neurosurgery 24(6):860-3.

Arenberg I.K., Murray J.P., Schenck N.L., Norback D.H.. (1981). Experimental endolymphatic hydrops in sharks. I. Histologic studies. Am JK Otol. 3:81-95.

Arlaschenko N.I., Pogosov AIu. (1984). Experimental model for the objective assessment of the degree of manifestation of a primary reaction to irradiation in rabbits. Izv Akad Nauk SSSR [Biol]. 3:428-32. (English Abstract) (Russian)

Arnold J., Bertrand J., Benyshek L. (1992). Animal model for genetic evaluation of multibreed data. J Anim Sci 70(11):3322-32.

Artlet J., Gedeon P. (1982). Experimental arthrosis. Rev Rhum Mal Osteoartic. 49:145-52. (French)

Asakawa H., Jeppsson B., Mack P., Hultberg B., Hagerstrand I., Bengmark S. (1989). Acute ischemic liver failure in the rat: a reproducible model not requiring portal decompression. Eur Surg Res 21(1):42-8.

Ash S.R., Thornhill J.A. (Eds) (1985). Animal Models of Renal Failure. CRC Press, Boca Raton. 232 pp.

Ash S.R., Thornhill J.A., Dhein C.R., Rebar A.H. (1982). Dialytic support of dogs with clinically occurring renal failure: a realistic model of acute renal failure in man. Clin Exp Dial Apheresis. 6:25-44.

Asher J. J., Friedman T. (1990). Mouse and hamster mutants as models for Waardenburg syndromes in humans. J Med Genet 27(10):618-26.

Ashhurst D.E., Hogg J., Perren S.M. (1982). A method for making reproducible experimental fractures of the rabbit tibia. Injury. 14:236-42.

Ashurmetov R., Khoroshaev V., Kasymov A., Bazhenov L. (1992). [The modelling of diffuse peritonitis] Modelirovanie razlitogo peritonita. Khirurgiia (Mosk) (4):77-80.

ASIH (1990). American Society of Ichthyologists and Herpetologists. Resolution - The importance of animals in biological research. 70th annual meeting, Charleston, SC.: IRAR News 32:(4):11.

Asplund S., Hjelmstedt A. (1983). Experimentally induced hip dislocation in vitro and in vivo. A study in newborn rabbits. Acta Orthop Scand [Suppl]. 199:1-57.

Assmann K.J., Tangelder M.M., Lange W.P., Schrijver G., Koene RY.A. (1985). Anti-GBM nephritis in the mouse: severe proteinuria in the heterologous phase. Virchows Arch. 406:285-99.

Aufdemorte T.B., Boyan B.D., Fox W.C., Miller D. (1993). Diagnostic tools and biologic markers: animal models in the study of osteoporosis and oral bone loss. J Bone Miner Res. 8(Suppl 2):S529-34.

Auricchio S., Cardelli M., De Ritis G., Vincenzi M., Latte F., Silano V. (1984). An in vitro animal model for the study of cereal components toxic in celiac disease. Pediatr Res. 18:1372-8.

Australian Code of Practice for the Care and Use of Animals for Scientific Purposes. (1990). Australian Government Printing Service, Canberra, ISBN 0-644-10292-6. 75 pp.

Avanzini G., Marescaux C. (1991). Genetic animal models for generalized non convulsive epilepsies and new antiepileptic drugs. Epilepsy Res Suppl 3:29-38.

Awrich P., Madge G.E., Wolf B. (1983). Fatty liver and kidney syndrome in chickens as an animal model for Reye's syndrome. J Pediatr Gastroenterol Nutr. 2:683-92.

Awrich P., Wolf N. (1983). Is fatty liver and kidney disease in chickens a suitable model for Reye's syndrome? Lancet. 5 (8319):306.

Azorin I., Minana M., Felipo V., Grisolia S. (1989). A simple animal model of hyperammonemia. Hepatology 10(3):311-4.

Bach J.F., Boitard C. (1986). Experimental models of type-I diabetes. Pathol Immunopathol Res. 5:384-415.

Bach P.H., Hardy T.L. (1985). Relevance of animal models to analgesic-associated renal papillary necrosis in humans. Kidney Int. 28:605-13.

Bafort J.M., Schmidt H. (1984). Experimental Tru anosoma (Nannomonas) congolense infection in microtus montanus. Ann Trop Med Parasitol. 78:355-61.

Bain O., Petit G., Vuong Ngoc P., Chabaud A. (1985). Filarise of rodents useful for the experimental study of human onchocerciasis. C.R. Acad Sci (III). 301:513-5. (English Abstract). (French)

Baird J.D., Aerts L. (1987). Research priorities in diabetic pregnancy today: the role of animal models. Biol Neonate. 51:119-27.

Baird S.M., Beattie G.M., Lennom R.A., Lipsick J.S., Jensen F.C., Kaplan N.O. (1982). Induction of lymphoma in antigenically stimulated athymic mice. Cancer Res. 42:198-206.

Baker C.C., Chaudry I.H., Gaines H.O., Baue A.E. (1983). Evaluation of factors affecting mortality rate after sepsis in a murine cecal ligation and puncture model. Surgery. 94:331-5.

Baker H.J., Walkley S.U., Ratazzi M.C., Singer H.S., Watson H.L., Wood P.A. (1982). Feline gangliosidoses as models of human lysosomal storage diseases. Prog Clin Biol Res. 94:203-12.

Bakir M.A., Eccles S., Babich J.W., Aftab A., Styles J., Dean C.J., Lambrecht R.M., Ott R.J. (1993). C-erB2 protein overexpression in breast cancer as a target for PET using iodine-124 labeled monoclonal antibodies. J Nucl Med. 34:290.

Bakker N., van E. M., Zurcher C., Faaber P., Lemmens A., Hazenberg M., Bontrop R., Jonker M. (1990). Experimental immune mediated arthritis in rhesus monkeys. A model for human rheumatoid arthritis? Rheumatol Int 10(1):21-9.

Baklanova O.V., Padeiskaia E.N., Kutchak S.N. (1987). Experimental Candida infection in mice due to intracerebral contamination. Antibiot Med Biotekhnol. 32:48-53. (English Abstract). (Russian)

Bakris G. (1991). Renal effects of calcium antagonists in diabetes mellitus. An overview of studies in animal models and in humans. Am J Hypertens 4(7 Pt 2):487S-493S.

Balaian M.S. (1986). The use of monkeys to study problems concerning viral hepatitis. Vestn Akad med Nauk SSR. 3:60-5. (English Abstract). (Russian)

Balk M.W. (1987). Emerging models in the U.S.A.: swine, woodchucks and the hairless guinea pig. Prog Clin Biol Res. 229:311-26.

Bamberg M., Budach V., Stuschke M., Gerhard L., Streffer C. (1988). [Heterotransplantation of a human glioma and brain metastases in the athymic nude mouse - a preclinical model for radiation oncology. 1. Basic principles and methodology] Heterotransplantation menschlicher Gliome und Hirnmetastasen auf die thymusaplastische Nacktmaus - ein präklinisches Modell für die Radioonkologie. 1. Mitteilung: Grundlagen und Methodik. Strahlenther Onkol 164(4):235-43.

Bankiewicz K., Mandel R.J., Sofroniew M.V. (1993). Trophism, transplantation, and animal models of Parkinson's disease. Exp Neurol. 124(1):140-9.

Bankiewicz K., Plunkett R., Mefford I., Kopin I., Oldfield E. (1990). Behavioral recovery from MPTP-induced parkinsonism in monkeys after intracerebral tissue implants is not related to CSF concentrations of dopamine metabolites. Prog Brain Res 82:561-71.

Bar-Joseph G., Safar P., Saito R., Stezoski S., Alexander H. (1991). Monkey model of severe volume-controlled hemorrhagic shock with resuscitation to outcome. Resuscitation 22(1):27-43.

Barany S., Haggstromj E., Gunne L.M. (1983). Application of a primate model for tardive dyskinesia. Acta Pharmacol Toxicol (Copenh). 52:86-9.

Barillo D.J./, Rush B.F. Jr., Dikdan G.S., Hsieh J.T., Machiedo W. (1985). Shock and starvation: similar metabolism in different energy-depletion states. Curr Surg. 42:204-7.

Barna B.P., Deodhar S.D., Chiang T., Gautam S., Edinger M. (1984). Experimental beryllium-induced lung disease. I. Differences in immunologic responses to beryllium compounds in strains 2 and 13 guinea pigs. Int Arch Allergy Appl Immunol. 73:42-8.

Barral A., Petersen E.A., Sacks D.L., Nova F.A. (1983). Late metastatic Leishmaniasis in the mouse. A model for mucocutaneous disease. Am J Trop Med Hyg. 32:277-85.

Barrio J.R., Satyamurthy N., Huang S.C. et al. (1989). 3-(2'-[^{18}F]fluoroethyl)spiperone: In vivo biochemical and kinetic characterization in rodents, non-human primates, and humans. J Cereb Blood Flow Metab. 9:830-9.

Barrios C., Tunon M.T., De Salis J.A., Beguiristain J.L., Canadell J. (1987). Scoliosis induced by medullary damage: an experimental study in rabbits. Spine. 12:433-9.

Barrs D., Trahan C., Casey K., Brooks D. (1991). The porcine model for intratemporal facial nerve trauma studies. Otolaryngol Head Neck Surg 105(6):845-56.

Barsanti J., Crowell W., Finco D., Shotts E., Beck B. (1982). Induction of chronic bacterial prostatitis in the dog. J Urol. 127:1215-9.

Barsoum N.J., Moore J.D., Gough A.W., Sturgess J.M., De La Iglesia F.A. (1986). Parkinson-like syndrome in nonhuman primates receiving a tetrahydropyridine derivative. Neurotoxicology. 7:119-26.

Barth E., Sullivan T., Berg E. (1990). Animal model for evaluating bone repair with and without adjunctive hyperbaric oxygen therapy: comparing dose schedules. J Invest Surg 3(4):387-92.

Barthold S.W., Moody K.D., Terwilliger G.A., Jacoby R.O., Steere A.C. (1988): An animal model for Lyme arthritis. Ann N Y Acad Sci. 539:264-73.

Bartlett M., Fishman J., Durkin M., Queener S., Smith J. (1989). An improved rat model to study efficacy of drugs for treatment or prophylaxis of Pneumocystis carinii pneumonia. J Protozool 36(1):77S-78S.

Bartlett M., Fishman J., Durkin M., Queener S., Smith J. (1990). Pneumocystis carinii: improved models to study efficacy of drugs for treatment or prophylaxis of Pneumocystis pneumonia in the rat (Rattus spp.). Exp Parasitol 70(1):100-6.

Bartlett M.S, Fishman J.A., Queener S.F., Durkin M.M., Jay M.A., Smith J.W. (1988): New rat model of Pneumocystis carinii infection. J Clin Microbiol. 26(6):1100-2.

Bartlett M.S., Durkin M.M., Jay M.A., Queener S.F., Smith J.W. (1987). Sources of rats free of latent Pneumocystis carinii J Clin microbiol. 25:1794-5.

Bartlett M.S., Queener S.F., Jay M.A., Durkin M.M., Smith J.W. (1987). Improved rat model for studying Pneumocystis carinni pneumonia. J Clin Microbiol. 25:480-4.

Bartoshuk L.M. (1993). Genetic and pathologic taste variation: what can we learn from animal models and human disease? Ciba Found Symp. 179:251-62; discussion 262-7.

Bartoszyk G.D., Hamer M. (1987). The genetic animal model of reflex epilepsy in the Mongolian gerbil: differential efficacy of new anticonvulsive drugs and prototype antiepileptics. Pharmacol Res Commun. 19:429-40.

Bashir R., Okano M., Kleveland K., Pirrucello S., Masih A., Sanger W., Fordyce-Boyer R., Purtilo D. (1991). SCID/human mouse model of central nervous system lymphoproliferative disease. Lab Invest 65(6):702-9.

Basile A., Gammal S., Mullen K., Jones E., Skolnick P. (1988). Differential responsiveness of cerebellar Purkinje neurons to GABA and benzodiazepine receptor ligands in an animal model of hepatic encephalopathy. J Neurosci 8(7):2414-21.

Basile A., Pannell L., Jaouni T., Gammal SH., Fales H., Jones E., Skolnick P. (1990). Brain concentrations of benzodiazepines are elevated in an animal model of hepatic encephalopathy. Proc Natl Acad Sci U S A, 87(14):5263-7.

Baskerville A., Newell D.G., (1988): Naturally occurring chronic gastritis and C pylori infection in the rhesus monkey: a potential model for gastritis in man. Gut. 29(4):465-72.

Baskin G.B., Gormus B.J., Martin L.N., Wolf R.H., Blanchard J.L., Malaty R., Walsh G.P., Meyers W.M., Binford C.H. (1987). Experimental leprosy in African green monkeys (Ceropithecus aethiops): a model for polyneuritic leprosy. Am J Trop Med Hyg. 37:385-91.

Basset-Seguin N., Cartier N., Demoly P., Guilhou J. (1992). [Transgenic mice] Souris transgeniques. Ann Dermatol Venereol 119(8):597-603.

Bastien P., Landau I., Baccam D. (1987). Inhibition of the infectivity of Plasmodium gametocytes by the serum of the parasite host. Perfecting an experimental model. Ann Parasitol Hum Comp. 62:195-208. (English Abstract) (French).

Bastos O de C., Sadigursky M., do Nascimento M. do D. et al. (1984). Holochilus brasiliensis nanus Thomas, 1897. Suggestion for an experimental model for filariasis, leishmaniasis and schistosomiasis. Rev inst Med Trop Sao Paulo. 26:307-15. (English Abstract). (Portuguese).

Bates T., Williams S., Kauppinen R., Gadian D. (1989). Observation of cerebral metabolites in an animal model of acute liver failure in vivo: a 1H and 31P nuclear magnetic resonance study [see comments]. J Neurochem 53(1):102-10.

Batra S., Rakusan K., Campbell S. (1991). Geometry of capillary networks in hypertrophied rat heart. Microvasc Res 41(1):29-40.

Batshaw M.L., Hyman S.L., Mellits E.D., Thomas G.H., De Muro R., Coyle J.T. (1986). Behavioral and neurotransmitter changes in the urease-infused rat: a model of congenital hyperammonemia. Pediatr Res. 20:1310-5.

Batt R.M., McLean L., Carter M.W. (1987). Sequential morphologic and biochemical studies of naturally occurring wheat-sensitive enteropathy in Irish setter dogs. Dig Dis Sci. 32:184-94.

Bauer J., Fung H. (1990). Effects of chronic glyceryl trinitrate on left ventricular haemodynamics in a rat model of congestive heart failure: demonstration of a simple animal model for the study of in vivo nitrate tolerance. Cardiovasc Res 24(3):198-203.

Baum R.M. (1990). Biomedical researchers work to counter animal rights agenda. Chemical and Engineering News, May 7. p 9-24.

Baumal R.l, Hooi C., McAvoy D., Broder I. (1983). Time course of morphometric changes after acute allergic bronchoconstriction in the guinea pig. Int Arch Allergy App Immuno. 71 131-6

Bawdon R., Fiskin A., Little B., Davis L., Vergarra G. (1989). Fibronectin and postpartum infection in rabbits: an animal model. Gynecol Obstet Invest 28(4):185-90.

Baylis C. (1987). Renal disease in gravid animal models. Am J Kidney Dis. 9:350-3.

Beardsley P.M., Balster R.L., Harris L.S. (1986). Dependence on tetrahydrocannabinol in rhesus monkeys. J Pharmacol Exp Ther. 239:311-9.

Beatty W. (1988). Preservation and loss of spatial memory in aged rats and humans: implications for the analysis of memory dysfunction in dementia. Neurobiol Aging 9(5-6):557-61.

Beauchamp G., Devito M., Bourgie J., Lamoureux C. (1986). Experimental models of gastroesophageal reflux. Union Med Can. 115:387-92. (English Abstract). (French)

Beaumanoir A., Naguet R., Virouroux R. (1982). Temporal lobe epilepsy: experimental reproduction. Electroencephalogr Clin Neurophysiol [Suppl]. 35:159-70.

Becker H., Hale R. (1993). Repeated episodes of ethanol withdrawal potentiate the severity of subsequent withdrawal seizures: an animal model of alcohol withdrawal "kindling". Alcohol Clin Exp Res 17(1):94-8.

Bedard P., Boucher R., DiPaolo T. (1988). [Animal models of tardive dyskinesia] Les modeles animaux de la dyskinesie tardive. Encephale, 14 Spec No:163-6.

Begin R., Rola-Pleszcznski M., Masse S. (1983). Asbestos-induced lung injury in the sheep model: the inital alveolitis. Environ Res. 30:195-210.

Bejui J., Harmand M.F., Duphil R., Roussouly P., Comtet J.J., Anamia. (1986). Experimental arthrosis by hyperpressure. Eng Med. 15:67-9.

Bekemeier H., Hirschelmann R.Y., Giessler A.J. (1985). Carrageenin-induced thrombosis in rats and mice: a model for testing antithrombotic substance. Agents Actions. 16:446-51.

Benavides J., Capdeville C., Dauphin F., Dubois A., Duverger D., Fage D., Gotti B., MacKenzie ET., Scatton B. (1990). The quantification of brain lesions with an omega 3 site ligand: a critical analysis of animal models of cerebral ischaemia and neurodegeneration. Brain Res 522(2):275-89.

Bendele A., Benslay D., Hom J., Spaethe S., Ruterbories K., Lindstrom T., Lee S., Naismith R. (1992). Anti-inflammatory activity of BF389, a Di-T-butylphenol, in animal models of arthritis. J Pharmacol Exp Ther 260(1):300-5.

Bendele A.M. (1987). Progressive chronic osteoarthritis in femorotibial joints of partial medial meniscectomized guinea pigs. Vet Pathol. 24:444-8.

Bendinelli M., Pistello M., Matteucci D., Lombardi S., Baldinotti F., et al. (1993). Small animal model of AIDS and the feline immunodeficiency virus. Adv Exp Med Biol. 335:189-202.

Benedict C.R., Mathew B., Rex K.A. (1986). Correlation of plasma serotonin changes with platelet aggregation in an in vivo dog model of spontaneous occlusive coronary thrombus formation. Circ Res. 58:58-67.

Benediktsson R., Lindsay R., Noble J., Seckl J., Edwards C. (1993). Glucocorticoid exposure in utero: new model for adult hypertension. Lancet 341(8841):339-41.

Benesova O., Pavlik A. (1986). Experiment study of neuro-psycho-behavioral deviations caused by perinatal disorders of brain development. Cesk Psychiatr. 82:106-12. (English Abstract). (Czechoslaovakian)

Benestad H.B., Iversen J.G. (1983). Haemorrhagic and haemolytic anaemias in the rabbit: a clinically relevant laboratory project in physiology. Med Educ. 17:186-92.

Benfield J.R., Shors E.C., Hammond W.G., Paladugu R.R., Cohen A.H., Jensen T., Fu P.C., Pak H.Y., Teplitz R.L. (1981). A clinically relevant canine lung cancer model. Ann Thorac Surg. 32:592-601.

Beniashvili D., Aleksandrov V., Bardadze K., Bespalov V., Petrov A., Sartaniia M. (1992). [Esophageal tumor induction in monkeys] Induktsiia opukholei pishchevoda u obez'ian. Vopr Onkol 38(4):458-64.

Benjamin I.S., Ryan C.J., Engelbrecht G.H., Campbell J.A., van Hoorn-Hickman R., Blumgart L.H. (1984). Portacaval transposition in the rat: definition of a valuable model for hepatic research. Hepatology. 4:704-8.

Berenson M., Kimura R., Samowitz W., Bjorkman D. (1992). Protoporphyrin overload in unrestrained rats: biochemical and histopathologic characterization of a new model of protoporphyric hepatopathy. Int J Exp Pathol 73(5):665-73.

Berger J. (1982). Current problems of evaluation of drug-induced anaemias using the laboratory rat as an experimental model. 121:941-3. (English Abstract) (Czechoslovakian)

Berger M.E., Golub M.S., Sowers J.R., Brickman A.S., Nyby M., Troyer H., Rude R K., Singer F.R., Horst R., Deftos L.J. (1982). Hypercalcemia in association with a Leydig cell tumor in the rat: a model for tumor-induced hypercalcemia in man. Life Sci. 30:1509-15.

Bergqvist D., Jensen N. (1985). Experimental models of graft studies. Acta Chir Scand. 529:29-34.

Bermejo A., Gonzalez O., Gonzalez J. (1993). The pig as an animal model for experimentation on the temporomandibular articular complex. Oral Surg Oral Med Oral Pathol 75(1):18-23.

Bermudez L., Petrofsky M., Kolonoski P., Young L. (1992). An animal model of Mycobacterium avium complex disseminated infection after colonization of the intestinal tract. J Infect Dis 165(1):75-9.

Bernstein S.E. (1987). Hereditary hypotransferrinemia with hemosiderosis, a murine disorder resembling human atransferrinemia. J Lab Clin Med. 110:690-705.

Berthet J., Pasquier D., Racinet C. (1992). [An original model of experimental endometriosis in the rabbit] Modele original d'endometriose experimentale chez la lapine. J Gynecol Obstet Biol Reprod (Paris) 21(6):625-8.

Berti M., Rossi E., Candiani G., Arioli V. (1982). A new model of experimental Bacteroides fragilis infection in mice and rats. Chemotherapy. 28:213-7.

Bertram M.A., Inderlied C.B., Yadegar S., Kolanoski P., Yamada J.K., Young L.S. (1986). Confirmation of the beige mouse model for study of disseminated infection with Mycobacterium avium complex. J Infect Dis. 154:194-5.

Berty R., Adler S. (1991). In vivo and in vitro rat model for cyclosporine-induced proximal tubular toxicity [see comments]. J Lab Clin Med 118(1):17-25.

Besser T., Potter K., Bryan G., Knowlen G. (1990). An animal model of the Marfan syndrome. Am J Med Genet 37(1):159-65.

Bhardwaj J.R., Kukreja R.S., Banerjee A.K., Datta B.N., Chakravarti R.N. (1984). A morphological study of experimental cerebral atherosclerosis in rhesus monkeys. Indian J Med Res. 79:86-92.

Bhol K., Mukherjee R., Mehra S., Maitra T., Jalan K. (1989). A model of hepatic amoebiasis in random bred mice. Trans R Soc Trop Med Hyg 83(3):346-8.

Bia F.J., Griffith B.P., Fong C.K., Hsiung G.D. (1983). Cytomegaloviral infections in the guinea pig: experimental models for human disease. Rev Infect Dis. 5:177-95.

Bianchi G., Ferrari P., Cusi D., Salardi S., Guidi E., Nutta E., Tripodi G.. (1986). Genetic and experimental hypertension in the animal model-similarities and dissimilarities to the development of human hypertension. J Cardiovasc Pharmacol. 5:S64-70.

Bignami G. (1988): Pharmacology and anxiety: inadequacies of current experimental approaches and working models. Pharmacol Biochem Behav. 29(4):771-4.

Bill D., Fletcher A., Glenn B., Knight M. (1992). Behavioural studies on WAY100289, a novel 5-HT3 receptor antagonist, in two animal models of anxiety. Eur J Pharmacol 218(2-3):327-34.

Birkenmeier E., Davisson M., Beamer W., Ganschow R., Vogler C., Gwynn B., Lyford K., Maltais L., Wawrzyniak C. (1989). Murine mucopolysaccharidosis type VII. Characterization of a mouse with beta-glucuronidase deficiency. J Clin Invest 83(4):1258-6.

Birkui P.J., Geogiopoulos G., Richie M.C., Perrault M., Puisleux F., Merland J.J., Saumont R. (1981). Closed-chest myocardial ischaemia in dog. Med Prog Technol. 8:121-7.

Birt D.F., Roebuck B.D. (1986). Enhancement of pancreatic carcinogenesis by dietary fat in the hamster and rat models. Prog Clin Biol Res. 222:331-55.

Bishop N., Civitico G., Wang Y., Guo K., Birch C., Gust I., Locarnini S. (1990). Antiviral strategies in chronic hepatitis B virus infection: I. Establishment of an in vitro system using the duck hepatitis B virus model. J Med Virol 31(2):82-9.

Bishop S. (1989). Animal models of vasculitis. Toxicol Pathol 17(1 Pt 2):109-17.

Bispen A., Aleksandrova A., Vakhmistrova T., Vinogradova T. (1992). [Effect of plasmapheresis on the course of experimental tuberculosis and the tolerance of chemotherapy by patients with renal tuberculosis] Vliianie plazmafereza na techenie eksperimental'nogo tuberkuleza i perenosimost' khimioterapii ftiziourologicheskimi bol'nymi. Probl Tuberk (7-8):53-5.

Bito L.Z. (1984). Species differences in the responses of the eye to irritation and trauma: a hypothesis of divergence in ocular defense mechanisms and the choice of experimental animals for eye research. Exp Eye Res. 39:807-29.

Bito L.Z., Kaufman P.L., De Rousseau C.J., Koretz J. (1987). Presbyopia: an animal model and experimental approaches for the study of the mechanism of accommodation and ocular ageing. Eye. 1 (Pt 2):222-30.

Bittleman D.B., Casale T.B. (1994). Allergic models and cytokines. Am J Respir Crit Care Med. 150(5 Pt 2):S72-6.

Biziere K., Chambon J.P. (1987). Animal models of epilepsy and experimental seizures. Rev Neurol (Paris) 143:329-40. (English Abstract).   (French)

Bjork J., Smedegard G. (1984).. The microvasculature of the hamster cheek pouch as a model for studying acute immune-comples-induced inflammatory reactions. Int Arch Allergy Appl Immunol. 73:77-85.

Bjorklund A., Stenevi U., Dunnett S.B., Gage F.H. (1982). Cross-species neural grafting in a rat model of Parkinson's disease. Nature. 298 (5875):652-4.

Black P., Markowitz R.S., Cooper V., Mechanic A., Kushner H., Damjanov I., Finkelstein S.D., Wachs K.C. (1986). Models of spinal cord injury: Part 1. Static load technique. Neurosurgery. 19:752-62.

Blaser M.J., Duncan D.J., Warren G.H., Wang W.L. (1983). Experimental Campylobacter jejuni infection of adult mice. Infect Immun. 39:908-16.

Blay R.A., Bigley N.J., Giron D.J. (1985). A murine model of insulin-dependent diabetes mellitus resulting from the cumulative effects of the nondiabetogenic strain of encephalomyocarditis virus and a single low dose of streptozocin. Diabetes. 34:1288-92.

Bleiberg R.M. (1989). Animal workshop, Barron's, February 13. p 11.

Blizard D.A. (1988): The locus ceruleus: a possible neural focus for genetic differences in emotionality. Experientia. 15;44(6):491-5.

Blomqvist P., Jiborn H., Zederfeldt B. (1984). Models for studying long-term recovery following forebrain ischemia in the rat. 1. Circulatory and functional effects of 4-vessel occlusion. Acta Neurol Scand. 69:376-84.

Bluethmann H., Ohashi P.S. (Ed.) (1994). Transgenesis and targeted mutagenesis in immunology. 2nd rev. ed. San Diego: Academic Press. 494 P.

Bo G.P., Mainardi P., Benassi E., Besio G., Faverio A., Scotto P.A., Laeb C. (1986). Parenteral penicillin model of epilepsy in the rat: a reappraisal. Methods Find Exp Clin Pharmacol. 8:491-6.

Bodnoff S., Suranyi-Cadotte B., Aitken D., Quirion R., Meaney MJ. (1988). The effects of chronic antidepressant treatment in an animal model of anxiety. Psychopharmacology (Berl) 95(3):298-302.

Bogers A.J., van der Laarse A., van der May K.H., Rasser van der May A.A., Holaar L. (1983). Experimental right-ventricular infarction in rats by abdominodiaphragmal access to the heart. A new technique in the study of infarcted myocardium. Res Exp Med (Berl). 182:105-9.

Boissier M.C., Feng X.Z., Cardioz A., Roudier R., Fournier C. (1987). Induction of flare-ups of chronic progressive polyarthritis in mice after injection of type II homologous collagen. Rev Rhum mal Osteoartic. 54:801-4. (English Abstract). (French)

Boissy R., Lamoreux M. (1988). Animal models of an acquired pigmentary disorder-vitiligo. Prog Clin Biol Res 256:207-18.

Bokk M., Stemparzhetskii O., Malakhovskii V. (1990). [Postradiation motor disorders in rodents as the equivalent of the clinical manifestations of a primary radiation reaction] Postluchevye motornye narusheniia u gryzunov kak ekvivalent klinicheskikh proiavlenii pervichnoi luchevoi reaktsii. Radiobiologiia 30(2):233-7.

Bond N.W. (Ed). (1985). Animal Models in Psychopathology. Academic Press, New York. 328 p.

Bonkovsky H.L., Healey J.F., Lincoln B., Bacon B.R., Bishop D.F., Elder G.H. (1987). Hepatic heme synthesis in a new model of experimental hemochromatosis: studies in rats fed finely divided elemental iron. Hepatology. 7:1195-203.

Boobis A.R., Murray S., Speirs C.J., Seddon C.E. et al. (1987). Drug Metabolism - from Molecules to Man. In: Bedford D.J., Bridges J.W., Gibson G.G. (Eds.) London: Taylor & Francis, pp 352-68.

Boogerd W., Peters A.C. (1986). A simple method for obtaining cerebrospinal fluid from a pig model of herpes encephalitis. Lab Anim Sci. 36:386-8.

Boone C., Kelloff G., Malone W. (1990). Identification of candidate cancer chemopreventive agents and their evaluation in animal models and human clinical trials: a review. Cancer Res 50(1):2-9.

Bormans G., Maes A., Langendries W., Nuyts J. et al. (1995). Metabolism of nitrogen-13 labeled ammonia in different conditions in dogs, human volunteers and transplant patients. Eur J Nucl Med. 22:116-21.

Bornman M.S., du Plessis D.J., Ligthelm A.J., Van Tonder H.J. (1985). Histological changes in the penis of the Chacma baboon - a model to study aging penile vascular impotence. J Med Primatol. 14:13-8.

Borodina N.P., Klenova A.V., Voskoboinik A.D., Shevliagin VIa. (1984). Pathogenic properties of the human papovavirusi in the golden hamster model. Vopr Onkol. 30:80-4. (English Abstract) (Russian)

Borsini F., Brambilla A., Cesana R., Donetti A. (1993). The effect of DAU 6215, a novel 5HT-3 antagonist, in animal models of anxiety. Pharmacol Res 27(2):151-64.

Bose R., Pinsky C., Glavin G. (1990). Sensitive murine model and putative antidotes for behaviorial toxicosis from contaminated mussel extracts. Can Dis Wkly Rep 16 Suppl 1E:91-8; discussion 99-100.

Bosland M. (1992). Animal models for the study of prostate carcinogenesis. J Cell Biochem Suppl, 16H:89-98.

Bossinger T.R., Powe T.A. (1988): Campylobacter jejuni infections in gnotobiotic pigs. Am J Vet Res 49(4):456-8.

Botros S.S., El-Badrawi N., El-Raziky E.H. (1986). Subcutaneous implantation of the spleen as a new technique for experimental induction of hepatic Schistosoma mansoni egg granulomas. Trans R Soc Trop Med Hyg. 80:515-6.

Boucher M., Duchene-Marullaz P. (1985). Methods for producing experimental complete atrioventricular block in dogs. J Pharmacol Methods. 13:95-107.

Boulton A.A., Baker G.B., Butterworth R.F. (Ed.) (1992). Animal models of neurological disease. Totowa, N.J.: Humana Press.

Boulton A.A., Baker G.B., Wu P.H. (Ed.) (1992). Animal models of drug addiction. Totowa, N.J.: Humana Press. 436 P.

Bourdelat D., Moulinoux J.P., Chambon Y., Babut J.M. (1983). Intrahepatic bile duct proliferation in the gestating rat treated with 4,4' -diaminodiphenylmethane (4, 4DDPM). Bull Assoc Anat. (Nancy). 67:375-82. (English Abstract). (French)

Bourque W., Gross M., Hall BK. (1992). A reproducible method for producing and quantifying the stages of fracture repair. Lab Anim Sci 42(4):369-74.

Bouteille B., Darde M.L., Dumas M., Catanzano G., Pestre-Alexandre M., Breton J.C., Nicolas A., N'Do D.C. (1988): The sheep (Ovis aries) as an experimental model for African trypanosomiasis I. Clinical study. Ann Trop Med Parasitol 82(2):141-8.

Bovee K.C., Littman M.P., Saleh F., Beeuwkes R., Pn W., Kinter L.B. (1986). Essential hereditary hypertension in dogs: a new animal model. J Hypertens [Suppl]. 4:S172-1.

Bowen D. (1989). Possible explanations for excess weight gains in pregnancy: an animal model. Physiol Behav 46(6):935-9.

Bowles E.A., Weaver D.S., Telewski F.W., Wakefield A.H., Jaffe M.J., Miller L.C. (1985). Bone measurement by enhanced contrast image analysis: ovariectomized and intact. Macaca fascicularis as a model for human postmenopausal osteoporosis. Am J Phys Anthropol. 67:99-103.

Bowman T.A., Hughes H.C. (1984). Ventriculoatrial conduction in swine during cardiac pacing: animal model for retrograde conduction. Am Heart J. 108:337-41.

Boyce E. (1992). Feline experimental models for control of periodontal disease. Vet Clin North Am Small Anim Pract 22(6):1309-21.

Boyce N.W., Holdsworth S.R. (1988): A new experimental model of in-situ immune complex disease of the lung. Clin Exp Immunol. 72(3):493-8.

Boyera N., Cavey D., Bouclier M., Burg G., Rossio P., Hensby C. (1992). Repeated application of dinitrochlorobenzene to the ears of sensitized guinea pigs: a preliminary characterization of a potential new animal model for contact eczema in humans. Skin Pharmacol 5(3):184-8.

Boysen S.T., Capaldi E.J. (Ed.) (1993). The development of numerical competence: animal and human models. Hillsdale, N.J.: L. Erlbaum Associates. 277 P.

Bozekkla B.E., Sestini P., Gaumer H.R., Hammad Y., Heather C.J., Salvaggio J.E. (1983). A murine model of asbestosis. Am J Pathol. 112:326-37. Also see: Chest. 83 (5 Suppl):95-105.

Braak H., Braak E., Strenge H., Koppang N. (1984). Canine ceroid lipofuscinosis, a model for ageing of the human isocortex. Gerontology. 30:215-7.

Braff D., Geyer M. (1990). Sensorimotor gating and schizophrenia. Human and animal model studies [see comments]. Arch Gen Psychiatry 47(2):181-8.

Brandt K.D. (1994). Insights into the natural history of osteoarthritis provided by the cruciate-deficient dog. An animal model of osteoarthritis. Ann N Y Acad Sci. 732:199-205.

Brandt W., Barth A. (1993). Is the analgesic activity of epibatidine caused by a chemical reaction with the morphine opioid receptor? Environment Research 1:345-8.

Brasseur P., Lemeteil D., Ballet J.J. (1988): Rat model for human cryptosporidiosis. J Clin Microbiol. 26(5):1037-9.

Breedveld F.C., Trentham D.E. (1987). Progress in the understanding of inducible models of chronic arthritis. Rheum Dis Clin North Am. 13:531-44.

Breeze R.G., Brown C.M., Turk M.A. (1984). 3-methylindole as a model of equine obstructive lung disease. Equine Vet J. 16:108-12.

Breeze R.G., Legreid W.W., Bayly W.M., Wilson B.J. (1984). Perilla ketone toxicity: a chemical model for the study of equine restrictive lung disease. Equine Vet J. 16:180-4.

Brem G. (1990). [Transgenic mice as disease models] Transgene Mäuse als Krankheitsmodelle. Arzneimittelforschung 40(3):335-43.

Brenna W.J., Clark G.M. (1985). An animal model of acute otitis media and the histopathological assessment of a cochlear implant in the cat. J Laryngol Otol. 99:851-6.

Brenowitz G., Yonas H. (1990). Selective occlusion of blood supply to the anterior perforated substance of the dog: a highly reproducible stroke model. Surg Neurol 33(4):247-52.

Brent R.L., Beckman D.A., (1986). Animal models of hydrocephalus: recent developements. Proc Soc Exp Bilo Med. 181:1-2.

Bresalier R., Niv Y., Byrd J., Duh Q., Toribara N., Rockwell R., Dahiya R., Kim Y. (1991). Mucin production by human colonic carcinoma cells correlates with their metastatic potential in animal models of colon cancer metastasis. J Clin Invest 87(3):1037-45.

Breza J., Abòseif S., Lue T., Tanagho E. (1990). Cavernous vein arterialization for vasculogenic impotence. An animal model. Urology 35(6):513-8.

Briand P. (1983). Hormone-dependent mammary tumors in mice and rats as a model for human breast cancer (review). Anticancer Res. 3:273-81.

Briand P. (1989). [Animal models of gene therapy] Modeles animaux de therapies geniques. J Genet Hum 37(4-5):289-97.

Brick D.C., Oh J.O., Sicher S.E. (1981). Ocular lesions associated with dissemination of type 2 herpes simplex virus from skin infection in newborn rabbits. Invest Ophthalmol Vis Sci. 21:681-8.

Brigham P., Cappas A., Uno H. (1988). The stumptailed macaque as a model for androgenetic alopecia: effects of topical minoxidil analyzed by use of the folliculogram. Clin Dermatol 6(4):177-87.

Brinkhous K., Reddick R., Read M., Nichols T., Bellinger D., Griggs T. (1991). von Willebrand factor and animal models: contributions to gene therapy, thrombotic thrombocytopenic purpura, and coronary artery thrombosis. Mayo Clin Proc 66(7):733-42.

Brinton M.A., Nathanson N. (1981). Genetic determinants of virus susceptibility: epidemiologic implications of murine models. Epidemiol Rev. 3:115-39.

Brissot P., Campion J.P.. Guillorizo A., Allain H., Messner M., Simon M., Ferrand B., Bourel M. (1983). Experimental hepatic iron overload in the baboon: of a two year study. Evolution of biological and morphologic hepatic parameters of iron overload. Dig Dis Sci. 28:616-24.

Briukhin G., Grachev A. (1990). [Phagocytic activity of peripheral blood monocytes and peritoneal macrophages in the progeny of animals with experimental chronic liver disease] Fagotsitarnaia aktivnost' monotsitov perifericheskoi krovi i peritoneal'nykh makrofagov u potomstva zhivotnykh s eksperi- mental'nym khronicheskim porazheniem pecheni. Fiziol Zh 36(6):97-100.

Broderson J.R., Chapman W.L. Jr., Hanson W.L. (1986). Experimental visceral Leishmaniasis in the owl monkey. Vet Pathol. 23:293-302.

Brodeur B.R., Tsang P.S., Hamel J., Larosey Montplaisir S. (1986). Mouse models of infection for Neisseria meningitidis B, 2b and Haemophilus influenzae type b diseases. Can J Microbiol. 32:33-7.

Broekhuyse R., Kuhlmann E., Winkens H. (1993). Experimental autoimmune anterior uveitis (EAAU). III. Induction by immunization with purified uveal and skin melanins. Exp Eye Res 56(5):575-83.

Brouwer E., Huitema M., Klok P., de W. H., Tervaert J., Weening J., Kallenberg C. (1993). Antimyeloperoxidase-associated proliferative glomerulonephritis: an animal model. J Exp Med 177(4):905-14.

Brown D., McCluskey R.T., Ausiello D.A. (1987). The cell biology of Heymann nephritis: a model of human membranous glomerulonephritis. Am J Kidney Dis. 10:74-6.

Browne K.F., Rosa R., Haider B., Regan T.J. (1983). Intra-aortic balloon counterpulsation in an experimental model of myocardial infarction. Chest. 83:899-903.

Brugada J., Lamar J., Boisson P., Masse C., Puech P., Sassine A. (1988). Electrophysiological effects of the new cardioactive drug CERM 4205: a comparative study in an animal model and in man. Drugs Exp Clin Res 14(5):355-60.

Brugman S., Larsen G., Henson P., Honor J., Irvin C. (1993). Increased lower airways responsiveness associated with sinusitis in a rabbit model. Am Rev Respir Dis 147(2):314-20.

Brumback R.A. (1983). Selective damage to type 2B muscle fibres in ethanol-fed rats. J Clin Pathol. 36:1416-6.

Brunner N., Boysen B., Romer J., Spang-Thomsen M. (1993). The nude mouse as an in vivo model for human breast cancer invasion and metastasis. Breast Cancer Res Treat 24(3):257-64.

Brunner N., Thompson E., Spang-Thomsen M., Rygaard J., Dano K., Zwiebel J. (1992). lacZ transduced human breast cancer xenografts as an in vivo model for the study of invasion and metastasis. Eur J Cancer 28A(12):1989-95.

Bryan J.H. (1983). The immotile cilia syndrome. Mice vs man. Virchows Arch [A]. 399:265-75.

Buchan G., Griffin J. (1990). Tuberculosis in domesticated deer (Cervus elaphus): a large animal model for human tuberculosis. J Comp Pathol 103(1):11-22.

Buchhalter J.R. (1993). Animal models of inherited epilepsy. Epilepsia 34(Suppl 3):S31-41.

Budiansky S. (1985). Animal experimentation. Alternatives neglected [news]. Nature. 315 (6014):9.

Bui H., del R. A., Sonbati H., Lee C., George M., Ross J. (1991). Helicobacter pylori affects the quality of experimental gastric ulcer healing in a new animal model. Exp Mol Pathol 55(3):261-8.

Buissy R.E., Moellmann G., Trainer A.T., Smyth J.R. Jr., Lerner A.B. (1986). Delayed-amelanotic (DAM or Smyth) chicken: melanocyte dysfunction in vivo and in vitro. J Invest Dermatol. 86:149-56.

Buja L., Clubb F. J., Bilheimer D., Willerson J. (1990). Pathobiology of human familial hypercholesterolaemia and a related animal model, the Watanabe heritable hyperlipidaemic rabbit. Eur Heart J 11 Suppl E:41-52.

Bukaeva I.A., Iakovleva L.A., Lapin B.A., Kove E.M. (1984). Ultrastructural characteristics of malignant non-Hodgkin's lymphoma in baboons. Arkh patol. 46:51-9. (English Abstract) (Russian)

Bullock L.P. (1986). Animal models of androgen insensitivity. Adv Exp Med Biol. 196:269-78.

Bullock L.P. (1986). Models of androgen insensitivity in the study of androgen action. Prog Clin Biol Res 94:369-79.

Bullock R., McCulloch J., Graham D., Lowe D., Chen M., Teasdale GM. (1990). Focal ischemic damage is reduced by CPP-ene studies in two animal models. Stroke 21(11 Suppl):III32-6.

Bunt-Milam A.H., Dennis M.B. Jr., Bensinger R.lE. (1987). Hereditary glaucoma and buphthalmia in the rabbit. Prog Clin Biol Res. 247:397-406.

Buoro I.B., Atwell R.B., (1984). Development of a model of caval syndrome in dogs infected with Dirofilaria immitis. Aust Vet J. 61:267-8.

Burashnikov A., Efimov I., Fast V., Karasaeva A., Pertsov A. (1991). [Isolated right ventricle after coronary perfusion as a model for the study of ischemic and reperfusion-induced arrhythmia in rats] Izolirovannyi koronarno-perfuziruemyi pravyi zheludochek krysy kak model' dlia issledovaniia ishemicheskikh i reperfuzionnykh aritmii. Kardiologiia 31(7):58-61.

Burd D., Longaker M., Adzick N., Harrison M., Ehrlich H. (1990). Foetal wound healing in a large animal model: the deposition of collagen is confirmed. Br J Plast Surg 43(5):571-7.

Burdmann E., Woronik V., Prado E., Abdulkader R., Saldanha L., Barreto O., Marcondes M. (1993). Snakebite-induced acute renal failure: an experimental model. Am J Trop Med Hyg 48(1):82-8.

Burenin I.S., Smirnova I.O., Valueva I.M. (1987). Modelling of ovarian tumors in rats. Biull Eksp Biol Med. 104:507-9. (English Abstract). (Russian)

Burkhardt H., Rosenthal S., Rosenthal H., Karge E., De C. E. (1989). Treatment of bovine leukaemia virus-infected sheep with suramin: an animal model for the development of antiretroviral compounds. Acta Virol (Praha) 33(4):305-13.

Burkle G., Burkle V., Grehn S., Schweinsberg F., Faiss W. (1981). Autochthonous bladder tumors in rats as test model for radio-and chemotherapy). Strahlentherapie. 157:581-99. (English Abstract). (German)

Burns J., Felsburg P., Wilson H., Rosen FS., Glickman L. (1991). Canine pain syndrome is a model for the study of Kawasaki disease. Perspect Biol Med 35(1):68-73.

Burov I., Metkalova S., Kustov A., Petrov G., Shul'govskii V. (1992). [The effect of amiridin on the MPTP-induced Parkinson-like syndrome in monkeys] Vliianie amiridina na MFTP-indutsirovannyi parkinsonpodobnyi sindrom u obez'ian. Biull Eksp Biol Med 114(11):495-7, 494.

Burov IuV., Liubimov B.I., Iavorskii A.N., Kampov-Polevoi A.B., Sorokina A.V. (1983). Toxicological characteristics of an experimental model of alcoholism in rats. Farmakol Toksikol. 46:112-7. (English Abstract) (Russian)

Burtis W.J., Broadus A.E., Insogna K.L. (1986). Two species of adenylate cyclase-stimulating activity in a murine squamous carcinoma model of humoral hypercalcemia of malignancy. Endocrinology. 118:1982-8.

Bush M., Verlangieri A. (1989). Clinical profile of a 4-year primate atherosclerosis model. Artery 17(1):32-48.

Busto R., Ginsberg M.D. (1985). Graded focal cerebral schemia in the rat by unilateral carotid artery occlusion and elevated intracranial pressure: hemodynamic and biochemical characterization. Stroke. 16:466-76.

Butler J.E., Richerson H.B., Swanson P.A., Svelzer M.T., Kopp W.C. (1983). Carrier requirement for development of acute experimental hypersensitivity pneumonitis in the rabbit. Int Arch Allergy Appl Immunol. 71:74-82.

Butler M., Colombo C., Hickman L., O'Byrne E., Steele R., Steinetz B., Quintavalla J., Yokoyama N. (1983). A new model of osteoarthritis in rabbits. III. Evaluation of anti-osteoarthritic of effects of selected drugs administered intraarticularly. Arthritis Rheum. 26: 1380-6.

Butler T., Rahman H., Al-Mahmud K.A., Islam M., Bardhan P., Kabir I., Rahman M.M. (1985). An animal model of haemolytic-uraemic syndrome in shigellosis: lipopolysaccharides of Shigella dysenteriae I and S. flexneri produce leucocyte-mediated renal cortical necrosis in rabbits. Br J Exp pathol.

Butovskaia M.L., Deriagina M.A., Chirkov A.M., Startsev V.G. (1986). Effect of stress-inducing factors on monkey behavior. II. Hormonal indices and their relation to behavior in the modelling of emotional stress in hamadryas baboons. Biol Nauki. 2:59-64. (English Abstract) (Russian)

Byhardt R.W., Almagro U.A., Fish B.L., Moulder J.E. (1984). Development of a rat lung cancer model. Int J Radiat Oncol Biol Phys. 10:2125-30.

Bykov V.L., Karaev Z.O. (1986). Experimental model of combined Candida lesions of the skin and mucous membranes. Vestn Dermatol Venerol. 2:21-4. (English Abstract) (Russian)

Bynum W. (1990). "C'est un malade": animal models and concepts of human diseases. J Hist Med Allied Sci 45(3):397-413.

Cabot, E., & Fox, J. (1990). Bile reflux and the gastric mucosa: an experimental ferret model. J Invest Surg, 3 (2):177-89.

Caiozzo, V., Ma, E., McCue, S., Smith, E., Herrick, R., & Baldwin, K. (1992). A new animal model for modulating myosin isoform expression by altered mechanical activity. J Appl Physiol, 73 (4):1432-40.

Calabrase E.J. (1986). Animal extrapolation and the challenge of human heterogeneity. J Pharm Science 75:1041-6.

Calabrese E.J. (1984). Suitability of animal models for predictive toxicology: theoretical and practical considerations. Drug metab Rev. 15:505-23.

Calabrese E.J. (1988): Comparative biology of test species. Environ Health Perspect. 77:55-62.

Calabrese E.J., Williams P.S., Moore G.S. (1983) An evaluation of the dorset sheep as a predictive animal model for the response of glucose-6-phosphate dehydrogenase-deficient human erythrocytes to a proposed systemic toxic ozone intermediate, methyl oleate ozonide. Ecotoxicol Environ Safety 7:416-22. Also: Vet Hum Toxicol. 25:241-6.

Caldwell M.B., Walker R.I. (1986). Adult rabbit model for Cambylobacter enteritis. Am J Pathol. 122:573-6.

Caldwell M.B., Walker R.I., Stewart S.D., Rogers J.E. (1983). Simple adult rabbit model for Cambylobacter jejuni enteritis. Infect Immun. 42:1176-82.

Calvino B., Crepon-Bernard M.O., Le Bars D. (1987). Parallel clinical and behavioural studies of adjuvant-induced arthritis in the rat: possible relationship with 'chronic pain'. Behav Brain Res. 24:11-29.

Calvino B., Maillet S., Pradelles P., Besson J., Couraud J. (1991). [Variation of substance P-like immunoreactivity in plasma and cerebrospinal fluid in the course of arthritis induced by Freund adjuvant in rats, a model for the study of chronic pain] Variation de l'immunoreactivite de type substance P dans le plasma et le liquide cephalo-rachidien au cours de l'evolution de l'arthrite induite par adjuvant de Freund chez le rat, un modele d'etude de douleur chronique. C R Acad Sci III 312(8):427-32.

Camilleri J.P., Joseph D., Fabiani J.N., Amat P., Gueniot C., Gorny P., Barres D., Deloche A. (1981). Experimental myocardial infarction in the rat as a quantitative model for the study of anti-ischemic interventions. Pathol Res Pract. 172:42-52.

Campbell B.A., Sananes C.B., Gaddy J.R. (1984). Animal models of infantile amnesia, benign senescent forgetfullness, and senile dementia. Neurobehav Toxicol Teratol. 6:467-71.

Campbell C.C., Collins W.E., Chin W., Roberts J.N., Broderson J.R. (1983). Studies of the Sal I strai of Plasmodium vivax in the squirrel monkey (Saimiri sciuresu). J Parasitol. 69:598-601.

Campbell C.C., Collins W.E., Milhous W.K., Roberts J.M., Armstead A. (1986). Adaptation of the Indochina I/CDC strain of Plasmodium falciparum to the squirrel monkey (Saimiri sciureus). Am J Trop Med Hyg. 35:472-5.

Campbell J.R., Marwoto H.A., Tirtokusumo S., Masbar S., Rusch J.T., Purnomo Trenggono B. (1987). The silvered leak monkey (resbytis cristata) as a model for human bancroftian filariasis. Lab Anim Sci. 37:502-4.

Campbell W.C., Blair L.S., Kuhng F.Y., Ewanciw P.V. (1982). Experimental Trichinella spiralis infection in the ferret, Mustela putorius furo. J Helminthol. 56:55-8.

Campos C.A., Campos R., Pereira L.H. (1984). Mastomys natalensis as an alternative model in studies on experimental schistosomiasis mansoni. Rev Inst Med Trop Sao Paulo. 26:19-24. (English Abstract). (Portugese)

Cannon E., Williams B. (1990). Raised vascular calcium in an animal model: effects on aortic function. Cardiovasc Res 24(1):47-52.

Cappeliez P., Moore E. (1990). Effects of lithium on an amphetamine animal model of bipolar disorder. Prog Neuropsychopharmacol Biol Psychiatry 14(3):347-58.

Caputo G., Delgado-Paredes C., Swedlow D., Fleisher G. (1985). Anoxic cardiopulmonary arrest in a pediatric animal model: clinical and laboratory correlates of duration. Pediatr Emerg Care. 1:57-60.

Carballal G., Oubina J.R., Molinas F.C., Nagle C., dela Vega M.T., Videla C., Elsner B. (1987). Intracerebral infection of Cebus apella with the XJ-Clone 3 strain of Junin virus. J Med Virol. 21:257-68.

Carbon C. (1988): Ceftazidime on animal experimental models. Presse Med. 26;17(37):1910-3 (16 ref.) (English Abstract). (French)

Carbonell M., Saiz M., Marti M., Queralt J., Mitjavila M. (1989). Iron mobilization in three animal models of inflammation. Rev Esp Fisiol 45(2):163-70.

Cardesa A., Ribalta T., Von S. B., Palacin A., Mohr U. (1989). Experimental model of tumors associated with neurofibromatosis. Cancer 63(9):1737-49.

Carey R. (1990). Dopamine receptors mediate drug-induced but not Pavlovian conditioned contralateral rotation in the unilateral 6-OHDA animal model. Brain Res 515 (1-2):292-8.

Carey R. (1991). Naloxone reverses L-dopa induced overstimulation effects in a Parkinson's disease animal model analogue. Life Sci 48(13):1303-8.

Carlson J., Glick S. (1991). Brain laterality as a determinant of susceptibility to depression in an animal model. Brain Res 550(2):324-8.

Carlton W., Engelhardt J. (1989). Experimental renal papillary necrosis in the Syrian hamster. Food Chem Toxicol 27(5):331-40.

Carney S. (1991). Cartilage research, biochemical, histologic, and immunohistochemical markers in cartilage, and animal models of osteoarthritis. Curr Opin Rheumatol 3(4):669-75.

Carnoy P., Soobrie P., Puech A.J., Simon P. (1986). Performance deficit induced by low doses of dopamine agonists in rats. Toward a model for approaching the neurobiology of negative schizophrenic symptomatology? Biol Psychiatry. 21:11-22.

Caroll S.M., Grove D.I. (1984). Parasitological, hematologic and immunologic responses in acute and chronic infections of dogs with Ancylostoma ceylanicum: a model of human hookworm infection. J Infect Dis. 150:284-94.

Carr E.A. (1983). The development of radiotracers that are substrates for (catecholamine) uptake$_1$ and uptake$_2$. In: Lambrecht R.M., Eckelman W.C. (Eds). Animal models in radiotracer design. Heidelberg: Springer Verlag. pp 35-60.

Carraway J.H., Malone J.B. (1985). Brugia pahangi: comparative susceptibility of the mongolian jird, Meriones unguiculatus, and the PD4 inbred hamster, Mesocricetus auratus. Exp parasitol. 59:68-73.

Carre F., Lessard Y., Coumel P., Ollivier L., Besse S., Lecarpentier Y., Swynghedauw B. (1992). Spontaneous arrhythmias in various models of cardiac hypertrophy and senescence of rats. A Holter monitoring study. Cardiovasc Res 26(7):698-705.

Carrier G.O., Aronstam R.S. (1987). Altered muscarinic receptor properties and function in the heart in diabetes. J Pharmacol Exp Ther. 242:531-5.

Carroll W.M., Jennings A.R., Mastaglia F.L. (1985). Galactocerebroside antiserum causes demyelination of cat optic nerve. Brain Res. 330:378-81.

Carter H., Partin A., Coffey D. (1989). Prediction of metastatic potential in an animal model of prostate cancer: flow cytometric quantification of cell surface charge. J Urol 142 (5):1338-41.

Carter R., Cooke TG., Hemingway D., McArdle C., Angerson W. (1992). The combination of degradable starch microspheres and angiotensin II in the manipulation of drug delivery in an animal model of colorectal metastasis. Br J Cancer 65(1):37-9.

Casey D.E. (1984). Tardive dyskinesia--animal models. Psychopharmacol Bull. 20:376-9.

Casey L.C., Ballantyne H.K., Fletcher J.R., Chernow B., Lake C.R. (1983). An experimental model of intraabdominal abscess in the rat. 2:7-11.

Cashin C.H. (1987). The induction of an erosive arthropathy in the guinea pig with copper II bisglycinate and its treatment with antirheumatic drugs. Br J Rheumatol. 26:251-8.

Caspi R., Chan C., Leake W., Higuchi M., Wiggert B., Chader GJ. (1990). Experimental autoimmune uveoretinitis in mice. Induction by a single eliciting event and dependence on quantitative parameters of immunization. J Autoimmun 3(3):237-46.

Castle C., Colca J., Melchior G. (1993). Lipoprotein profile characterization of the KKA(y) mouse, a rodent model of type II diabetes, before and after treatment with the insulin-sensitizing agent pioglitazone. Arterioscler Thromb 13(2):302-9.

Cavalheiro E.A., Riche D.A., Le Gal La Salle G. (1982). Long-term effects of intrahippocampal kainic acid injection in rats: a method for inducing spontaneous recurrent seizures. Electroencephalogr Clin Neurophysiol. 53:581-9.

Cavallo T., Goldman M., Lambert P.H. (1984). Animal model of human disease Proliferative glomerulonephritis associated with polyclonal B-cell activation. Am J pathol. 114:346-8.

Cavanagh D., Rao P.S., Knuppel R.A., Desai U., Balis J.U. (1985). Pregnancy-induced hypertension: development of a model in the pregnant primate (Papio anubis). Am J Obstet Gynecol. 15:987-99.

Ceballos-Picot I., Nicole A., Briand P., Grimber G., Delacourte A., Defossez A., Javoy-Agid F., Lafon M., Blouin J., Sinet P. (1991). Neuronal-specific expression of human copper-zinc superoxide dismutase gene in transgenic mice: animal model of gene dosage effects in Down's syndrome. Brain Res 552(2):198-214.

Chabel C., Russell L., Lee, R. (1990). Tourniquet-induced limb ischemia: a neurophysiologic animal model. Anesthesiology 72(6):1038-44.

Chader G.J., Fletcher R.T., Barbehenn E., Aguirre G., Sanyal S. (1987). Studies on abnormal cyclic GMP metabolism in animal models of retinal degeneration: genetic relationships and cellular compartmentalization. Prog Clin Biol Res. 247:289-307.

Chahinian A., Kirschner P., Gordon R., Szrajer L., Holland J. (1991). Usefulness of the nude mouse model in mesothelioma based on a direct patient-xenograft comparison. Cancer 68:558-60.

Chalon S., Guimbal C., Guilloteau D., Mayo W., Huguet F., Schmitt M., Desplanches G., Baulieu J., Besnard J. (1990). Iodobenzamide for in vivo exploration of central dopamine receptors: evaluation in animal models of supersensitivity. Life Sci 47(8):729-34.

Chandler M.J., DeLeo J., Carney J.M. (1985). An unanesthetized-gerbil model of cerebral ischemia-induced behavioral changes. J Pharmacol Methods. 14:137-46.

Chandler R.L., Turfrey B.A., Smith K. (1982). Development of a laboratory animal model for infectious bovine keratoconjunctivitis. Res Vet Sci. 32:128-30.

Chang J.C., Jagirdar J., Lesser M. (1986). Long-term evolution of BCG- and CFA-induced granulomas in rat lungs. Correlation of histologic features with cells in bronchoalveolar lavage samples. Am J Pathol. 125:16-27.

Chang L., Mercer R., Pinkerton K., Crapo J. (1991). Quantifying lung structure. Experimental design and biologic variation in various models of lung injury. Am Rev Respir Dis 143(3):625-34.

Chanh P.H., Kaiser R., Lasserre B., Navarro-Delmasure C., Moutier R. (1988): Creation of a strain of genetically obese-hypertensive rats. Int J Obes. 12(2):141-7.

Chaouat G., Menu E., Bonneton C., Kinsky R. (1989). Immunological manipulations in animal pregnancy and models of pregnancy failure. Curr Opin Immunol 1(6):1153-6.

Chapman C.B., Mitchell G.F. (1982). Fasciola hepatica: comparative studies of fascioliasis in rats and mice. Int J Parasitol. 12:81-91.

Chapman W.L. Jr., Hanson W.L. (1981). Visceral leishmaniasis in the squirrel monkey (Saimiri sciurea). J Parasitol. 67:740-1.

Chappel C.I., Chappel W.R. (1983). The discovery and development of the BB rat colony: an animal model of spontaneous diabetes mellitus. Metabolism. 32 (7 Suppl 1):8-10.

Charlton H., Wood M. (1992). Animal models for brain and pituitary gonadal disturbances. Prog Brain Res 93:321-31; discussion 331-2.

Chateauvert J., Grynpas M., Kessler M., Pritzker K. (1990). Spontaneous osteoarthritis in rhesus macaques. II. Characterization of disease and morphometric studies [see comments]. J Rheumatol 17(1):73-83.

Chen S. (1990). [Experimental research on 1-methyl-4-phenyl-1,2,3,6-tetrahydropyriqine- induced parkinsonian animal models in the rhesus monkey and C57 black mouse]. Chung Hua I Hsueh Tsa Chih 70(5):252-4, 18.

Chen S. (1990). [Study of an MPTP-induced parkinsonian animal model in the rhesus monkey and the mechanism of the action of MPTP]. Chung Hua Shen Ching Ching Shen Ko Tsa Chih 23(1):23-6, 62.

Chen S., Xu D., Yu H., Tang Q., Xu X., Wang Z., Liang P. (1988). Study on MPTP-induced parkinsonian animal model in rhesus monkey and the mechanism of MPTP. Chin Med J (Engl) 101(12):879-83.

Chen S.T., Hso C.Y., Hogan E.L., Marieq H., Balentine J.D. (1986). A model of focal ischemic stroke in the rat: reproducible extensive cortical infarction. Stroke. 17:738-43.

Chen X., Fang Y., Xiong W., Su Z., Hu K., Wu W., Liu Z. (1988). Comparative effects of captopril, nitroprusside, dopamine and lanatoside C on a new model of rabbit congestive heart failure. Chung Kuo Yao Li Hsueh Pao 9(5):402-8.

Chengappa M.M., Carter G.R., Chang T.S. (1983). Hemoglobin enhancement of experimental infection of mice with Pasteurella haemolytica. Am J Vet Res.. 44:1545-6.

Chester J., Norris M., Lever J., Turnbull A., Britton D. (1989). Experimental pancreatic cancer in the Syrian hamster: effect of cholecystectomy. Digestion 44(1):36-40.

Cheung P.H., Pugsley M.K., Walker M.J. (1993). Arrhythmia models in the rat. J Pharmacol Toxicol Methods 29(4):179-84.

Chezalviel-Guilbert F., Weissenburger J., Davy J., Vernhet L., Guhennec C., Cheymol G. (1993). Reproducibility of the model of induced ventricular tachycardia in conscious dogs with infarction. J Pharmacol Toxicol Methods 29(1):45-57.

Chi L., Mu D., Lucchesi B. (1991). Electrophysiology and antiarrhythmic actions of E-4031 in the experimental animal model of sudden coronary death. J Cardiovasc Pharmacol 17(2):285-95.

Chiba S., Edamura M., Ito M., Kikuchi S., Matsumoto H. (1985). Experimental pyridoxine neuropathy- an electrophysiological and histological study in rabbits. Rinsho Shinkeigaku. 25:939-43. (English Abstract) (Japanese)

Chiesa C., Joseph-Francios A., Alonso J.M., Pacifico L., Mollaret H.H. (1987). Yersinia enterocolitica infection in pregnant mice and their offspring. Ann Rech Vet. 18:241-4.

Chilaia S., Khodeli N. (1990). [Left-ventricular bypass: characteristics of homeostasis] Levozheludochkovyi obkhod: osobennosti gomeostaza. Grud Serdechnososudistaia Khir (1):30-4.

Chiou R. (1991). The impact of tumor size on the efficacy of monoclonal antibody-targeted radiotherapy: studies using a nude mouse model with human renal cell carcinoma xenografts. J Urol 146(1):232-7.

Chisari F.V., Pinkert C.A., Millich D.R., Filippi P., McLachlan A., Palmiter R.D., Brinster R.L. (1985). A transgenic mouse model of the chronic hepatitis B surface antigen carrier state. Science. 230:1157-60.

Chiu D., Chen L., Chen Z. (1990). Rat ear reattachment as an animal model. Plast Reconstr Surg 85(5):782-8.

Chizhow N.P., Luk'ianova R.I. (1985). Model of experimental Pixuna infection in white mice. Vopr Virusol. 30:214-5. (English Abstract).

Chkhikvishvili TsSh., Somundzhian A.A. (1984). Informational neuroses. Zh Vyssh Nerv Deiat. 34:175-80.

Chole R.A., Henry K.R. (1985). Ossicular and Otic capsular lesions in LP/J mice. Ann Otol Rhinol Laryngol. 94 (4 Pt1):366-72.

Chole R.A., Henry K.R., McGinn M.D. (1981). Cholesteatoma: spontaneous occurrence in the Mongolian gerbil Meriones unguiculatis. Am J Otol. 2:204-10.

Chong L.J., Smith T.D., Porzhitkow M.M. (1985). A new model of congestive heart failure in anesthetized dogs. Proc West Pharmacol Soc. 28:81-5.

Chowdhury J.R., Kondapalli R., Chowdhury N.R. (1993). Gunn rat: a model for inherited deficiency of bilirubin glucuronidation. Adv Vet Sci Comp Med. 37:149-73.

Chrisp C., Reid W., Rush H., Suckow M., Bush A., Thomann M. (1990). Cryptosporidiosis in guinea pigs: an animal model. Infect Immun 58(3):674-9.

Christensen S., Ottosen P.D. (1983). Lithium-induced uremia in rats - a new model of chronic renal failure. Pflugers Arch. 399:208-12.

Chrousos G.P., Loriaux D.L., Tomita M., Brandon D.D., Renquist D., Albertson B., Lipsett M.B. (1986). The new world primates as animal models of gluococorticoid resistance. Adv Exp Med Biol. 196:129-44.

Chubb C., Nolan C. (1985). Animal models of male infertility: mice bearing single-gene mutations that induce infertility. Endocrinology. 117:338-46.

Chudler E.H., Dong W.K. (1981). Adjuvant-induced arthritis in rats: a possible model of chronic pain. Pain. 11:407-8.

Chudwin D.S., Artip S.G., Odgen J.D., Schiffman G. (1987). Tamarin model of pneumococcal bacteremia. J Med Primatol. 16:249-60.

Chung L.W., Auble K. (1985). An experimental model for mouse prostatic hyperplasia: characterization of hormonal, age and tissue specificities. Proc West Pharmacol Soc. 28:35-9.

Chung L.W., Matsuura J., Rocco A.K., Thompson T.C., Miller G.J., Runner M.N. (1984). A new mouse model for prostatic hyperplasia: induction of adult prostatic overgrowth by fetal urogenital sinus implants. Prog Clin Biol Res. 145:291-306.

Chung T., O'Rear E., Whitsett T., Hinshaw L., Smith M. (1991). Survival factors in a canine septic shock model. Circ Shock 33(3):178-82.

Claman H. (1990). Graft-versus-host disease and animal models for scleroderma. Curr Opin Rheumatol 2(6):929-31.

Claman H.N., Jaffee B.P. (1983). Desensitization of contact allergy to DNFB in mice. Description of a model system. J Immunol. 131:2682-6.

Claoue C. (1986). A new look at experimental herpes simplex eye disease: preliminary results of clinical disease in the NIH mouse after zosteriform spread. Trans Ophthalmol Soc UK. 105: (Pt 4):401-3.

Clapp N.K., Lushbaugh C.C., Humason G.L., Gangaware B.L., Henke M.A., McArthur A.H. (1985). The marmoset as a model of ulcerative colitis and colon cancer. Prog Clin Biol Res. 186:247-61.

Clapp, N.K. (Ed.) (1993). A primate model for the study of colitis and colonic carcinoma: the cotton top tamarin (Saguinus oedipus). Boca Raton: CRC Press. 339 P.

Clark I., MacMicking J., Gray K., Rockett K., Cowden W. (1992). Malaria mimicry with tumor necrosis factor. Contrasts between species of murine malaria and Plasmodium falciparum. Am J Pathol 140(2):325-36.

Clarke A.R. (1994). Murine genetic models of human disease. Curr Opin Genet Dev. 4(3):453-460.

Clarke C.E., Sambrook M.A., Mitchell I.J., Crossman A.R. (1987). Lavodopa-induced dyskinesia and response fluctuations in primates rendered parkinsonian with 1-methyl-4-phenyl-1,2-3,6-tetrahydropyridine (MPTP). J Neurol Sci. 78:273-80.

Clarkson A.B. Jr., Bacchi C.J., Mellow G.H., Nathan H.C., McCann P.P., Sjoerdsma A. (1983). Efficacy of combinations of difluoromethylornithine and bleomycin in a mouse model of central nervous system African trypanosomiasis. Proc Natl Acad Sci USA.. 80:5729-33.

Clarkson T.B., Koritnik D.R., Weingaud K.W., Miller L.C. (1985). Nonhuman primate models of atherosclerosis: potential for the study of diabetes mellitus and hyperinsulinemia. Metabolism. 34 (12 Suppl):51-9.

Clarren S.K., Bowden D.M. (1984). Measures of alcohol damage in utero in the pigtailed macaque) (Macaca nemestrina). Ciba Found Symp. 105:157-72.

Clator G.M., Klapper P.E., Sharma H., Longson M. (1987). A rat model of herpes encephalitis with special reference to its potential for the development of diagnostic brain imaging. J Neurol Sci. 79:55-66.

Clay M., Hopkins G., Ehnholm C., Barter P. (1989). The rabbit as an animal model of hepatic lipase deficiency. Biochim Biophys Acta 1002(2):173-81.

Clayman R.V., Bithartz L.E., Buja L.M., Spady D.K., Dietschy J.M. (1986). Renal cell carcinoma in the Wistar-Lewis rat: a model for studying the mechanisms of cholestrol acquisition by a tumor in vivo. Cancer Res. 46:2958-63.

Cleator G., Klapper P., Lewis A., Sharma H., Longson M. (1988). Specific neuro-radiological diagnosis of herpes encephalitis in an animal model. Arch Virol 101(1-2):1-12.

Clerc J., Mardon K., Galons H., Loc'h C., Lumbroso J., Merlet P., Zhu J., Jeusset J., Syrota A., Fragu P. (1995). Assessing intratumor distribution and uptake with MBBG versus MIBG imaging and targeting xenografted PC12-pheochromocytoma cell line. J Nucl Med. 36:859-66.

Coderre T.J., Wall P.D., (1987). Ankle joint urate arthritis (AJUA) in rats: an alternative animal model of arthritis to that produced by Freund's adjuvant. Pain. 28:379-93.

Coenen H.H., Wienhard K., Stöcklin G. et al. (1988). PET measurement of D2 and S2 receptor binding of 3-N-([2'-^{18}F]fluoroethyl)spiperone in baboon brain. Eur J Nucl Med. 14:80-7.

Coggeshall J.W., Lefferts P.L., Butterfield M.J., Bernard G.R., Carroll F.E., Pou N.A., Snapper J.R. (1987). Perilla ketone: a model of increased pulmonary microvascular permeability pulmonary edema in sheep. Am Rev Respir Dis. 136:1453-8.

Coggle J. (1991). The role of animal models in radiation lung carcinogenesis. Radiat Environ Biophys 30(3):239-41.

Cohen A., Geller S.A., Horowitz I., Toth L.S., Werther J.L. (1984). Experimental models for gastric leiomyosarcoma. Cancer. 53:1088-92.

Cohen B.I., Mosbach E.H. (1993). Cholesterol cholelithiasis. Adv Vet Sci Comp Med. 37:289-312.

Cohen J.R., Leal J., Pillari G., Chang J.B., Ilardi C. (1987). Superior mesenteric artery balloon occlusion. A non-operative model of small bowel ischemia in dogs. Invest Radiol. 22:871-4.

Cohen N.J., Eichenbaum, H. (1993). Memory, amnesia, and the hippocampal system. Cambridge, Mass.: MIT Press. 330 P.

Cohen S.B., Weetman A.P. (1987). Characterization of different types of experimental autoimmune thyroiditis in the Buffalo strain rat. Clin Exp Immunol. 69:25-32.

Coker S. (1989). Anesthetized rabbit as a model for ischemia- and reperfusion-induced arrhythmias: effects of quinidine and bretylium. J Pharmacol Methods 21(4):263-79.

Cole J., Forte L., Thorne P., Poelling R., Krause W. (1989). Autotransplantation of avian parathyroid glands: an animal model for studying parathyroid function. Gen Comp Endocrinol 76(3):451-60.

Coleman D. L. (1982). Other potentially useful rodents as models for the study of human diabetes mellitus. Diabetes. 31 (Suppl 1 Pt 2):24-5.

Coleman D.L. (1982). Diabetes-obesity syndromes in mice. Diabetes. 31 (Suppl 1 Pt 2):1-6.

Coleman D.L. (1983). Lessons from studies with genetic forms of diabetes in the mouse. Metabolism. 32 (7 Suppl 1):162-4.

Collins A.C., Wehner J.M., Wilson W.R. (1993). Animal models of alcoholism: genetic strategies and neurochemical mechanisms. Biochem Soc Symp. 59:173-91.

Collins W.E., Skinner J.C., Broderson J.R., Huong A.Y., Mehaffey P.C., Stanfill P.S., Sutton B.B. (1986). Infection of Aotus azarae boliviensis monkeys with different strains of Plasmodium falciparum. J Parasitol. 72:525-30.

Collins W.E., Skinner J.C., Mehaffey P. (1985). Infection of Aotus azarae boliviensis monkeys with the RO strain of Plasmodium cynomolgi. J Parasitol. 71:848-9.

Collins W.E., Skinner J.C., Pappaioanou M., Broderson J.R., McClure H.M., Strobert E., Sutton B.B., Stanfill P.S., Filipski V., Campbell C.C. (1987). Chesson strain Plasmodium vivax in Saimiri sciureus boliviensis monkeys. J Parasitol. 73:929-34.

Colombo C., Butler M., O'Byrne E., Hickman L., Swatzendruber D., Selwyn M., Steneitz B. (1983). A new model of osteoarthritis in rabbits. I. Development of knee joint pathology following lateral meniscectomy and section of the fibular ocllateral and sesamoid ligaments. Arthritis Rheum. 26:875-86.

Colpaert F.C. (1987). Evidence that adjuvant arthritis in the rat is associated with chronic pain. Pain 28:201-22.

Conder G., Jen L., Marbury K., Johnson S., Guimond P., Thomas E., Lee B. (1990). A novel anthelmintic model utilizing jirds, Meriones unguiculatus, infected with Haemonchus contortus. J Parasitol 76(2):168-70.

Conley F.K. (1984). Metastatic brain tumor model in mice that mimics the neoplastic cascade in humans. Neurosurgery. 14:187-92.

Connelly D., Taberner P. (1989). Characterization of the spontaneous diabetes obesity syndrome in mature male CBA/Ca mice. Pharmacol Biochem Behav 34(2):255-9.

Constantopoulos G., Shull R.M., Hastings N., Neufeld E.F. (1985). Neurochemical characterization of canine alpha-L-iduronidase deficiency disease (model of human mucopolysaccharidosis I). J Neurochem. 45:1213-7.

Cooley B., Li X., Dzwierzynski W., Gruel S., Hall R., Wright R., O'Brien E., Fagan D., Hanel D., Gould J. (1992). The de-endothelialized rat carotid arterial graft: a versatile experimental model for the investigation of arterial thrombosis. Thromb Res 67(1):1-14.

Cooper H., Herbin M., Nevo E. (1993). Visual system of a naturally microphthalmic mammal: the blind mole rat, Spalax ehrenbergi. J Comp Neurol 328(3):313-50.

Cooper J., Petty R., Hayes D., Challiss R., Brosnan M., Shoubridge E., Radda G., Morgan-Hughes J., Clark J. (1988). An animal model of mitochondrial myopathy: a biochemical and physiological investigation of rats treated in vivo with the NADH-CoQ reductase inhibitor, diphenyleneiodonium. J Neurol Sci 83(2-3):335-47.

Cooper J., Petty R., Hayes D., Morgan-Hughes J., Clark J. (1988). Chronic administration of the oral hypoglycaemic agent diphenyleneiodonium to rats. An animal model of impaired oxidative phosphorylation (mitochondrial myopathy). Biochem Pharmacol 37(4):687-94.

Cooper J.F. (1985). Pyrogen testing: Practical considerations. In: Warbick-Cerone A., Johnston L.G. (Eds.) Quality assurance of pharmaceuticals manufactured in the hospital. Dublin: Pergamon Press. p 123-132.

Cooper J.F., Harbert J.C. (1975). Endotoxin as a cause of aseptic meningitis after radionuclide cisternography. J Nucl Med. 16:809-13.

Cooper M., Allen T., O'Brien R., Papazoglou D., Clarke B., Jerums G., Doyle AE. (1990). Nephropathy in model combining genetic hypertension with experimental diabetes. Enalapril versus hydralazine and metoprolol therapy. Diabetes 39(12):1575-9.

Copp A.J. (1994). Genetic models of mammalian neural tube defects. Ciba Found Symp. 181:118-34; discussion 134-43.

Corbeil L.B., Strayer D.S., Skaletsky E., Wunderlich A., Sell S. (1983). Immunity to pasteurellosis in compromised rabbits. Am J Vet Res. 44:845-50.

Cornelius C.E. (1993). Fasting hyperbilirubinemia in Bolivian squirrel monkeys with a Gilbert's-like syndrome. Adv Vet Sci Comp Med. 37:127-47.

Cornelius C.E. (Ed.) (1993). Animal models in liver research. San Diego: Academic Press. 479 P.

Cornelius C.E., Rosenberg D.P. (1985). Neonatal biliary atresia. Am J pathol. 118:168-71.

Corominas M., Sloan S., Leon J., Kamino H., Newcomb E., Pellicer A. (1991). ras activation in human tumors and in animal model systems. Environ Health Perspect 93:19-25.

Corris P.A., Odom N.J., Jackson G., McGregor C.G. (1987). Reimplantation injury after lung transplantation in a rat model. J Heart Transplant. 6:234-7.

Cosgriff T., Morrill J., Jennings G., Hodgson L., Slayter M., Gibbs P., Peters C. (1989). Hemostatic derangement produced by Rift Valley fever virus in rhesus monkeys. Rev Infect Dis 11 Suppl 4:S807-14.

Costall B., Domeney A., Kelly M., Tomkins D., Naylor R., Wong E., Smith W., Whiting R., Eglen R. (1993). The effect of the 5-HT3 receptor antagonist, RS-42358-197, in animal models of anxiety. Eur J Pharmacol 234(1):91-9.

Costello L., Combs D., Dempsey RJ. (1990). Unilateral carotid artery ligation in the Mongolian gerbil as a model for testing infarction-reducing therapies. Neurol Res 12(4):237-42.

Coulais Y., Marcelon G., Cros J., Guirand R. (1983). An experimental model osteoarthritis. I. induction and ultrastructural study. Pathol Biol (Paris). 31:577-82. (English Abstract) (French)

Coulter D.M., Papine T., Gooch W.M. 3d. (1984). Intraventricular hemorrhage in the premature rabbit pup. Limitations of this animal model. J Neurosurg. 60:1243-5.

Counsell R.E., Yu T., Ranade V.V., Buswink A.A., Carr Jr. E.A., Caroll M. (1974). Radioiodinated bretylium analogs for myocardial scanning. J Nucl Med. 15:991-6.

Court J.P., Lees G.M, Coop R.L., Angus K.W., Beesley J.E. (1988): An attempt to produce Ostertagia circumcincta infections in Mongolian gerbils. Vet Parasitol. 28(1-2):79-91.

Couser W.G., Salant D.J., Adler S., Madaio M.p. (1982). Studies of experimental membranous nephropathy. Transplant Proc. 14:474-81.

Cousins S., Gonzalez A., Atherton S. (1989). Herpes simplex retinitis in the mouse. Clinicopathologic correlations. Invest Ophthalmol Vis Sci 30(7):1485-94.

Cova L., Fourel I., Vitvitski L., Lambert V., Chassot S., Hantz O., Trepo C. (1993). Animal models for the understanding and control of HBV and HDV infections. J Hepatol 17 Suppl 3:S143-8.

Cox D.R., Smith S.A., Epstein L.B., Epstein C.J. (1984). Mouse trisomy 16 as an animal model of human trisomy 21 (Down syndrome): production of viable trisomy 16 diploid mouse chimeras. Dev Biol. 101:416-24.

Cox R. (1991). Exercise training and response to stress: insights from an animal model. Med Sci Sports Exerc 23(7):853-9.

Crabbe J.C., Belknap J.K., Buck K.J. (1994). Genetic animal models of alcohol and drug abuse. Science 264(5166):1715-23.

Craft J.C. (1982). Experimental infection with Giardia lamblia in rats. J Infect Dis. 145:495-8.

Craig W. (1993). Relevance of animal models for clinical treatment. Eur J Clin Microbiol Infect Dis. 12(Suppl 1):S55-7.

Craighead J., Huber S., Sriram S. (1990). Animal models of picornavirus-induced autoimmune disease: their possible relevance to human disease. Lab Invest 63(4):432-46.

Cramer D.V., Podesta L.G., Makowka L. (Ed.) (1994). Handbook of animal models in transplantation research. Boca Raton, Fla: CRC Press. 352 P.

Cramer H.B., Chole R.A. (1986). Dynamics of otosclerosis-like lesions in LP/J mice. Ann Otol Rhinol Laryngol. 95:169-72.

Crandall R.B., Thompson J.P., Cannor D.H., McGreevy P.B., Crandall C.A. (1984). Pathology of experimental infection with Brugia malayi in ferrets: comparison with occult filariasis in man. Acta Trop (Basel). 41:373-81.

Crawley J.N. (1984). Evaluation of a proposed hamster separation model of depression. Psychiatry Res. 11:35-47.

Crawley J.N., Sutton M.E., Pickar D. (1985). Animal models of self-destructive behavior and suicide. Psychiatr Clin North Am. 8:299-310.

Crewther S.G., Crewther D.P., Cleland B.G. (1985). Convergent strabismic amblyopia in cats. Exp Brain Res. 60:1-9.

Croese J.W., Vas Nunes C.M., Radl J., Van den Enden-Vieveen M.H., Brondijk R.J., Boersma W.J. (1987). The 5T2 mouse multiple myeloma model: characterization of 5T2 cells within the bone marrow. Br. J Cancer. Novel. 56:555-60.

Cross A.S., Opal S.M., Sadoff J.C., Gemski P. (1993). Choice of bacteria in animal models of sepsis. Infect Immun. 61(7):2741-7.

Crossman A.R. (1987). Primate models of dyskinesia: the experimental approach to the study of basal gangilia-related involuntary movement disorders. Neuroscience. 21:1-40.

Crouthamel W., Sarupu A. (Eds). (1983). Animal Models for Oral Drug Delivery in man: In Situ and In Vivo Approaches. American Pharmaceutical Association. Washington D.C. 192 pp.

Crouzel C., Guillaume M., Barré L., Lemaire C., Pike V.W. (1992). Ligands and tracers for PET studies of the 5-HT system - current status. Nucl Med Biol. 19:857-70.

Croy B.A., Percy D.H., Smith A.L. (1993). What are SCID mice and why is it timely to devote a special topic issue to them? Lab Anim Sci. 43(2):120-2.

Cruickshank J.K., Price K.M., MacKenzie C.D., Spry C.J., Denham D.A. (1983). Infection of inbred and nude (athymic) rats with Brugia spp. Parasite Immunol. 5:527-37.

Cryz S.J. Jr., Furer E., Germanier R. (1983). Simple model for the study of Psedomonas aeruginoas infections in leukopenic mice. Infect Imun. 39:1067-71.

Cummings J.F., de Lahunta A., Braund K.G., Mitechll W.J. Jr. (1983). Hereditary sensory neuropathy. Nociceptive loss and acral mutilation in pointer dogs: canine hereditary sensory neuropathy. Am J Pathol. 112:136-8.

Cunningham S.G., Mitchell P.H. (1982). The use of animals in nursing research. ANS. 4:72-84.

Curran E., Becker J. (1991). Changes in blood-brain barrier permeability are associated with behavioral and neurochemical indices of recovery following intraventricular adrenal medulla grafts in an animal model of Parkinson's disease. Exp Neurol 114(2):184-92.

Curtis M.J., Macleod B.A., Walker M.J. (1987). Models for the study of arrhythmias in myocardial ischaemia and infarction: the use of the rat. J Mol Cell Cardiol. 19:399-419.

Cutler L.S., Bullis D., Christian C.P., Rendell J.R., Greiner D.L. (1987). Animal models of Sjogren's syndrome. J Dent Res. 66:590-1.

Cutler P.D., Cherry S.R., Hoffman E.J., Digby W.M., Phelps M.E. Design features and performance of a PET system for animal research. J Nucl Med. 33:595-604.

Cywes R., Greig P., Morgan G., Sanabria J., Clavien P., Harvey P., Strasberg S. (1992). Rapid donor liver nutritional enhancement in a large animal model. Hepatology 16(5):1271-9.

D'Amato R. (Ed.) (1992). Relevance of animal studies to the evaluation of human cancer risk: proceedings of a symposium held December 5-8, 1990. New York: Wiley-Liss. 457 P.

Daemen B.J.G., Elsinga P.H., Mooibroek J., Paans A.M.J., Wieringa A.R., Konings A.W.T., Vaalburg W. (1991). PET measurement of hyperthermia induced supression of protein synthesis in tumors in relation to effects on tumor growth. 32:1587-92.

Dahlberg E., Snochowski M., Gustafsson J.A. (1980). Comparison of the R-3327H rat prostatic adenocarcinoma to human benign prostatic hyperplasia and metastatic carcinoma of the prostate with regard to steroid hormone receptors. Prostate. 1:61-70.

Dai S. (1982). The production of ventricular arrhythmias in the guinea-pigs isolated heart using hypoxic perfusion fluids containing adrenaline. Clin Exp Pharmacol Physiol. 9:1-9.

Dailey J.W., Jobe P.C. (1985). Anticonvulsant drugs and the genetically epilepsy-prone rat. Fed Proc. 44:2640-4.

Daley G.Q. (1993). Animal models of BCR/ABL induced leukemias. Leuk Lymphoma 11(Suppl 1):57-60.

Dalhoff A., Frank G., Luckhaus G. (1983). The granuloma pouch: an in vivo model for pharmacokinetic and chemotherapeutic investigations. II. microbiological characterization. Infection. 11:41-6.

Daniel S., James S., Stark R., Tropper P. (1989). Prevention of the normal expansion of maternal plasma volume: a model for chronic fetal hypoxaemia. J Dev Physiol 11(4):225-33.

Danpure C., Jennings P., Mistry J., Chalmers R., McKerrell R., Blakemore W., Heath M. (1989). Enzymological characterization of a feline analogue of primary hyperoxaluria type 2: a model for the human disease. J Inherit Metab Dis 12(4):403-14.

Daristotle,L. (1992). AIDS research: from apes to cats [news]. J Am Vet Med Assoc 201(9):1334.

Darling S., Gossler A. (1994). A mouse model for Fraser syndrome? Clin Dysmorphol. 3(2):91-5.

Das M., Asokan P., Don P.S., Krueger G.G., Bickers D.R., Mukhtar H. (1986). Carcinogen metabolism in human skin grafted onto athymic nude mice: a model system for the study of human skin carcinogenesis. Biochem Biphys Res Commun. 138:33-9.

Davey G.C. (Ed). (1983). Animal Models of Human Behavior: Conceptual Evolutionary and Neurobiological Perspectives. John Wiley, New York. 371 pp.

Davidoff A.J., Gwathmey J.K. (1994). Pathophysiology of cardiomyopathies: Part I. Animal models and humans. Curr Opin Cardiol. 9(3):357-68.

Davidson M.K., Lindsey J.R., Davis J.K. (1987). Requirements and selection of an animal model. Isr J Med Sci. 23:551-5.

Davidson T., Wallace J. (1986). The rabbit as an experimental model for regional chemotherapy. 2. Isolated perfusion of hindlimbs. Lab Anim. 20:347-50.

Davidson, R. (1988). Strongyloides stercoralis infection in the ferret [published erratum appears in J Parasitol (1988) Feb;74(1):177]. J Parasitol, 74 (1):177-9.

Davin J., Dechenne C., Mahieu P. (1989). [Acute experimental glomerulonephritis induced by the glomerular deposition of circulating polymeric IgA-concanavalin A complexes] Glomerulonephrite aigue experimentale induite par le depot glomerulaire de complexes circulants IgA polymerique-concanavaline A. Nephrologie 10(3):151-5.

Davis C.P., Cohen M.S., Anderson M.D., Reinarz J.A., Warren M.M. (1987). Total and specific immunoglobulin response to acute and chronic urinary tract infections in a rat model. J Urol. 138:1308-17.

Davis L.E., Cole L.L., Lockwood S.J., Kornfield M. (1983). Experimental influenza B virus toxicity in mice. A possible model for Reye's syndrome. Lab Invest. 48:140-7.

Davis L.E., Kornfeld M. (1986). Mouse influenza B virus model of Reye's syndrome. Encephalopathy and microvascular fatty metamorphosis of the liver by influenza B virus following intravenous administration in mice. Am J Pathol. 122:190-2.

Davisson M., Schmidt C., Akeson EC. (1990). Segmental trisomy of murine chromosome 16: a new model system for studying Down syndrome. Prog Clin Biol Res 360:263-80.

Davisson M.T., Schmidt C., Reeves R.H., Irving N.G., Akeson E.C., Harris B.S. et al. (1993). Segmental trisomy as a mouse model for Down syndrome. Prog. Clin Biol Res. 384:117-33.

Davson H. (1993). An introduction to the blood-brain barrier. Houndmills, Basingstoke, Hampshire: Macmillan. 335 P.

Daws L., Schiller G., Overstreet D., Orbach J. (1991). Early development of muscarinic supersensitivity in a genetic animal model of depression. Neuropsychopharmacology 4(3):207-17.

De Boer K., McKnight M. (1988). Surgical model of a chronic subluxation in rabbits. J Manipulative Physiol Ther 11(5):366-72.

De Bruin D., Dormehl I.C., Du Plessis D.J., Jacobs L., Hugo N., Maree M. (1991). Prostaglandin E1 and Papaverine: A Comparative Study on the Ability to Increase the Penile Bloodpool as Measured by the ^{99m}Tc-Penogram in the Baboon Model. Amer J Physiologic Imaging 6:129-132.

De Carneri I., Trane F. (1983). A chemotherapy model of human giardiasis. Unsuccessful attachment of Lombardy and Pakistani strains of Giardia intestinalis in rabbits, rats and pathogen-free immunodepressed mice. Parassitologia. 25:113-9. (Italian)

De Castro Costa M., De Sutter P., Gybels J., van Hees J. (1982). Adjuvant-induced arthritis in rats: a possible model of chronic pain. Pain 13:205-6.

De Foe G, Lisciani R., Capezzone d. J. A., Mazzanti G., Tolu L., Pace S. (1989). A total body hyperthermia animal model for pharmacological studies. In Vivo 3(5):295-9.

De Groot G.H., Reuvers C.B., Schalm S.W., Boks A.L., Terpstra O.T., Jeekel H., ten Kate F.W., Bruinvels J. (1987). A reproducible model of acute hepatic failure by transient ischemia in the pig. J Surg Res. 42:92-100.

De Koning P., Brakkee J.H., Gispen W.H. (1986). Methods for producing a reproducible crush in the sciatic and tibial nerve of the rat and rapid and precise testing of return of sensory function. J Neurol Sci. 74:237-46.

De Lemos R.A., Kuehl T.J. (1987). Animal models for evaluation of drugs for use in the mature and immature newborn. Pediatrics. 79:275-80.

DeBoer L.W.V., Rude R.E., Klower R.A., Ingwall J.S., Maroko P.R., Davis M.A., Braunwald E. (1983). A flow- and time-dependent index of ischemic injury after experimental coronary occlusion and reperfusion. Proc Nat Acad Sci USA 80:5784-8.

Decker M.W., Majchrzak M.J., Anderson D.J. (1992). Effects of nicotine on spatial memory deficits in rats with septal lesions. Brain Res. 572:281-5.

Dedrick R.L. (1986). Interspecies scaling in regional drug delivery. J Pharm Science 75:1046-52.

Dedushkin V., Dulaev A., Khomutov V., Erokhov A. (1990). [Experimental substantiation of the mechanism of adaptive disintegration in the pathogenesis of traumatic disease] Eksperimental'noe obosnovanie mekhanizma adaptatsionnoi dezintegratsii v patogeneze travmaticheskoi bolezni. Vestn Khir 145(9):92-6.

Deems R., Friedman M. (1988). Macronutrient selection in an animal model of cholestatic liver disease. Appetite 11(2):73-80.

Deerberg F., Kaspareit J. (1987). Endometrial carcinoma in BD II/Han rats: model of a spontaneous hormone-dependent tumor. JNCI. 78::1245-51.

DeGrado T.R., Turkington T.G., Williams J.J., Stearns C.W., Hoffman J.M., Coleman R.E. (1994). Performance characteristics of a whole-body PET scanner. J Nucl Med. 35:1398-406.

Dehmlow E.V. (1995). Review article: The epibatidine competition: Synthetic work on a novel natural analgetic. J Praktische Chemie 337:167-74.

Dehring D.J., Crocker S.H., Wismer B.L., Steinberg S.M., Lowery B.D., Cloutier C.T. (1983). Comparison of live bacteria infusions in a porcine model of acute respiratory failure. J Surg Res. 34:151-8.

Dehring D.J., Lowery B.D., Flynn J., Reithy G., Steinberg S., Carey S., Clontier C.T. (1983). Indomethacin improvement of septic acute respiratory failure in a porcine model. J Trauma. 23:725-9.

Deitrich R.A., Baker R.C. (1984). Initial sensitivity of rat inbred strains to acute alcohol. Alcoholism (NY). 8:487-90.

Dejana E., Villa S., Heiss W.D. (1982). Bleeding time in rats: a comparison of different experimental conditions. Thromb Haemost. 48:108-11.

Del Portillo H.A., Damian R.T. (1986). Experimental Schistosoma mansoni infection in a small New World monkey, the saddle-back tamarin - (Saguinus fuscicollis). Am J Trop Med Hyg. 35:515-22.

Del Soldato P. (1982). A rat model based on the histamine H2-receptor-activation-induced gastric pathology. Pharmacol Res Commun. 14:175-85.

Delbarre B., Delbarre G. (1988). Effect of indapamide on an experimental model of cerebral ischemia in hypertensive rats. Am J Med. 84:20-5.

Delbarre G., Delbarre B., Barrau Y. (1987). A suitable method to select gerbils with incomplete circle of Willis. Stroke. 19:126.

Delgado-Zygmunt T., Arbab M., Shiokawa Y., Svendgaard N. (1992). A primate model for acute and late cerebral vasospasm: angiographic findings. Acta Neurochir (Wien) 118(3-4):130-6.

Della Penta D. (1982). Immune responses to mouse neuroblastoma C1300, II. Cell-mediated kinetics and specificity studies. Int. Arch. Allergy Appl. Immunol. 69:322-9.

Demaria Pesce V.H., Stupfel M., Gourlet V., Lemercerre C. (1987). Age and survival of an acute carbon monoxide intoxication an animal model. Sci Total Environ. 65:41-51.

Demeter J., De J. S., Oslapas R., Ernst K., Hessel P., Jarosz H., Smith M., Nayyar R., Lawrence A., Paloyan E. (1991). High phosphate diet-induced primary hyperparathyroidism: an animal model. Surgery 110(6):1053-60.

Den Hartog Jager W.A. (1985). Experimental amyotrophic lateral sclerosis in the guinea-pig. J Neurol Sci. 67:113-42.

Den Ottolander G.J., te Velde J., Veenhof W., Kleiverda K., Haak H.L., Spaander P.J. (1982). Busulphan aplasia in rabbits: a model for human aplastic anaemia. Br J Haematol. 51:265-76.

Denham D., Midwinter I., Shipley M. (1990). Brugia pahangi adults implanted into mice: a possible screen for filaricidal activity. Trop Med Parasitol 41(2):223-4.

Deshmukh D.R. (1985). Animal models of Reye's syndrome. Rev Infect Dis. 7:31-40.

Deshmukh D.R., Thomas P.E. (1985). Arginine deficiency, hyperammonemia and Reye's syndrome in ferrets. Lab Anim Sci. 35:242-5.

Desjardins S., Mueller R., Cauchy M. (1988). A pressure overload model of congestive heart failure in rats [see comments]. Cardiovasc Res 22(10):696-702.

Desnick R.J., McGovern M. M., Schuchman E.H., Hasins M.E. (1982). Animal analogues of human inherited metabolic diseases: molecular pathology and therapeutic studies. Prog Clin Biol Res. 94:27-65.

Desnick R.J., Patterson D.F. (Eds). (1982). Animal Models of Inherited Metabolic Diseases (Progress in Clinical and Biological Research Ser. Vol. 94). A R Liss, New York. 544 pp.

Desowitz R., Shida K., Pang L., Buchbinder G. (1989). Characterization of a model of malaria in the pregnant host: Plasmodium berghei in the white rat. Am J Trop Med Hyg 41(6):630-4.

Deutch A., Rosin D., Goldstein M., Roth R. (1989). 3-Acetylpyridine-induced degeneration of the nigrostriatal dopamine system: an animal model of olivopontocerebellar atrophy-associated parkinsonism. Exp Neurol 105(1):1-9.

Deutsch E., Bushong W., Glavan K.A., Elder R.C., Sodd V.J., Scholz K.L., Fortman D.L., Lukes S.J. (1981). Heart imaging with cationic complexes of technetium. Science 214:85-86.

Deutsch E., Glavan K.A., Bushong W., Sodd V.J. (1982). The inorganic chemistry of ^{99m}Tc myocardial imaging agents. In: Lambrecht R.M., Morcos N.A. (Eds.). Applications of Nuclear and Radiochemistry. New York: Pergamon Press. pp 139-151.

Deutsch E., Ketring A.R., Libson K., Vanderheyden J.-L., Hirth W.W. (1989). The Noah's Ark experiment: Species dependent biodistributions of cationic ^{99m}Tc complexes. Int J Nucl Med Biol. 16:191-232.

Dewanjee M.K. (1992). Radioiodinated oligonucleotide probes for in vitro and in vivo hybridization. In: Dewanjee M.K. (Ed.). Radioiodination: Theory, practice, and biomedical applications. Boston: Kluwer Academic Publishers. p 484-91.

Dewanjee M.K. (1995). Intracellular communications. In: Wagner H.N., Szabo Z., Buchanan J. (Eds.) (1995). Principles of Nuclear Medicine. 2nd ed. Philadelphia: W.B. Saunders.

Dewanjee M.K., Ghafouripour A.K., Kapadvanjwala M. et al. (1993). Radiolabeled antisense oligonucleotides: In vitro and in vivo applications. J Clin Immunoassay 16:276-89.

Dewanjee M.K., Ghafouripour A.K., Kapadvanjwala M., Dewanjee S., Serafini A.N., Lopez D.M., Sfakianakis G.N. (1994). Noninvasive imaging of c-myc oncogene messenger RNA with indium-11-antisense probes in a mammary tumor-bearing mouse model. J Nucl Med. 35:1054-63.

Dewanjee M.K., Ghaouripour A.K., Werner R.K., Serafini A.N., Sfakianakis G.N. (1991). Development of sensitive radioiodinated anti-sense oligonucleotide probes by conjugation technique. Bioconj Chem. 2:195-200.

Dewey S.L., MacGregor R.R., Brodie J.D. et al. (1990). Mapping muscarinic receptors in human and baboon brain using [N-^{11}C-methyl]benztropine. Synapse 5:213-23.

Diamond B.I., Reyes M.G., Borison R. (1982). A new animal model for Tourette syndrome. Adv Neurol. 35:221-5.

Diamond T., Dolan S., Rowlands B. (1991). An improved technique for choledochoduodenostomy in a rat model of obstructive jaundice. Lab Anim Sci 41(1):82-3.

Dib M., Vitqal A., Vital C., Georgescault D.,k Baquay A., Bazian J. (1987). The C57BL mice: an animal model for inflammatory demyelinating polyneuropathy. J Neurol Sci. 81:101-11.

Dick J. (1991). Immune-deficient mice as models for human hematopoietic disease. Mol Genet Med 1:77-115.

Dick-Hegedus E., Lee A. (1991). Use of a mouse model to examine anti-Helicobacter pylori agents. Scand J Gastroenterol 26(9):909-15.

Dickinson J., Meyer B., Chmielowiec S., Palmer S. (1991). Streptozocin-induced diabetes mellitus in the pregnant ewe. Am J Obstet Gynecol 165(6 Pt 1):1673-7.

Dickneite G., Schorlemmer H.U., Sedlacek H.H. (1984). Chronic bacterial infection models for BRM screening. Behring Inst. Mitt. 74:174-82.

Dickson C., Vanderwolf C. (1990). Animal models of human amnesia and dementia: hippocampal and amygdala ablation compared with serotonergic and cholinergic blockade in the rat. Behav Brain Res 41(3):215-27.

Dieter M., Jameson C., Maronpot R., Langenbach R., Braun A. (1990). The chemotherapeutic potential of glycol alkyl ethers: structure-activity studies of nine compounds in a Fischer-rat leukemia transplant model. Cancer Chemother Pharmacol 26(3):173-80.

Dietrich W.D., Watson B.D., Busto R., Ginsberg M.D., Bethea J.R. (1987). Photochemically induced cerebral infarction. I. Early microvascular alterations. Acta Neuropathol. 72:315-25.

Dilley A., Dy D., Warlters A., Copeland S., Gillies AE., Morris R., Gibb D., Cook T., Morris D. (1993). Laboratory and animal model evaluation of the Cryotech LCS 2000 in hepatic cryotherapy. Cryobiology 30(1):74-85.

Dilworth J., Neal D. J., Fussell E., Roberts J. (1990). Experimental prostatitis in nonhuman primates: I. Bacterial adherence in the urethra. Prostate 17(3):227-31.

Dima V., Petrovici M., Lacky D. (1989). Reaction and response of newborn guinea pigs to experimental Salmonella typhi infection. Arch Roum Pathol Exp Microbiol 48(4):299-321.

Ding Y.S., Fowler J.S., Dewey S.L., Wolf A.P., Logan J., Gatley S.J., Volkow N.D., Shea C., Taylor D.P. (1993). Synthesis and PET studies of fluorine-18-BMY 14802: A potential antipsychotic drug. J Nucl Med. 34:246-54.

Dirnagl U., Thoren P., Villringer A., Sixt G., Them A., Einhaupl K. (1993). Global forebrain ischaemia in the rat: controlled reduction of cerebral blood flow by hypobaric hypotension and two-vessel occlusion. Neurol Res 15(2):128-30.

Dix R.D., McKendall P.R., Baringer J.R. (1983). Comparative neurovirulence of herpes simplex virus type 1 strains after peripheral or intracerebral inoculation of BALB/c mice. Infect immun. 40:103-12.

Dixit V., Chang T. (1990). Brain edema and the blood brain barrier in galactosamine-induced fulminant hepatic failure rats. An animal model for evaluation of liver support systems. ASAIO Trans 36(1):21-7.

Dixon C.E., Lyeth B.G., Povlishock J.T., Findling R.L., Hamm R.J., Marmarou A., Young H.F., Hayes R.L. (1987). A fluid percussion model of experimental brain injury in the rat. J Neurosurg. 67:110-9.

Dixon M.D., Merz W.G., Elliott H.L., MacLeay S. (1987). Experimental central nervous system phaeochyphomycosis following intranasal inoculation of Xylohypha bantiana in cortisone-treated mice. Mycopathologia. 100:145-53.

Dodds W.J. (1982). An effective mass-screening program for animal models of the inherited bleeding disorders. Prog Clin Biol Res. 94:117-32.

Dodds W.J. (1983). Learning from animal models of bleeding disorders. Ann NY Acad Sci. 406:59-61.

Doherty P.C., Kaufmann S.H. (1994). Novel insights and new models in a time of rapid technological change [editorial]. Curr Opin Immunol. 6(4):515-7.

Dole V.P. (1986). On the relevance of animal models to alcoholism in humans. Alcoholism (NY). 10:361-3.

Dole V.P., Gentry R.T. (1984). Toward analogue of alcoholism in mice: scale factors in the model. Proc Natl Acad Sci USA. 81:3543-6.

Dole V.P., Ho A., Gentry R.T. (1985). Toward an analogue of alcoholism in mice: criteria for recognition of pharmacologically motivated drinking . Proc Natl Acad Sci USA.. 82:3469-71.

Dole V.P., Ho A., Gentry R.T., Chin A. (1988). Toward an analogue of alcholism in mice: analysis of nongenetic variance in consumption of alcohol. Proc Natl Acad Sci USA. 85:827-30.

Dombroski R., Woodard D., Harper M., Gibbs R. (1990). A rabbit model for bacteria-induced preterm pregnancy loss. Am J Obstet Gynecol 163(6 Pt 1):1938-43.

Domino E.F., Kovacic B. (1983). Monkey models of tardive dyskinesia. Mod Probl Pharmacopsychiatry. 21:21-33.

Donahoe R.M., Byrd L.D., McClure H.M., Fultz P., Brantley M. et al. (1993). Consequences of opiate-dependency in a monkey model of AIDS. Adv Exp Med Biol. 335:21-8.

Donham K.J., Leininger J.R. (1984). Animal studies of potential chronic lung disease of workers in swine confinement buildings. Am J Vet Res. 45:926-31.

Dooley T., Stamp-Cole M., Ouding R. (1993). Evaluation of a nude mouse tumor model using beta-galactosidase-expressing melanoma cells. Lab Anim Sci 43(1):48-57.

Dormehl I.C., Jacobs D.J., de Plessis M., Goosen D.J. (1983). Standardization of radiorenography in dehydrated and rehydrated primates under laboratory conditions. J Med Primatol. 12:68-76.

Dormehl I.C., Jacobs D.J., Pretorius J.P., Maree M., Franz R.C. (1987). Baboon (Papio ursinus) model to study deep vein thrombosis using 111-indium-labeled autologous platelets. J Med Primatol. 16:27-38.

Dormehl I.C., Kilian J., Pretorius J.P., van Gelder A.L., Hugo N. (1991). The Effect of Fluid Resuscitation on Cardiac Function Changes Monitored by RadionuclideVentriculography in the Septic Shock Baboon Model. Amer J Physiologic Imaging 6:29-33.

Doskocil M., Starka L., Obenberger J. (1985). Experimental caractogenesis in chick embryos. Intra-amniotic injections of glucocorticoids and mineralocorticoids. Cesk Oftalmol. 41:90-4.

Doudet D., Gross C., Lebrun-Gradie P., Bioulac B. (1985). MPTP primate model of Parkinson's disease: a mechanographic and electromyographic study. Brain Res. 335: 19-49.

Downs N.S., Britton K.T., Gidds D. M., Koob G.F., Swerdlow N.R. (1986). Supersensitive endorcrine response to physostigmine in dopamine-depleted rats: a model of depression? Biol Psychiatry. 21:775-86.

Dragan, Y., Xu, Y., & Pitot, H. (1991). Tumor promotion as a target for estrogen/antiestrogen effects in rat hepatocarcinogenesis. Prev Med, 20 (1):15-26.

Draganescu N., Girjabu E., Grosser F., Cajal N. (1985). Data on the experimental transmission in the guinea pig of some human chronic degenerative diseases: Creutzfeldt-Jakob and Alzheimer's disease. Virologie. 36:255-9.

Draganescu N., Girjabu E.k, Petrescu A., Anghelescu N., Marcutiu V., Ionescu M., Antipa C. (1981). Laboratory data on the experimental transmission of Creutzfeld-Jakob disease in the guinea pig. Virologie. 32:207-9.

Drago J.R.(1984). The Noble rat bladder cancer model. FAFT-induced tumors. Cancer 53:1093-9.

Drago J.R., Nesbitt J.A. (1987). NB rat bladder cancer model: evaluation of the subrenal capsular assay system. J Surg Oncol. 36:5-7.

Drago J.R., Weed P., Fralisch A. (1983). Nb rat prostate adenocarcinoma and model androgen-sensitive tumor: metastasis control. J Surg Oncol. 24:33-5.

Driscoll C., Streissguth A., Riley E. (1990). Prenatal alcohol exposure: comparability of effects in humans and animal models. Neurotoxicol Teratol 12(3):231-7.

Driscoll P. (Ed.) (1992). Genetically defined animal models of neurobehavioral dysfunctions. Boston: Birkhaeuser. 304 P.

Druet P. (1990). Experimental models of autoimmune diseases. Curr Eye Res 9 Suppl:139-44.

Drugan R., Skolnick P., Paul S., Crawley JN. (1989). A pretest procedure reliably predicts performance in two animal models of inescapable stress. Pharmacol Biochem Behav 33(3):649-54.

Drummond G.S., Kappas A. (1982). The cytochrome P-450-depleted animal: an experimental model for in vivo studies in chemical biology. Proc Natl Acad Sci USA. 79:2384-8.

Du Toit D.F., Heydenrych J.J., Low G., Zuurmond T., Laker L., Smith B., Els D., Weideman A., Davids H., Wolfe-Coote S. (1987). Diabetes in pancreatectomized baboons: a model for pancreatic transplantation studies. J Surg Oncol 35:213-6.

Dubach M.F., Bowden D.M. (1983). Response to intracerebral dopamine injection as a model of schizoprenic symptomatology. Prog Clin Biol Res. 131:157-84.

Duff K. (1994). Modeling Alzheimer's disease in transgenic mice. J Fla Med Assoc. 81(9):625-8.

Dumont A.E. (1983). Experimental models of splenic dysfunction. Lymphology. 16:56-9.

Duncan B., Adzick N., Moelleken B., Chua J., Bradley S., Longaker M., Levinsohn D., Harrison M., Kaban L. (1992). An in utero model of craniosynostosis. J Craniofac Surg 3(2):70-8.

Duncan C.C., Lambrecht R.M., Bennett G.W., Ment L.R. (1984). Observations of dynamics of ionic potassium in brain. Stroke 15:145-8.

Dunn C.D., Smith L.N., Leonard J.I., Andrews R.B. et al. (1980). Animal and computer investigations into the murine erythroid response to chronic hypoxia. Exp Hematol. 8 Suppl 8:259-82.

Dunn D. (1988). Antibody immunotherapy of gram-negative bacterial sepsis in an immunosuppressed animal model. Transplantation 45(2):424-9.

Dunningan A., Noren G.R., Einzig S., Benditt D.G., Staley N.A., Benson D.W. Jr. (1984). Inducible ventricular arrhythmias in a naturally occurring model of cardiomyopathy. Cardiovasc Res. 18:645-50.

Dunnington D.J., Buscarino C., Gennaro D., Greig R., Poste G. (1987). Characterization of an animal model of metastatic colon carcinoma. Int J Cancer. 39:248-54.

Dunselman G., Willebrand D., Land J., Bouckaert PX., Evers J. (1989). A rabbit model of endometriosis. Gynecol Obstet Invest 27(1):29-33.

Durnova G.N., Vorotnikova E.V., Prodan N.G. (1987). Comparative evaluation of the stress reaction of rats under different methods of simulating the effects of weightlessness. Kosm Biol Aviakosm Med. Seot-Oct; 21:79-81. (Russian)

Dutta G.P., Singh P.P., Saibaba P. (1981). Presbytis entellus as a new host for experimental Plasmodium knowlessi infection. Indian J Med Res. 73:Suppl:63-6.

Dutton G.N., Hay J., Hair D.M., Raiston J. (1986). Clinicopathological features of a congenital murine model of ocular toxoplasmosis. Graefes Arch Clin Exp Ophthalmol. 224:256-64.

Dwivedi S., Chansouria J.P., Somani P.N. (1987): An experimental model for myocardial ischaemia in rabbits. Indian J Exp Biol. 25(11):753-7.

Dymecki J., Markiewicz D., Poltorak M., Pucilowski O., Kobtowski W., Bidzinski. (1985). Effects of intracerebral transplantation of immature substantia nigra in rats with experimentally induced Parkinson's disease. I. Comparative evaluation of two models of Parkinson's disease induced by unilateral stereotaxic lesion of the substantia nigra with electrocoagulation and with 6-hydroxidopamine. Neuropathol Pol. 23:167-79.

Dzhalogoniia ShL., Uzunian L.A., Vavilova V.P., Babaiants B.S. (1983). Method of creating a conflict situation based on feeding behavior in the monkey. Zh Vyssh Nerv Deiat. 33:776-9.

Dzhikidze E.K. (1986). Modelling bacterial infections in monkeys. Vestn Akad Med Nauk SSSR. 3:54-6. (English Abstract) (Russian)

Dzhikidze E.K., Shaginian S.A., Psopelova V.V., Rakhimova N.G., Khaleneva M.P. (1986). Use of monkeys as a model to evaluate the efficacy of microbial biopreparations in disease related to dysbacteriosis. Vestn Akad Med Nauk SSSR. 3:74-7. (English Abstract). (Russian)

Eberhard M., Dickerson J., Boyer A., Tsang V., Zea-Flores R., Walker E., Richards F., Zea-Flores G., Strobert E. (1991). Experimental Onchocerca volvulus infections in mangabey monkeys (Cercocebus atys) compared to infections in humans and chimpanzees (Pan troglodytes). Am J Trop Med Hyg 44(2):151-60.

Eby T.L. (1986). Experimental cochlear hydrops in cats. Am J Otol. 7:414-6.

Eckholm E. (1985). Fight over animal experiment gains intensity on many fronts. New York Times, May 7. p C1, C6.

Eddy A.A., Falk R.J., Sibley R.K., Hostetter T.H. (1986). Subtotal nephrectomy in the rabbit: a model of chronic hypercalcemia, nephrolithiasis, and obstructive nephropathy. J Lab Clin med. 107:508-16.

Eder G., Kaiser E., King F.A., (Ed) (1994). The role of the chimpanzee in research. Symposium, Vienna, May 22-24. Basel; New York: Karger. 203 P.

Edmond J.C., Capron-Laudereau M., Meriggi F., Reynes M., Houssin D. (1988): Acute liver failure after subtotal hepatectomy in the rat: failure of testosterone pretreatment and hepatocyte transplantation to improve survival. Curr Surg. 45(3):200-3.

Edwards B.R. (1982). Water balance in the Brattleboro rat: single or multiple defects? 394:414-23.

Edwards E., Harkins K., Wright G., Henn F. (1991). 5-HT1b receptors in an animal model of depression. Neuropharmacology 30(1):101-5.

Edwards E., Harkins K., Wright G., Henn F. (1991). Modulation of [3H]paroxetine binding to the 5-hydroxytryptamine uptake site in an animal model of depression. J Neurochem 56(5):1581-6.

Edwards E., Kornrich W., van H. P., Henn F. (1992). In vitro neurotransmitter release in an animal model of depression. Neurochem Int 21(1):29-35.

Edwards J.F., Slauson D.O. (1983). Complete Freund's adjuvant-induced pneumonia in swine: a model of interstitial lung disease. J Comp Pathol. 93:353-61.

Edwards S., Small J., Geratz JD., Alexander L. et al. (1992). An experimental model for myocarditis and congestive heart failure after rabbit coronavirus infection. J Infect Dis 65(1):134-40.

Egwang T., Kazura J. (1990). The BALB/c mouse as a model for immunological studies of microfilariae-induced pulmonary eosinophilia. Am J Trop Med Hyg 43(1):61-6.

Eichberg J.W., Lee D.R., Allan J.S., Cobb K.E., Barbosa L.H., Nemo G.J., Prince A.M. (1988): In utero infection of an infant chimpanzee with HIV. N Engl J Med. 15;319(11):722-3.

Eisenberg J., Brecher-Fride E., Weizman R., Ebstein R.P., Belmaker R.H. (1982). Dopamine receptors in a rat model of minimal brain dysfunction. Neuropsychobiology. 8:151-5.

Eison M.S. (1984). Use of animal models: toward anxioselective drugs. Psychopathology. 17 Suppl 1:37-44.

El Kouri D., Dupas B., Peltier P., de F. P., Planchon B. (1992). Experimental venous thrombosis: what animal model? Int Angiol 11(4):304-8.

El Sinnary K.A., Bianco A.E., Williams J.F. (1987). Implantation of adult Onchocerca gutturosa into laboratory rodents. Parasitology. 95:(Pt 1):155-8.

Eletskii Iu. K., Tsibulevskii A.Iu., Zimatkin S.M., Ettinger A.P. (1985). An improved experimental model for studying post-vagotomy complications in patients with duodenal ulcer. Vestn Akad Med Nauk SSSR. 7:61-8. (English Abstract). (Russian)

Ellias P.M., Lampe M.A., Chung J.C., Williams M.L. (1983). Diazacholesterol-induced ichthyosis in the hairless mouse. I. Morphologic, histochemical, and lipid biochemical characterization of a new animal model. Lab Invest. 48: 565-77.

Elliott E., Watson A., Walker-Smith J., Farthing M. (1991). Search for the ideal oral rehydration solution: studies in a model of secretory diarrhoea. Gut 32(11):1314-20.

Elmazar M., Vogel R., Spielmann H. (1988). Amniotic fluid cholinesterase of valproate-induced exencephaly in the mouse: an animal model for prenatal diagnosis of neural tube defects. Arch Toxicol 61(6):501-3.

Elovskaia L.T., Kapitano I.uT., Iaglov V.V. (1986). Models of experimental pneumoconiosis and dust-induced bronchitis via inhalational exposure to dust. Gig Sanit. 6:19-22. (English Abstract).

Elsner J. (1991). Tactile-kinesthetic system of rats as an animal model for minimal brain dysfunction. Arch Toxicol 65(6):465-73.

Emini E.A., Luka J., Armstrong M.E., Banker F.S., Provost P.J., Pearson G.R. (1986). Establishment and characterization of a chronic infectious mononucleosislike syndrome in common marmosets. J Med Virol. 18:369-79.

Emmett-Oglesby M.W., Spencer D.G.Jr., Eklmersallamy F., Lal H. (1983). The pentylenetetrazol model of anxiety detects withdrawal from diazepam in rats. Life Sci. 33:161-8.

Emslie K.R., Nade S. (1986). Pathogenesis and treatment of acute hematogenous osteomyelitis: evaluation of current views with reference to an animal model. Rev Infect Dis. 8:841-9.

Engel J. J. (1992). Experimental animal models of epilepsy: classification and relevance to human epileptic phenomena. Epilepsy Res Suppl 8:9-20.

Engel S., Bollmann R., Sokolowska-Kohler W., Audring H., Klug H. (1988). Ureaplasma urealyticum and male infertility: an animal model. I. Artificial infection, breeding experiments and histological preparation of organs. Andrologia 20(6):467-71.

Engelhardt J., Appel S., Killian J. (1989). Experimental autoimmune motoneuron disease. Ann Neurol 26(3):368-76.

Engels F., Carstairs J., Barnes P., Nijkamp F. (1989). Autoradiographic localization of changes in pulmonary beta-adrenoceptors in an animal model of atopy. Eur J Pharmacol 164(1):139-46.

Engerman R.L., Kramer J.W. (1982). Dogs with induced or spontaneous diabetes as models for the study of human diabetes mellitus. Diabetes 31 (Suppl 1 Pt 2):26-9.

Enriquez de Salamanca R., Mas Andres V., Catalan Beltran T., Molina Ferragut C., Chinarro Familiar S. Olmos Andres A. (1982). Induction of experimental porphyria by hexachlorobenzene in rats. Rev Esp Enferm Apar Dig. 62:1-14. (English Abstract) (Spanish)

Epstein C.J., Avraham K.B., Lovett M., Smith S., Elroy-Stein O., Rotman G., Bry C., Groner Y. (1987). Transgenic mice with increased Cu/Zn-superoxide dismutase activity: animal model of dosage effects in Down syndrome. Proc Natl Acd Sci. USA. 94:8044-8.

Epstein J. (1992). Experimental models for primary melanoma. Photodermatol Photoimmunol Photomed 9(3):91-8.

Erdman M.D., Verley F.A., Dondari K. (1987). Effects of the sex-linked prenatal lethal gene tortoise (Moto) on reproduction and growth in the mouse. Growth, Summer; 51:189-97.

Erickson R.P. (1988): Creating animal models of genetic disease. Am J Hum Genet. 43(5):582-6.

Eriksson K. (Ed). Animal Models in Alcohol Research: (1980). Proceedings International Conference, June 4-8, 1979. Academic Press, Helsinki.

Erlebacher J.A. (1985). Ventricular remodeling in myocardial infarction-the rat and the human. Am J Cardiol. 56:910

Escajadillo A., Frenkel J. (1991). Experimental toxoplasmosis and vaccine tests in Aotus monkeys. Am J Trop Med Hyg 44(4):382-9.

Escrich E. (1987): Validity of the DMBA-induced mammary cancer model for the study of human breast cancer. Int J Biol Markers. 2(3):197-206 (70 ref.)

Esper E., Chan EK., Buchwald H. (1993). Natural history of atherosclerosis and hyperlipidemia in heterozygous WHHL (WHHL-Hh) rabbits. I. The effects of aging and gender on plasma lipids and lipoproteins. J Lab Clin Med 121(1):97-102.

Esper E., Runge W., Gunther R., Buchwald H. (1993). Natural history of atherosclerosis and hyperlipidemia in heterozygous WHHL (WHHL-Hh) rabbits. II. Morphologic evaluation of spontaneously occurring aortic and coronary lesions. J Lab Clin Med 121(1):103-10.

Espinal C., Moreno E., Umana J., Ramirez J., Montilla M. (1984). Susceptibility of different populations of Colombian Aotus monkeys to the FCB-1 strain of Plasmodium falciparum. Am J Trop Med Hyg. 33:777-82.

Essnan W.B., Essman E.J. (1982). Comparative features of an animal model for behavioral and neurochemical change. Adv Neurol. 35:227-32.

Estourgie R.J., Tinnemans J.G. (1983). The clinical and histopathological effects of pancreatic duct occlusion in experimental acute pancreatitis in dogs. J Surg Res. 34:164-70.

Ettenberg A., Geist T. (1991). Animal model for investigating the anxiogenic effects of self-administered cocaine. Psychopharmacology (Berl) 103(4):455-61.

Evans E.F., Wilson J.P., Borerwe T.A. (1981). Animal models of tinnitus. Ciba Found Symp. 85:108-38.

Evans M.I., Mukherjee A.B., Schulaman J.D. (1983). Animal models of intrauterine growth retardation. Obstet Gynecol Surv. 38:183-92.

Evans R.M., Swanson L., Rosenfeld M.G. (1985). Creation of transgenic animals to study development and as models for human disease. Recent Prog Horm Res. 41:317-37.

Eveson J.W. (1981). Animal models of intra-oral chemical carcinogenesis: a review. J Oral Pathol. 10:129-46. Also: J Oral Pathol. 10:322-31. Also J Oral Pathol. 10:332-41.

Ezer E. (1989). Effect of cytoprotective and antiulcer drugs on the healing process of subacute gastric ulcer in rat (a new model). Acta Physiol Hung 73(2-3):233-40.

Fabry M.E. (1993). Transgenic animal models of sickle cell disease. Experimentia 49(1):28-36.

Fabry M.E., Kaul D.K., Davis L., Gore J.C., Brown M., Nagel R.L. (1987). An animal model for sickle cell vaso-occlusion: a study using NMR and technetium imaging. Prog Clin Biol Res. 240: 297-304.

Fadem B.H., Hill H.Z. (1985). The gray opossum. (Monodelphis domestrica): a marsupial model for xenogenic neoplasms. Cancer Lett. 27:233-8.

Faggiotto A. (1986). Experimental atherogenesis. G. Ital Cardiol. 16:350-65. (English Abstract).

Fahr A., Hiestand P., Ryffel B. (1990). Studies on the biologic activities of Sandimmun metabolites in humans and in animal models: review and original experiments. Transplant Proc 22(3):1116-24.

Fajfar-Wheostne C.J., Collins W.E., Ristic M. (1987). In vitro and in vivo adaptation of the Geneve/SGE-1 strain of Plasmodium falciparum to growth in a squirrel monkey (Saimiri sciureus) model. Am J Trop Med Hyg. 36:221-7.

Faraco P., Hewitson T., Kincaid-Smith P. (1991). An animal model for the study of the microangiopathic form of cyclosporine nephrotoxicity. Transplantation 51(5):1129-31.

Faraj B.A., Caplan D.B., Malveaux E.J., Camp V.M., Ali F.M. (1983). Similarity between tyramine-induced neurotoxicity and the coma of Reye's syndrome. J Pharmacol Exp Ther. 226:608-15.

Farde L., Halldin E., Nagren K., Suhara T., Karlsson P. et al. (1994). Positron emission tomography shows high specific uptake of racemic carbon-11 labeled norepinephrine in the primate heart. Eur J Nucl Med. 21:345-7.

Fariello R., Garant D. (1992). Neurotransmitter pharmacology of the epilepsies: discrepancies between animal models and human conditions. Epilepsy Res Suppl 8:21-6; discussion 26-7.

Faure J.P., Phuc L.H., Takano S., Sterkers M., Thillaye B., de Kozak Y. (1981). Experimental uveoretinitis induced in monkeys by retinal S antigen. Induction, histopathology. J Fr Ophtalmol. 4:465-72. (English Abstract). (French)

Fein F.S., Capasso J.M., Aronson R.S., Cho S., Nordin C., Miller-Green B., Sonnenblick E.H., Factor S.M. (1984). Combined renovascular hypertension and diabetes in rats: a new preparation of congestive cardiomyopathy. Circulation. 70:318-30.

Feinberg S.E. (1983). An animal model to investigate the interaction between the immune system and oral carcinomas. J Oral Maxillofac Surg. 41:578-85.

Feitelson M., DeTolla L., Zhou X. (1988). A chronic carrier-like state is established in nude mice injected with cloned hepatitis B virus DNA. J Virol 62(4):1408-15.

Fekete I., Hegedus K., Molnar L. (1988). Cerebral ischaemia produced by homologous blood clot emboli in rabbit. J Neurol 235(5):314-7.

Fekete S. (1993). Animal models in experimental atherosclerosis: a critical review. Acta Vet Hung. 41(1-2):3-9.

Feldenzer J.A., McKeever P.E., Schaberg D.R., Cambell J.A., Hoff J.T. (1987). Experimental spinal epidural abscess: a pathophysiological model in the rabbit. Neurosurgery. 20:859-67.

Feldon J., Weiner I. (1992). From an animal model of an attentional deficit towards new insights into the pathophysiology of schizophrenia. J Psychiatr Res 26(4):345-66.

Ferenci P., Covell D., Schafer D.F., Waggover J.G., Shrager R., Jones E.A. (1983).. Metabolism of the inhibitory neurotransmitter gamma-aminobutyric acid in a rabbit model of fulminant hepatic failure. Hepatology. 3:507-12.

Fergusson R.J., Carmichael J., Smyth J.F. (1986). Human tumour xenografts growing in immunodeficient mice: a useful model for assessing chemotherapeutic agents in bronchial carcinoma. Thorax. 41:376-80.

Ferrick D.A., DiMolfetto-Landon L., Ohashi P.S. (1994). Transgenic mice as an in vivo model for self reactivity. Austin: R.G. Landes Co. 98 P.

Fettman M.J. (1986). Endotoxemia in Yucatan miniature pigs: metabolic derrangements and experimental therapies. Lab Anim Sci. 36:370-4.

Fichtner I., Becker M., Lemm M., Arndt D. (1987). Characterization of a new tumor in NMRI-mice suitable for chemotherapeutic experiments. Arch Geschwulstforsch. 57:105-14.

Fidler I., Naito S., Pathak S. (1990). Orthotopic implantation is essential for the selection, growth and metastasis of human renal [correction of real] cell cancer in nude mice. Cancer Metastasis Rev 9(2):149-65.

Fiebig H.H., Schuchhardt C., Henss H., Fiedler L., Lohr G.W. (1984). Comparison of tumor response in nude mice and in the patients. Behring Inst Mitt. 74:343-52.

Field H., Brown G. (1989). Animal models for antiviral chemotherapy. Antiviral Res 12:165-80.

Figueiredo M., Baffa O., Barbieri N. J., Zago M. (1993). Liver injury and generation of hydroxyl free radicals in experimental secondary hemochromatosis. Res Exp Med (Berl) 193(1):27-37.

File S.E. (1984). The validation of animal tests of anxiety--pharmacological implications. Pol J Pharmacol Pharm. 36:505-12.

Filice G., Cereda P.M., Varnier O.E. (1988): Infection of rabbits with human immunodeficiency virus. Nature. 22;335(6188):366-9.

Fineman R.M., Schoenwolf G.C. (1987). Animal model sysmorphogenesis and death in a chicken embryo model. Am J Med Genet. 27:543-52.

Fish R.E., Spitzer J.A. (1984). Continous infusion of endotoxin from an osmotic pump in the conscious, unrestrained rat: a unique model of chronic endotoxemia. Circ Shock. 12:135-49.

Fisher A., Brandeis R., Karton I., Pittel Z., Gurwitz D., Haring R. et al. (1991). (+-)-cis-2-methyl-spiro(1,3-oxathiolane-5,3')quinuclidine, an M1 selective cholinergic agonist, attenuates cognitive dysfunctions in an animal model of Alzheimer's disease. J Pharmacol Exp Ther 257(1):392-403.

Fisher-Hoch S.P., Platt G.S., Lloyd G., Simpson D.I., Neild G. H., Barrett A.J. (1983). Haematological and biochemical monitoring of Ebola infection in rhesus monkeys: implications for patient management. Lancet. 2:1055-8.

Fisler J.S., Lupien J.R., Wood R.D., Bray G.A., Schemmel R.A. (1987). Brown fat thermogenesis in a rat model of dietary obesity. Am J. Physiol. 253 (5 Pt 2):R756-62.

Fitzgeorge R.B., Backerville A., Broster M., Hambleton P., Dennis P.J. (1983). Aerosol infection of animals with strains of Legionella pneumophila of different virulence: comparison with intraperitoneal and intra-nasal routes of infection. J Hyg (Lond). 90:81-9.

Fitzgerald N., Papadimitriou J., Shellam G. (1990). Cytomegalovirus-induced pneumonitis and myocarditis in newborn mice. A model for perinatal human cytomegalovirus infection. Arch Virol 115(1-2):75-88.

Fitzsimons E., Lange C. (1991). Hybridomas to specific streptococcal antigen induce tissue pathology in vivo; autoimmune mechanisms for post-streptococcal sequelae. Autoimmunity, 10(2):115-24.

Flameng W., Vanhaecke J., Vandeplassche G. (1986). Studies on experimental myocardial infarction: dogs or baboons? Cardiovasc Res. 20:241-7.

Fleisher G.R., Templeton J., Delgado-Paredes C. (1987). An animal model for the study of hemorrhagic shock from abdominal trauma in children. Pediatr Emerg Care. 3:18-21.

Fleming J.O. (1985). Animal models of multiple sclerosis [editorial]. Mayo Clin proc. 60:490-2.

Fletcher J., Dryden M., Munro R., Xu J., Hehir MD. (1990). Establishment of a vascular graft infection model in the sheep carotid artery. Aust N Z J Surg 60(10):801-3.

Flood J.F., Cherkin A. (1986). Scopolamine effects on memory retention in mice: a model of dementia? Behav Neural Biol. 45:169-84.

Florczyk A.P., Schuring J.E., Bradner W.T. (1982). Cisplatin-induced emesis in the Ferret: a new animal model. Cancer Treat Rep. 66:187-9.

Floth A., Paick J., Suh J., Lue T. (1991). Hemodynamics of revascularization of the corpora cavernosa in an animal model. A preliminary report. Urol Res 19(5):281-4.

Flower R. (1990). Perinatal ocular physiology and ROP in the experimental animal model. Doc Ophthalmol 74(3):153-62.

Flower R.W., Blake D.A. (1981). Retrolental fibroplasia: evidence for a role of the prostaglandin cascade in the pathogenesis of oxygen-induced retionopathy in the newborn beagle. Pediatr Res. 15:1293-1302.

Foa EB., Zinbarg R., Rothbaum B. (1992). Uncontrollability and unpredictability in post-traumatic stress disorder: an animal model. Psychol Bull 112(2):218-38.

Fodstad O., Aamdal S., McMenamin M., Nesland J., Pihl A. (1988). A new experimental metastasis model in athymic nude mice, the human malignant melanoma LOX. Int J Cancer 41(3):442-9.

Fohlmeister I., Fischer R., Schaefer H.E. (1981). Experimental induction of preleukemic myelopoietic dysplasias by dimethylbenz (a) anthrazene (DMBA). A rat model for investigation of human 'preleukemia'. Pathol Res Pract. 171:389-410. (English Abstract). (German)

Folds J.D., Rauchback A.S., Shores E., Saunders J.M. (1983). Evaluation of the inbred mouse as a model for experimental Treponema pallidum infection. Scand J Immunol. 18:201-6.

Ford R.W. (1983). A reproducible spinal cord injury model in the cat. J Neurosurg. 59:268-75.

Foreman J.W., Bowring M.A., Lee J., States B., Segal S. (1987). Effect of cystine dimethylester on renal solute handling and isolated renal tubule transport in the rat: a new model of the Fanconi syndrome. Metabolism. Dec. 36:1185-91.

Formby B., Schmid-Formby F., Jovanovic L., Peterson C.M. (1987). The offspring of the female diabetic "non-obese diabetic" (NOD) mouse are large for gestational age and have elevated pancreatic insulin content: a new animal model of human diabetic pregnancy. Proc Soc Exp Biol Med. 184:291-4.

Fourré C., Halpern S., Jeusset J., Clerc J., Fragu P. (1992). Significance of secondary ion mass spectrometry microscopy for technetium-99m mapping in leukocytes. J Nucl Med. 33:2162-6.

Fourtanier A., Berrebi C. (1989). Miniature pig as an animal model to study photoaging. Photochem Photobiol 50(6):771-84.

Fowler J.S., Volkow N.D., Wolf A.P. et al. (1989). Mapping cocaine binding sites in human and baboon brain in vivo. Synapse 4:371-7.

Fowlis D.J., Balmain A. (1993). Oncogenes and tumour suppressor genes in transgenic mouse models of neoplasia. Eur J Cancer 29A(4):638-45.

Fox J., Correa P., Taylor N., Lee A., Otto G., Murphy J., Rose R. (1990). Helicobacter mustelae-associated gastritis in ferrets. An animal model of Helicobacter pylori gastritis in humans. Gastroenterology 99(2):352-61.

Fox J., Lee A., Otto G., Taylor N., Murphy J. (1991). Helicobacter felis gastritis in gnotobiotic rats: an animal model of Helicobacter pylori gastritis. Infect Immun 59(3):785-91.

Fox J.G., Ackerman J.I., Taylor N., Claps M., Murphy J.C. (1987). Campylobacter jejuni infection in the ferret: an animal model of human campylobacteriosis. Am J Vet Res. 48:85-90.

Fox R.I. (1994). Epidemiology, pathogenesis, animal models, and treatment of Sjogren's syndrome. Curr Opin Rheumatol. 6(5):501-8.

Fragu P. Biançon C., Fourré C., Clerc J., Jeusset J., Halpern S. (1993). How can SIMS microscopy be used in biomedicine? Microbeam Analysis 2:199-207.

Franch H.A., Dixon R.A., Blaine E.H., Siegl P.K. (1988). Ventricular atrial natriuretic factor in the cardiomyopathic hamster model of congestive heart failure. Circ Res. 62:31-6.

Francis D.P., Feorino P.M., Broderson J.R., McClure H.M., Getchell J.P., McGrath C.R., Swenson B., McDougal F.S., Palmer E.L., Harrison A.K. (1984). Infection of chimpanzees with lymphadenopathy-associated virus. Lancet. 2:1276-7.

Frazee J.G., (1982). A primate model of chronic cerebral vasospasm. Stroke. 13:612-4.

Freed W., Geller H., Poltorak M., Cannon-Spoor H., Cottingham S., LaMarca M., Schultzberg M., Rehavi M., Paul S., Ginns EI. (1990). Genetically altered and defined cell lines for transplantation in animal models of Parkinson's disease. Prog Brain Res 82:11-21.

Frey H.H. (1987): Induction of seizures by air blast in gerbils: stimulus duration/effect relationship. Epilepsy Res. 1(4):262-4.

Fricke R., Bartel M. (1982). Animal experimental model of lung contusion. Z Exp Chir. 15:172-6. (English Abstract). (German)

Friedman A.L., Mehls O., Kleinknecht C., Laouari D., Dodu C., Aperia A. et al. (1986). Animal models of chronic renal failure: influence of nutrition on growth. Am J Kidney Dis. 7:335-9.

Friedman A.M., Huang C.C., Kulmala H.A., Dinerstein R., Navone J., Brundsen B., Gawlas D., Cooper M. (1982). The use of radiobrominated p-bromospiroperiodol for gamma-ray imaging of dopamine receptors. Int J Nucl Med Biol. 9:57-61.

Friedman R. (1988): Environmental-genetic interactions in experimental hypertension: the Dahl rat model. Health Psychol. 7(2):149-58.

Friedrich R., Muller W. (1988). [Preliminary results with a rabbit model of ocular toxoplasmosis] Erste Erfahrungen mit einem Kaninchenmodell der Augentoxoplasmose. Z Versuchstierkd 31(1):27-31.

Fritzberg A.R. (1995). Tissue perfusion of copper-62-PTSM: Relevance of studies in animal models as predictors of clinical radiopharmaceutical performance. J Nucl Med. 36:1456-7.

Fritzberg A.R., Bloedow D.C. (1983). Animal models in the study of hepatobiliary radiotracers. In: Lambrecht R.M., Eckelman W.C. (Eds). Animal models in radiotracer design. Heidelberg: Springer Verlag. pp 179-210.

Frohlich M., Henke E., Arnold W., Naundorf H. (1986). Experimental research following intratumor bleomycin use in the nude mouse model of oral mucosa cancer and the clinical pilot study. Arch Geschwulstforsch. 56:125-34. (English Abstract). (German)

Fromtling R.A, Abruzzo G.K., Ruiz A. (1988): Cryptococcus neoformans: a central nervous system isolate from an AIDS patient that is rhinotropic in a normal mouse model. Mycopathologia. 102(2):79-86.

Fry D.E., Garrison R.N., Rink R.D., Casey J., DeComp M.M., Richardson J.D. (1982). An experimental model of intraabdominal abscess in rat. Adv. Shock Res. 7:7-11.

Fry J.L.Jr., Koch W.E., Jennette J.C., McFarland E., Fried F.A., Mandell J. (1985). A genetically determined murine model of infantile polycystic kidney disease. J Urol.. 134:828-33.

Fu X., Hoffman R. (1993). Human ovarian carcinoma metastatic models constructed in nude mice by orthotopic transplantation of histologically-intact patient specimens. Anticancer Res 13:283-6.

Fukuda K., Matsumoto S., Kage M., Arakawa M., Nakashima T. (1985). The pathogenesis of idiopathic portal hypertension (so-called Banti's disease)- an experimental study. Kurume Med. J. 32:255-61.

Fulghum R.S., Brinn J.E., Smith A.M. , Daniel H.J. 3rd, Loesche P.J. (1982). Experimental otitis media in gerbils and chinchillas with Streptococcus pneumoniae, Haemophilus influenzae, and other aerobic and anaerobic bacteria. Infect Immun. 36:802-10.

Fulghum R.S., Hoodmoed R.P., Brinn J.E., Smith A.M. (1985). Experimental pneumococcal otitis media: longitudinal studies in the gerbil model. Int J Pediatr Otorhinolaryngol. 10:9-20.

Fuller R.W., Yen T.T. (1987). The place of animal models and animal experimentation in the study of food intake regulation and obesity in humans 499:167-78.

Fulmer J.D., Fliut A., Law D.E. (1983). Experimental disease in guinea pigs. Morphology and Collagan Analysis. Lung. 161:287-300.

Fultz P. (1989). Nonhuman primates and the acquired immunodeficiency syndrome: a union of necessity. J Med Primatol 18(2):73-83.

Fultz P.N., Greene C., Switzer W., Swenson B., Anderson D., McClure H.M. (1987). Lack of transmission of human immunodeficiency virus from infected to uninfected chimpanzees. J Med Primatol. 16:341-7.

Furlow T.W. Jr. (1982). Experimental air embolism of the brain: an analysis of the technique in the rat. Stroke. 13:847-52.

Furness P.N., Harris K. (1994). An evaluation of experimental models of glomerulonephritis. Int J Exp Pathol. 75(1):9-22.

Gabbai F.B., Gushva L.C., Wilson C.B., Blantz R.C. (1987). An evaluation of the developemnt of experimental membranous nephropathy. Kidney Int. 31:1267-78.

Gabel H., Bitter-Suermann H., Henriksson C., Save-Soderbergh J., Lundholm K., Brynger H. (1985). Streptozotocin diabetes in juvenile pigs. Evaluation of an experimental mode. Horm Metab Res. 17:275-80.

Gad S.C., Chengelis C.P. (Ed.) (1992). Animal models in toxicology. New York: Marcel Decker. 884 P:

Gagnon C., Bedard P.J., Di Paolo T. (1994). Grafts in the treatment of Parkinson's disease: animal models. Rev Neurosci. 4(1):17-40.

Gagnon R.F., Duguid W.P. (1983). A reproducible model for chronic renal failure in the mouse. Urol. Res. 11:11-4.

Gal D., Rongione A., Slovenkai G., DeJesus S., Lucas A., Fields C., Isner J. (1990). Atherosclerotic Yucatan microswine: an animal model with high-grade, fibrocalcific, nonfatty lesions suitable for testing catheter-based interventions. Am Heart J 119(2 Pt 1):291-300.

Galaburda A.M. (1994). Developmental dyslexia and animal studies: at the interface between cognition and neurology. Cognition 50(1-3):133-49.

Galikeyev K.L., Shevchenko T.F. (1982). Experimental model of dysentery. J Hyg Epidemoil Microbiol Immunol. 26:37-43.

Gallagher B.M. (1983). Monoclonal antibodies: The design of appropriate carrier and evaluation systems. In: Lambrecht R.M., Eckelman W.C. (Eds). Animal models in radiotracer design. Heidelberg: Springer Verlag. pp 60-106.

Gallagher M., Nicolle M.M. (1993). Animal models of normal aging: relationship between cognitive decline and markers in hippocampal circuitry. Behav Brain Res. 57(2):155-62.

Galleti G., Gavicchi G., Ussia G. (1982). Replication of Mycobacterium leprae in hibernating ground squirrels. (Citellus tridecemlineatus). 88:23-31.

Gamerman L.C., Rosenkrauz A., Schor N., Ghiraldini M.A., Jurkiewiez A., Ajzen H., Romos O.L. (1985). Characteristics of spontaneously hypertensive, Wistar Kyoto and Munich Wistar rats bred in Brazil. Braz J Med Biol Res. 18:513-8.

Gammal S., Basile A., Geller D., Skolnick P., Jones E. (1990). Reversal of the behavioral and electrophysiological abnormalities of an animal model of hepatic encephalopathy by benzodiazepine receptor ligands. Hepatology 11(3):371-8.

Gangadharan P.R., Edwards C.K. 3rd., Murphy P.S., Pratt P.F. (1983). An acute infection model for mycolobacterium intracellulare disease using beige mice: preliminary results. Am Rev Respir Dis. 127:648-9.

Gao Y., van A. H., Kamphorst W. (1990). Observations on experimental saccular aneurysms in the rat after 2 and 3 months. Neurol Res 12(4):260-3.

Garavilla L, Babbs C.F., Tacker W.A. (1984). An experimental circulatory arrest model in the rat to evaluate calcium antagonists in cerebral resuscitation. Am J Emerg. 2:321-6.

Garcia J.H. (1984). Experimental ischemic stroke: a review. Stroke. 15:5-14.

Garcia-Dorado D., Theroux P., Elizaga J., Galinanes M., Salares J., Riesgo M., Gomes M.J., Garcia-Dorado A., Fernandez-Aviles F. (1987). Myocardial reperfusion in the pig heart model: infarct size and duration of coronary occlusion. Cardiovasc Res. 21:537-44.

Gardner K.D. Jr., Reed W.P., Evan A.P., Zadaliz J., Hylarides M.D., Leon A.A. (1987). Endotoxin provocation of experimental renal cystic disease. Kidney Int. 32:329-43.

Gardner M. (1989). SIV infected rhesus macaques: an AIDS model for immunoprevention and immunotherapy. Adv Exp Med Biol 251:279-93.

Gardner M.B. (1987). Naturally occurring leukaemia viruses in wild mice: how good a model for human? Cancer Surg. 6:55-71.

Gardner W.A., Culberson D.E., Scimeca J.M., Brady A.G., Pindak F.F., Abee C.R. (1987). Experimental genital trichomoniasis in the squirrel monkey (Saimiri sciureus). Genitourin Med. June: 63:188-91.

Garlepp M.J., Kay P.H., Farrow B.R., Dawkins R.L. (1984). Autoimmunity in spontaneous myasthenia gravis in dogs. Clin Immunol Immunopthol. 31:301-6.

Garnett R., Fairman R.P., Glauser F.L. (1987). Ethchlorvynol-induced pulmonary edema: a chronically instrumented, awake sheep model mimicking human disease. Am J Med Sci. 294:317-23.

Garside P., Behnke JM., Rose R. (1989). The immune response of male DSN hamsters to a primary infection with Ancylostoma ceylanicum. J Helminthol 63(3):251-60.

Garson A. Jr. (1984). Ventricular dysrhythmias after congenital heart surgery: a canine model. Pediatr Res. 18:1112-20.

Gartner L.M., Allonso E. (1993). Physiologic jaundice of the newborn: animal models of perinatal development. Adv Vet Sci Comp Med. 37:61-86.

Gauntt C., Higdon A., Bowers D., Maull E., Wood J., Crawley R. (1993). What lessons can be learned from animal model studies in viral heart disease? Scand J Infect Dis Suppl 88:49-65.

Gause E.M., Mendez V., Geller I. (1985). Exploratory studies of a rodent model for inhalant abuse. Neurobehav Toxicol Teratol. 7:143-8.

Gay W.I. (1984). The dog as a research subject. Physiologist. 27:133-41.

Genin C., Laurent B., Sabatier J.C., Colon S., Berthoux F.C. (1986). IgA mesangial deposits in C3H/HeJ mice after oral immunization with ferritin or bovine serum albumin. Clin Exp Immunol. 63:385-94.

Gennarelli T.A., Thibault L.E., Adams J.H., Graham D.I., Thompson C.J., Marcincin R.R. (1982). Diffuse axnol injury and traumatic coma in the primate. Ann neurol. 12:564-74.

Genta R.M., Harper J.S.3d., Gam A.A., London W.I. et al. (1984). Experimental disseminated strongyloidiasis in Erythrocebus patas. II. Immunology Am J Trop med Hyg. 33:444-50.

Gerberding J.L., Sande M.A. (1986). Limitations of animal models in predicting beta-lactam efficacy for endocarditis and meningitis. Rev Infect Dis. 3:S315-8.

Gerberick G., Ryan C. (1990). A predictive mouse ear-swelling model for investigating topical photoallergy. Food Chem Toxicol 28(5):361-8.

Gericke D. (1988): AIDS also an experimental problem. Selection of experimental animals is difficult - no new therapeutic approaches in view. Fortschr Med. 30;106(25):19-20. (German)

Gerin J.L., Tennant B.C., Ponzetto A., Purcell R.H. (1983). The woodchuck animal model of hepatitis B-like virus infection and disease. Prog Clin Biol Res. 143:23-8.

Gerovich L.M., Vinnik E.M., malkin Vishnevetskii F.E. (1985). Pathogenetic aspects of papain-induced emphysema in rabbits. Patol Fiziol Eksp Ter. May-June (3):47-9. (English Abstract) (Russian)

Gerritsen G.C. (1982). The Chinese hamster as a model for the study of diabetes mellitus. Diabetes. 31 (Suppl 1 Pt 2):14-23.

Gerrity L.W., Friedman J.M. (1982). Choosing animal models of human inborn errors of metabolism. Prog Clin Biol Res. 94:459-61.

Gerundini P., Savi A., Giraldi M.C. et al. (1986). Evaluation in dogs and humans of three potential technetium-99m myocardial perfusion agents. J Nucl Med. 27:409-16.

Gessman L.J., Agarwal J.B., Endo T., Helpant R.H. (1983). Localization and mechanism of ventricular tachycardia by ice mapping 1 week after the onset of myocardial infarction in dogs. Circulation. 68:657-66.

Ghafoor S.Y., Smith H.V., Lee W.R., Quinn R., Girwood R.W. (1984). Experimental ocular toxocariasis: a mouse model. Br J Ophthalmol. 68:89-96.

Gherezghiher T., Koss M. (1989). Argon laser-induced ocular hypertension: animal model of ocular inflammation. J Ocul Pharmacol 5(1):7-17.

Gherezghiher T., March W.F., Nordquist R.E., Koss M.C. (1986). Laser-induced glaucoma in rabbits. Exp Eye Res. 43:885-94.

Ghonien G.M., Shoukry M.S., VandenBerg T.L., Roberts J.A. (1994). Monkey as an animal model. Neurourol Urodyn. 13(2):181-98.

Ghosh A.K., Gosh D.K. (1987). Infection pattern of leishmaniasis in hamster produced by recent isolates from kala-azar patients in India. Indian J Med Res. 86:14-9.

Ghosh P., Armstrong S., Read R., Numata Y., Smith S., McNair P., Marshall R. (1993). Animal models of early osteoarthritis: their use for the evaluation of potential chondroprotective agents. Agents Actions Suppl 39:195-206.

Gibson R.E., Schneidau T.A., Cohen V.I., Sood V., Ruch J., Melograna J., Eckelman W.C., Reba R.C. (1989). In vitro and in vivo characteristics of I-125(R)-3-quinuclidinyl (S)-4-iodobenzilate. J Nucl Med. 30:1079-87.

Giebink G. (1989). Studies of Streptococcus pneumoniae and influenza virus vaccines in the chinchilla otitis media model. Pediatr Infect Dis J 8(1 Suppl):S42-4.

Gilbert F., Tsao K.L., Lalatta F., Xu L., Potluri V..R., LaBadie G. (1988): Human neuroblastoma metastases in a nude mouse model: tumor progression and onc gene amplication. Prog Clin Res. 271:17-29.

Gilbert J.M. (1987). Experimental colorectal cancer as a model of human disease. Ann R Coll Surg Engl. 69:48-53.

Giles A.R. (1994). Functional, biochemical, and morphological evaluations of experimental hemophilia therapies in animal models. Semin Hematol. 31(2 Suppl 4):56-9.

Gill N.J., Ganguly N.K., Muhajan R.C., Bhusnurmath S.R., Dilawari J.B. (1983). Progesterone-induced amoebic liver abscess in guinea-pigs - a new model. Trans R Soc Trop Med Hyg. 77:53-8.

Gillet P., Bannwarth B., Charriere G., Leroux P., Fener P., Netter P., Hartmann DJ., Pere P., Gaucher A. (1989). Studies on type II collagen induced arthritis in rats: an experimental model of peripheral and axial ossifying enthesopathy. J Rheumatol 16(6):721-8.

Gimenez-Conti I.B., Slaga T.J. (1993). The hamster cheek pouch carcinogenesis model. J Cell Biochem Suppl. 17F:83-90.

Gingras J., Weese-Mayer D. (1990). Maternal cocaine addiction. II: An animal model for the study of brainstem mechanisms operative in sudden infant death syndrome. Med Hypotheses 33:231-4.

Ginsberg M.D., Reivich M., Giandomenico A., Greenberg J.H. (1977). Local glucose utilization in acute focal cerebral ischemia: Local dysmetabolism and diaschisis. Neurology 27:1042-8.

Girlia V., Danilenko A. (1991). [Acute experimental enzymatic cholecystitis (clinico-morphological comparisons)] Ostryi eksperimental'nyi fermentativnyi kholetsistit (kliniko-morfologicheskie sopostavleniia). Klin Khir (4):24-6.

Gisvold S.E., Safar P., Rao G., Moossy J., Kelseys Alexander H. (1984). Multifaceted therapy after global brain ischemia in monkeys. Stroke. 15:803-12.

Githure J.I., Reid G.D., Binhazim A.A., Anjili C.O., Shatry A.M. (1987). Leishmania major: the suitability of East African nonhuman primates as animal models for cutaneous leishmaniasis. Exp parasitol. 64:438-47.

Gitsu G.A., Kovalenko F.P. (1983). Susceptibility of djungarian hamsters, cotton rats and white rats to experimental Opisthorchis infection. Med Parasitol (Mosk). 5:63-4. (English Abstract). (Russian)

Gkonos P.J., Hayes T., Burtis W., Jacoby R., McGuire J., Baron R. et al. (1984). Squamous carcinoma model of humoral hypercalcemia of malignancy. Endocrinology. 115:2384-90.

Glaser T., Lane J., Housman D. (1990). A mouse model of the aniridia-Wilms tumor deletion syndrome. Science 250(4982):823-7.

Glauser M.P., Francoili P. (1987). Relevance of animal models of the prophylaxis of infective endocarditis. J Antimicrob Chemother. 20 Suppl A:87-98.

Glavin G., Pinsky C., Bose R. (1990). Domoic acid-induced neurovisceral toxic syndrome: characterization of an animal model and putative antidotes. Brain Res Bull 24(5):701-3.

Gleicher N. (1987). A potential animal model for autoimmune reproductive failure [editorial]. Am J Reprod Immunol Microbiol. 14:122.

Glockner R. (1986). Mortality rate and body mass development of premature rats delivered by caesarean section. Z Versuchstierkd,. 28:147-52.

Gluckert K., Koch-Kallnbach M., Liebig K., Weseloh G. (1983). Comparison of biochemical studies in experimental and human arthrosis. Z Rheumatol. 42:195-8. (German)

Goa T.L. (1981). Experimental arrrhythmic models in mice and the factors affecting them. Chung Hua Hsin Hsueh Kuan Ping Tsa Chih. 9:223-7. (English Abstract) (Chinese)

Goetz C.G., Klawans H.L., Carvey P. (1983). Animal models of tardive dyskinesia: their use in the search for new treatment methods. Mod Probl Pharamacopsychiatry. 21:5-20.

Goke B. (1990). A critical appraisal of studies of the pancreas. Animal models used in pancreas research: studies on feedback regulations of the pancreas. Int J Pancreatol 6(3):181-8.

Golan A. (1987). Surgical induction of endometriosis in the rat. Fertil Steril. 47:359-60.

Golan A., Winston R.M., Dargenio R. (1984). Experimental endometriosis: a microsurgical animal model in rats. Isr J Med Sci. 20:1094-6.

Golda V., Petr R. (1988). Genetically based animal model of depression: cholinergic supersensitivity. Act Nerv Super (Praha) 30(4):292-4.

Golda V., Petr R. (1990). Animal model of anxiety: the effect of methyldopa in the genetically hypertensive non-obese rats of Koletsky type and in the rats of Wistar strain. Sb Ved Pr Lek Fak Karlovy Univerzity Hradci Kralove 33(5):529-37.

Golda V., Petr R. (1990). Validation of aversion towards open space and height as a measure of anxiety in the genetically based animal model of depression. Sb Ved Pr Lek Fak Karlovy Univerzity Hradci Kralove 33(5):513-27.

Golden J.G., Hughes H.C., Lang C.M. (1980). Experimental toxemia in the pregnant guinea pig. (Cavia porcellus). Lab Anim Sci. 30 (2 Pt 1):174-9.

Goldin R. (1994). Rodent models of alcoholic liver disease. Int J Exp Pathol. 75(1):1-7.

Goldman M., Frame B., Singal DP., Blajchman M. (1991). Effect of blood transfusion on survival in a mouse bacterial peritonitis model. Transfusion 31(8):710-2.

Goldstein L., Davis J. (1990). Beam-walking in rats: studies towards developing an animal model of functional recovery after brain injury. J Neurosci Methods 31(2):101-7.

Goldstein M., Kuga S., Kusano N., Meller E., Dancis J. Schwarez R. (1986). Dopamine agonist induced self-multilative biting behavior in monkeys with unilateral ventromedial tegmental lesions of the brainstem: possible pharmacological model for Leach-Nyhan syndrome. Brain Res. 367:114-20.

Gole G., Browning J., Elts S. (1990). The mouse model of oxygen-induced retinopathy: a suitable animal model for angiogenesis research. Doc Ophthalmol 74(3):163-9.

Gomez C.M., Wollmann R.L., Richman D.P. (1984). Induction of the morphologic changes of both acute and chronic experimental myasthenia by monoclonal antibody directed against acetylcholine receptor. Acta Neuropathol (Berl). 63:131-43.

Gomez S., Vicente V. (1988). Epithelial cutaneous lesions induced in Dunkin-Hartley albino guinea-pigs by means of 7,12-dimethyl-benzanthracene. Br J Dermatol 119(6):743-50.

Gomita Y., Ogawa N., Ueki S. (1985). Effects of psychotropic drugs on discrimination conditioning in olfactory bulbectomized rats. Pharmacol Biochem Behav. 22:717-22.

Gomoll A., Lekich R. (1990). Use of the ferret for a myocardial ischemia/salvage model. J Pharmacol Methods 23(3):213-23.

Gonczol E., Danczig E., Baldogh I., Toth T., Vaczi L. (1985). In vivo model for the acute, latent and reactivated phases of cytomegalovirus infection. Acta Microbiol Hung. 32:39-47.

Gonda M., Oberste M., Garvey K., Pallansch L., Battles J., Pifat D., Bess J., Nagashima K. (1990). Development of the bovine immunodeficiency-like virus as a model of lentivirus disease. Dev Biol Stand 72:97-110.

Gonzales-Crussi F., Hsueh E. (1983). Experimental model of ischemic bowel necrosis. The role of platelet-activating factor and endotoxin. Am J Pathol. 112:127-35.

Gonzalez Reimers C.E., Santolaria Fernandez F.T., Batista Lopez N., Gonzalez Hernandez T., Hernandez Garcia M., Essardas Daryanani H., Rodriquez Moreno F., Ferres Torres R. (1988): Histomorphometric analysis of hepatocyte changes in hypothyroidism: experimental study in male albino mice. Rev Esp Enferm Apar Dig. 73(4):341-3. (English Abstract). (Spanish)

Goosen C. (1981). Abnormal behavior patterns in rhesus monkeys: symptoms of mental disease. Biol Psychiatry. 16:697-716.

Gopalakrishnakone P. (1985). Idiopathic toricollis. Torticollis in white Pekin ducks. Am J Pathol. 118:500-1.

Gopalakrishnakone P. (1986). Muscular dystrophy in white pekin ducks. Am J Pathol. 125:218-9.

Gordon J.R., Quigley J.P. (1986). Early spontaneous metastasis in the human epidermoid carcinoma HEp3/chick embryo model: contribution of incidental colonization. Int J Cancer. 38:437-44.

Gordon T.P., Reid C., Rozenbilds M.A., Ahern M. (1986). Crystal shedding in septic arthritis: case reports and in vivo evidence in an animal model. Aust NZ J Med. 16:336-40.

Gorin B., Krutovskikh V. (1988). [A method for inducing gallbladder cancer in Syrian hamsters] Metodika indutsirovaniia raka zhelchnogo puzyria u siriiskikh khomiakov. Eksp Onkol 10(6):60-1.

Goriunova A.G., Savinov A.P. (1987). Persistent infection caused by the Coxackie B3 virus in adult mice. Vopr Virusol. 32:213-6. (English Abstract). (Russian)

Gorka Z., Earley B., Leonard B.E. (1985). Effect of bilateral olfactory bulbectomy in the rat, alone or in combination with antidepressants, on the learned immobility model of depression. Neuropsychobiology. 13:26-30.

Gotoff S.P., Odell C., Papierniak C.K., Klegerman M.E., Boyer K.M. (1986). Human IgG antibody to group b Streptococcus type III: comparison of protective levels in a murine model with levels in infected human neonates. J Infect Dis. 153:511-9.

Goudsmit J., Van der Wools F.W. (1986). Scrapie and its association with amyloid-like fibrils and glycoproteins encoded by cellular genes: an animal model for human dementia.. Prog Brain Res. 70:391-8.

Goulbourne I.A., Davies G.C. (1986). Bacteriology of the closed duodenal loop model of acute pancreatic ultrastructural changes induced in the lungs. J Surg. Res 41:600-8.

Gould E., Bres M. (1986). Regurgitation in gorillas: possible model for human eating disorders (rumination/bulimia). J Dev Behav Pediatr. 7:314-9.

Gould M.N. (1993). The introduction of activated oncogenes to mammary cells in vivo using retroviral vectors: a new model for the chemoprevention of premalignant and malignant lesions of the breast. J Cell Biochem Suppl. 17G:66-72.

Gould S.F., Powell D., nett T., Globe L.M. (1983). A rat model for chemotherapy-induced male infertility. Arch Androl. 11:141-50.

Gower A.J., Lamberty Y. (1993). The aged mouse as a model of cognitive decline with special emphasis on studies in NMRI mice. Behav Brain Res. 57(2):163-73.

Gracia R. J., Ferrandez L. A., Guallart L. A., Moros G., Alvarez A. R., Garcia J. G. (1990). [Experimental cryptorchism in the Wistar rat] Criptorquidia experimental en rata Wistar. Cir Pediatr 3(3):97-102.

Graf T. (1984). Mechanism of virus-induced leukemogenesis in an animal model system. Klin Padiatr. 196:125-9. (English Abstract).

Graf W., Sundin A., Glimelius B., Ahlstrom H., Carlsson J. (1992). Induction and quantification of hepatic metastases from a human colonic cancer in the nude rat. Eur J Surg Oncol 18:608-14.

Graham L., Vasil A., Vasil M., Voelkel N., Stenmark K. (1990). Decreased pulmonary vasoreactivity in an animal model of chronic Pseudomonas pneumonia. Am Rev Respir Dis 142(1):221-9.

Graham W., Clarke C., Boyce S., Sambrook M., Crossman A., Woodruff G. (1990). Autoradiographic studies in animal models of hemi-parkinsonism reveal dopamine D2 but not D1 receptor supersensitivity. II. Unilateral intra-carotid infusion of MPTP in the monkey (Macaca fascicularis). Brain Res 514(1):103-10.

Graham W., Crossman A., Woodruff G. (1990). Autoradiographic studies in animal models of hemi-parkinsonism reveal dopamine D2 but not D1 receptor supersensitivity. I. 6-OHDA lesions of ascending mesencephalic dopaminergic pathways in the rat. Brain Res 514(1):93-102.

Grana D., Beigelman R., Milei J. (1989). [Genetically hypertensive rats: a model for essential arterial hypertension] Ratas geneticamente hipertensas: modelos de hipertension arterial esencial. Medicina (B Aires) 49(4):379-86.

Grant K.A., Samson H.H. (1985). Oral self administration of ethanol in free feeding rats. Alcohol. 2:317-21.

Grashchenkova O.V., Zykov M.P. (1985). Evaluation of Mycobacterium tuberculosis virulence by the intracerebral infection of guinea pigs. Probl. Tuberk. 8:56-9. (English Abstract). (Russian)

Grau M., Balasch J. (1985). Protective effects of cerebroactive drugs in a model of acute hypoxia. Gen Pharmacol. 16:37-41.

Green M.A. (1987). A potential copper radiopharmaceutical for imaging the heart and brain: Copper-labeled pyrunvaldehyde Bis(N⁴-methylthiosemicarbazone). Nucl Med Biol. 14:59-61.

Green M.T., Rosborough J.P., Dunkel E.C. (1982). In vivo reactivation of herpes simplex virus in rabbit trigeminal ganglia: electrode model. Infect Immun. 34:69-74.

Green S.T., Green F.A. (1987): The Manx cat: an animal model for neural tube defects. Mater Med Pol. 19(4):219-21.

Greene B.M. (1987). Primate model for onchocerciasis research. Ciba Found Symp. 127:236-43.

Gregory D.W., Cardella M.A., Myers L.L. (1983). Lamb model in the study of immunity to enteropathogenic Escherichia coli infections. Am J Vet Res. 44:2073-7.

Grencis R.K. (1993). Cytokine-mediated regulation of intestinal helminth infections: the Trichuris muris model. Ann Trop Med Parasitol. 87(6):643-7.

Gretz N., Meisinger E., Strauch M. (1988). Partial nephrectomy and chronic renal failure: the 'mature' rat model. Contrib Nephrol 60:46-55.

Gretz N., Meisinger E., Waldherr R., Strauch M. (1988). Acute renal failure after 5/6 nephrectomy: histological and functional changes. Contrib Nephrol 60:56-63.

Gretz N., Strauch M. (Ed.) (1993). Experimental and genetic rat models of chronic renal failure. Basel; New York: Karger. 343 P.

Grieve R.B., Griffing S.A., Goldschmidt M.H., Abraham D. (1985). Transplantation of adult Dirofilaria immitis into Lewis rats: parasitologic and serologic findings. J. Parasitol. 71:391-2.

Griez E. (1984). Experimental models of anxiety. Problems and perspectives. Acta Psychiatr Belg. 84:511-32.

Griffeth J.K., Gallagher T.J., Packer D.L. (1988): Hemodynamic effects of nifedipine in a canine model of acid aspiration. Anesth Analg. 67(12):1166-8.

Griffith B.P., McCormick S.R., Booss J., Huiung G.D. (1986). Inbred guinea pig model of intrauterine infection with cytomegalovirus. Am J Pathol. 122:112-9.

Griffiths-Johnson D., Karol M. (1991). Validation of a non-invasive technique to assess development of airway hyperreactivity in an animal model of immunologic pulmonary hypersensitivity. Toxicology 65(3):283-94.

Groffen J., Voncken J.W., Kaartinen V., Morris C., Heisterkamp N. (1993). Ph-positive leukemia: a transgenic mouse model. Leuk Lymphoma 11(Suppl 1):19-24.

Gross D.R. (1994). Animal models in cardiovascular research. 2nd rev. ed. Dordrecht; Boston: Kluwer Academic Publishers.

Gruys E., Snel F.W. (1994). Animal models for reactive amyloidosis. Baillieres Clin Rheumatol. 8(3):599-611.

Grynpas M.D., Simmons E.D., Carnes D., Gundberg C., Pritzker K.P. (1987). Bone mineral in the castrated rat model of osteopenia. J Orthop Res. 5:586-91.

Guan Z., Ricard G., Charest-Boule L., Neilson K., Kiruluta G. (1990). Augmentation cystoplasty in rats: development of an animal model. J Urol 144(2 Pt 2):461-5; discussion 474.

Gudnodottir M. (1981). Slow viral infections of animals: experimental models for human disease. M Med Biol Res. 59:77-84.

Guerreiro D., Lennox S., Anderson RH. (1988). Experimental ventricular hypertrophy in growing pigs. Int J Cardiol 21(3):311-22.

Guinee P.A., Jensen W.H., Petes P.W. (1985). Vibrio cholerae infection and acquired immunity in an adult rabbit model. Zentralbl Bakteriol Mikrobiol. Hyg. 259:118-31.

Gündisch D., Lambrecht R.M. (1995). unpublished.

Gurguis G., Klein E., Mefford I., Uhde T. (1990). Biogenic amines distribution in the brain of nervous and normal pointer dogs. A genetic animal model of anxiety. Neuropsychopharmacology 3(4):297-303.

Gushchin I.S., Zebrev A.I., Bogush N.L., Aleshkin V.A., Ponomareva A.M. (1986). An experimental model for the elaboration and evaluation of the methods of control of immediate allergy. Patol Fiziol Eksp Ter. 4:18-23. (English Abstract). (Russian)

Guthke R., Veckenstedt A., Guttner J., Stracke R., Bergter F. (1987). Dynamic model of the pathogenesis of Mengo virus infection in mice. Acta Virol (Praha). 31:307-20.

Gutschik E. (1983). Experimental Staphylococcal endorcarditis: an overview. Scand J. Infect Dis [Suppl]. 41:87-94.

Guy-Grand B. (1988): Value of animal models for understanding human obesity. Journ Annu Diabetol Hotel Dieu. 55-61. (French).

Gysin J., Aikawa M., Tourneur N., Tegoshi T. (1992). Experimental Plasmodium falciparum cerebral malaria in the squirrel monkey Saimiri sciureus. Exp Parasitol 75(4):390-8.

Gysin J., Fandeur T. (1983). Saimiri sciureus (karyotype 14-7): an alternative experimental model of Plasmodium falciparum infection. Am J Trop Med Hyp. 32:461-7.

Haas K. (1993). Lest we forget: our investment in animal research. J Am Vet Med Assoc 202(7):1061-2.

Habenicht U.F., Schwarz K., Neumann F., el Etreby M.F. (1987). Induction of estrogen-related hyperplastic changes in the prostate of the cynomolgus monkey (Macaca Fascicularis) by androstenedione and its antagonization by the aromatase inhibitor 1-methyl-androsta-1-4-diene-3-17-dione. Prostate: 11:313-26.

Hackett R., Huang T., Berger R. (1988). Experimental Escherichia coli epididymitis in rabbits. Urology 32(3):236-40.

Hafner H., Behrens S., De V. J., Gattaz WF. (1991). An animal model for the effects of estradiol on dopamine-mediated behavior: implications for sex differences in schizophrenia. Psychiatry Res 38(2):125-34.

Hagan M., Moss D. (1991). An animal model of bulimia nervosa: opioid sensitivity to fasting episodes. Pharmacol Biochem Behav 39(2):421-2.

Hagenbeck A., Martens A. (1990). Minimal residual disease in acute leukemia: lessons learned from animal models. Hamatol Bluttransfus 33:31-5.

Hale S.L., Kloner R.A. (1994). Experience from experimental models in the quest to protect myocardium from ischemic damage: update on preconditioning strategies. Curr Opin Cardiol. 9(4):411-6.

Halldin C., Farde L., Högberg T., Mohell N., Hall H., Suhara T., Karlsson P., Nakashima Y., Swahn C.G. (1995).Carbon-11-FLB 457: A radioligand for extrastriatal D2 dopamine receptors. J Nucl Med. 36:1275-81.

Hamada E., Iwano T., Ushiro K., Tada N., Kinoshita T., Kumazawa T. (1993). Animal model of otitis media with effusion. Acta Otolaryngol Suppl (Stockholm) 500:70-4.

Hamaguchi F., Hamaguchi Y., Juhn S., Sakakura Y. (1988). The relationship between antigen levels and middle ear inflammation in antigen-induced otitis media in the chinchilla. Arch Otorhinolaryngol 245(1):42-6.

Hamm B., Taupitz M. (1993). [A liver tumor model in the rat suitable for experimental MRT] Ein für die experimentelle MRT geeignetes Lebertumormodell der Ratte. Rofo Fortschr Geb Röntgenstr Neuen Bildgeb Verfahr 158(4):332-6.

Hammarstrom L., Abedi M.R., Hassan M.S., Smith C.I. (1993). The SCID mouse as a model for autoimmunity. J Autoimmun. 6(6):667-74.

Hammer R., Maika S., Richardson J., Tang J., Taurog J. (1990). Spontaneous inflammatory disease in transgenic rats expressing HLA-B27 and human beta 2m: an animal model of HLA-B27-associated human disorders. Cell 63(5):1099-112.

Hammock B., Beale A., Work T., Gee SJ., Gunther R., Higgins R., Shinka T., Castagnoli N. J. (1989). A sheep model for MPTP induced Parkinson-like symptoms. Life Sci 45(17):1601-8.

Hammond W., Teplitz R., Benfield J. (1991). Lung cancer model for study of the metastatic process. Ann Thorac Surg 52(4):732-6; discussion 737.

Hammond W.G., Benfield J.R. (1993). Hamster bronchial carcinogenesis induced by carcinogen-containing sustained release implants placed endobronchially: a clinically relevant model. J Cell Biochem Suppl. 17F:104-17.

Hanauer G. (1989). [Radioiodine administration for the production of an athyreotic animal model] Radioiodapplikation zur Herstellung eines athyreoten Modelltieres. Z Versuchstierkd 32(1):7-15.

Handa Y., Hayashi M., Takeuchi H., Kobayashi H., Kawano H., Kabuto M. (1991). Effect of cyclosporine on the development of cerebral vasospasm in a primate model. Neurosurgery 28(3):380-5; discussion 385-6.

Handley S.L., McBlane J.W. (1993). Serotonin mechanisms in animal models of anxiety. Braz J Med Biol Res. 26(1):1-13.

Hanel H., Braun B., Loschhorn K. (1990). Experimental dermatophytosis in nude guinea pigs compared with infections in Pirbright White animals. Mycoses 33(4):179-89.

Hankins G., Snyder R., Clark S., Schwartz L., Patterson W., Butzin C. (1993). Acute hemodynamic and respiratory effects of amniotic fluid embolism in the pregnant goat model. Am J Obstet Gynecol 168(4):1113-29; discussion 1129-30.

Hannigan J., Abel E., Kruger M. (1993). "Population" characteristics of birthweight in an animal model of alcohol-related developmental effects. Neurotoxicol Teratol 15(2):97-105.

Hansen J., Bing G., Notter M., Kordower J., Fiandaca M., Gash D. (1989). Adrenal chromaffin cells as transplants in animal models of Parkinson's disease. J Electron Microsc Tech 12:308-15.

Hansen R.J., Walzem R.L. (1993). Avian fatty liver hemorrhagic syndrome: a comparative review. Adv Vet Sci Comp Med. 37:451-68.

Hantraye P., Leroy-Willig A., Denys D., Riche D., Isacson O., Maziere M., Syrota A. (1992). Magnetic resonance imaging to monitor pathology of caudate-putamen after excitotoxin-induced neural loss in the nonhuman primate brain. Exp Neurol. 118:18-23.

Hantraye P., Loc'h C., Maziere B., Khalili-Varasteh M., Crouzel C., Fournier D., Yorke JC. et al. (1992). 6-[^{18}F]fluoro-L-dopa uptake and [^{76}Br]bromolisuride binding in the excitotoxically lesioned caudate-putamen of nonhuman primates studied using positron emission tomography. Exp Neurol. 115:218-27.

Hantraye P., Varastet M., Peschanski M., Riche D., Cesaro P., Willer J.C., Maziere M. (1993). Stable Parkinsonian syndrome and uneven loss of striatal dopamione fibres following chronic MPTP administration in baboons. Neuroscience 53(1):169-78.

Hardy S., Gough M. (1991). Pharmacological manipulation of gastrocnemius muscle blood flow in an animal model of reperfusion injury. J Biomed Eng 13(3):263-6.

Hargens A., Millard R., Petterson K., Hässle AB., Johansen K. (1987) Nature Sept. 3 p. 59.

Harkema J.R., Hotchkiss J.A. (1993). Ozone- and endotoxin-induced mucous cell metaplasias in rat airway epithelium: novel animal models to study toxicant-induced epithelial transformation in airways. Toxicol Lett. 68(1-2):251-63.

Harris J. (1989). Experimental animal modeling of depression and anxiety. Psychiatr Clin North Am 12(4):815-36.

Harris M., Douglas S. (1990). Nutritional influence on neonatal infections in animal models and man. Ann N Y Acad Sci 587:246-56.

Harris S., Davis N.K., Jowett M.I., Rees E.S., Topps S. (1993). Transgenic animals as tools in drug development. Agent Actions 38(Spec No.):C57-8.

Hart D., Garlepp M., Fritzler M. (1989). Plasma proteinase regulation during disease progression in murine models of SLE. J Clin Lab Immunol 30(1):27-34.

Hart H.L.A. (1980). Are There Any Natural Rights? D. Lyons (ed.), Wadsworth, Belmont, California.

Hartley P., Neill D., Hagler M., Kors D., Vogel G. (1990). Procedure- and age-dependent hyperactivity in a new animal model of endogenous depression. Neurosci Biobehav Rev 14:69-72.

Hartman A., Powell C., Schultz C., Oaks E., Eckels K. (1991). Small-animal model to measure efficacy and immunogenicity of Shigella vaccine strains. Infect Immun 59(11):4075-83.

Hartvig P., Nagren K., Lundberg P.O., Muhr C., Terenius L., Lundqvist H., Langstrom B. (1986). Kinetics of four carbon-11 labelled enkephalen peptides in the brain pituitary and plasma of Rhesus monkeys. Regulat Peptides 16:1-13.

Harvey S. (1990). "Paradoxical" growth hormone secretion in acromegaly: an avian model? J Exp Zool Suppl 4.195-9.

Hasey G., Hanin I. (1991). The cholinergic-adrenergic hypothesis of depression reexamined using clonidine, metoprolol, and physostigmine in an animal model. Biol Psychiatry 29(2):127-38.

Haskins M., Aguirre G., Jezyk P., Schuchman E., Desnick R., Patterson D. (1991). Mucopolysaccharidosis type VII (Sly syndrome). Beta-glucuronidase-deficient mucopolysaccharidosis in the dog. Am J Pathol 138(6):1553-5.

Hatazawa J., Hatano K., Ishiwala K., Itoh M., Ido T. et al. (1991). Measurement of D_2 dopamine receptor-specific carbon-11 YM-09151-2 binding in the canine brain by PET: Importance of partial volume correction. J Nucl Med. 32:713-8.

Hatch G.E., Raub J.A., Graham J.A. (1984). Functional and biochemical indicators of pneumoconiosis in mice: comparison with rats. J Toxicol Environ Health. 13:487-97.

Hathaway S.C., Blackmore D.K., Marshall R.B. (1983). Leptospirosis and the maintenance host: a laboratory mouse model. Rest Vet Sci. 34:82-9.

Hatton D.C., McCarron D.A. (1994). Dietary calcium and blood pressure in experimental models of hypertension. A review. Hypertension 23(4):513-30.

Hauer-Jensen M., Poulakos L., Osborne JW. (1988). Effects of accelerated fractionation on radiation injury of the small intestine: a new rat model. Int J Radiat Oncol Biol Phys 14:1205-12.

Havel R.J., Kita T., Kotite L., Kane J.P., Hamilton R.L., Goldstein J.L., Brown M.S. (1982). Concentration and composition of lipoproteins in blood plasma of the WHHL rabbit. An animal model of human familial hypercholesterolemia. Arteriosclerosis. 2:467-74.

Hawkins R., Choi Y., Scates S., Rege S., Hoh CK., Glaspy J., Phelps M. (1993). An animal model for in vivo evaluation of tumor glycolytic rates with positron emission tomography. J Surg Oncol 53(2):104-9.

Hawthorne J.D., Lorenz D., Albrecht P. (1982). Infection of marmosets with para-influenza virus types 1 and 3. Infect immun. 37:1037-41.

Hay J., Graham D.I., Hutchison W.M., Siim J.C. (1985). Meningo-encephalitis accompanying retinochoroiditis in a murine model of congenital toxoplasmosis. Ann Trop med Parasitol. 79 21-9.

Hay J., Lee W.R., Dutton G.N., Hutchinson W.M., Siim J.C. (1984). Congenital toxoplasmic retinochoroiditis in a mouse model. Ann Trop Med Parasitol. 78:109-16.

Hay J.B. (Ed). (1982). Animal models of Immunological Processes. Academic Press, New York.

Hay R.J., Calderson R.A., Collins M.J. (1983). Experimental dermatophytosis: the clinical and histopathologic features of a mouse model using Trichophyton quinckeanum (mouse favus). J Invest Dermatol. 81:270-4.

Hayashi T., Dorko M. (1988). A rat model for the study of intrauterine growth retardation. Am J Obstet Gynecol 158(5):1203-7.

Hayashi Y., Kurashima C., Utsuyama M., Hirokawa K. (1989). An animal model of autoimmune sialadenitis in aged mice. Pathol Immunopathol Res 8(2):118-24.

Hayek T., Ito Y., Azrolan N., Verdery R., Aalto-Setala K., Walsh A., Breslow J. (1993). Dietary fat increases high density lipoprotein (HDL) levels both by increasing the transport rates and decreasing the fractional catabolic rates of HDL cholesterol ester and apolipoprotein (Apo) A-I. Presentation of a new animal model and mechanistic studies in human Apo A-I transgenic and control mice. J Clin Invest 91(4):1665-99.

Hayes J., Daniel R., Tee R., Barnes P., Taylor A., Chung K. (1992). Bronchial hyperreactivity after inhalation of trimellitic anhydride dust in guinea pigs after intradermal sensitization to the free hapten. Am Rev Respir Dis 146(5 Pt 1):1311-4.

Hazama F., Hashimoto N. (1987). An animal model of cerebral aneurysms. Neuropathol Appl Neurobiol. 13:77-90.

Healy C., Martin L., Roberts E., Rubin A. (1989). Experimental arthropathy induced in rhesus monkeys and DBA/1 mice by a novel method: intraperitoneal implantation of type II collagen adsorbed onto nitrocellulose filters. Lab Invest 60(3):462-70.

Hecker E. et al. (Ed.) (1993). Skin carcinogenesis in man and in experimental models. Berlin; New York: Springer Verlag. 364 P.

Hector R., Yee E., Collins M. (1990). Use of DBA/2N mice in models of systemic candidiasis and pulmonary and systemic aspergillosis. Infect Immun 58(5):1476-8.

Heesemann J., Gaede K., Autenrieth I.B. (1993). Experimental Yersinia enterocolitica infection in rodents: a model for human yersiniosis. APMIS 101(6):417-29.

Hegreberg G.A. (1982). Animal models of collagen disease. Prog Clin Biol Res. 94:229-44.

Heidemann H.T., Jackson E.K., Gerkens J.F., Workman R.J., Brough R.A. (1985). Unilaterally nephrectomized rat with aortic ligation: a uremic model of severe hypertension. Clin Exp Hypertens. 7:1109-20.

Heikkila R.E., Sonsalla P.K. (1987). The use of the MPTP-treated mouse as an animal model of parkinsonism. Can J Neurol Sci. Aug. 14 (3 Suppl):436-40.

Heine J., Moon H.W., Woodmansee O.B. (1984). Persistent Cryptosporidium infection in congenitally athymic (nude) mice. Infect Immun. 43:856-9.

Heininger K., Liebert U.G., Toyka K.V., Haneveld F.T., Schwendemann G., Kolb-Bachofen V. et al. (1984). Chronic inflammatory polyneuropathy. Reduction of nerve conduction velocities in monkeys by systemic passive transfer of immunoglobulin G. J Neurol Sci. 66:1-14.

Heiss W.D., Wienhard K., Graf R., Löttgen J., Pietrzyk U., Wagner R. (1995). High-resolution PET in cats: Application of a clinical camera to experimental studies. J Nucl Med. 36:493-8.

Hellerstrom C., Swenne I., Eriksson U.J. (1985). Is there an animal model for gestational diabetes? Diabetes. 34 Suppl 2:28-31.

Hendley E.D., Wessel D.J., Van Houten J. (1986). Inbreeding of Wistar-Kyoto rat strain with hyperactivity but without hypertension. Behav Neural Biol. 45:1-16.

Hendrich C.E., Jackson W.J., Porterfield S.P. (1984). Behavioral testing of progenies of Tx (hypothyroid) and growth hormone-treated Tx rats: an animal model for mental retardation. Neuroendocrinology. 38:429-37.

Hendricks J.C., Kline L.R., Kovalski R.J., O'Brien J.A., Marrison A.R., Pack A.I. (1987). The English bulldog: a natural model of sleep-disordered breathing. J App Physiol. 63:1344-50.

Hendrickson E.A. (1993). The SCID mouse: relevance as an animal model system for studying human disease. Am J Pathol. 143(6):1511-22.

Hendrickx A., Tarara R. (1990). Triamcinolone acetonide-induced meningocele and meningoencephalocele in Rhesus monkeys. Am J Pathol 136(3):725-7.

Hendrikson C.F.M., Koeter (Eds.) (1991). Animals in biomedical research. Replacement, reduction and refinement: Present possibilities and future prospects. New York: Elsevier. 290p.

Henne-Bruns D., Artwohl J., Broelsch C., Kremer B. (1988). Acetaminophen-induced acute hepatic failure in pigs: controversial results to other animal models. Res Exp Med (Berl) 188(6):463-72.

Henne-Bruns J.C., Gramminger K., Kruger U., Kremer B. (1987). Hepatocyte transplantation-development of a clinical model. Z Gastroenterol [Verh]. 22:61-5.

Henningsen G.M., Koller L.D., Exon J.H., Talcott P.A., Osborne C.A. (1984). A sensitive delayed-type hypersensitivity model in the rat for assessing in vivo cell-mediated immunity. J Immunol Methods. 70:153-65.

Henriques M.G., Silva P.M., Martins M.A., Flores C.A., Cunha F.Q., Assreuy-Filho J., Cardeiro R. (1987). Mouse paw edema. A new model for inflammation? Braz J Med Biol Res. 20:243-9.

Henry G.A., Jarnot B.M., Steinhoff M.M., Bigazzi P.E. (1988): Mercury-induced renal autoimmunity in the MAXX rat. Clin Immunol Immunopathol. 49(2):187-203.

Henry K.R., Chole R.A. (1987). Genetic and functional analysis of the otosclerosis-like condition of the LP/J mouse. Audiology. 26: 44-55.

Henry M.A., Sweet R.S., Tange J.D. (1983). A new reproducible experimental model of analgesic nephropathy. J Pathol. 139:23-32.

Hepp A., Schier H., Kochsiek K. (1984). Is the rat a suitable model for studying alcoholic cardiomyopathy. Hemodynamic studies at various stages of chronic alcohol ingestion. Basic Res Cardiol. 79:230-7.

Heraief E., Glauser M.P., Freedman L.R. (1982). Natural history of aortic valve endocarditis in rats. Infect Immun. 37:127-31.

Herr M.D., McInerney J.J., Copenhaver G.L., Morris D.L. (1988): Coronary artery embolization in closed-chest canines using flexible radiopaque plugs. J Appl Physiol. 64(5):2236-9.

Herrera C. (1982). Mice with persistent gastrointestinal Candida albicans as a model for antifungal therapy. Antimicrob Agents Chemother. 21:51-3.

Herring S., Abildgaard C., Shitanishi K., Harrison J., Gendler S., Heldebrant C. (1993). Human coagulation factor IX: assessment of thrombogenicity in animal models and viral safety. J Lab Clin Med 121(3):394-405.

Herrmann T., Voigtmann L., Knorr A., Lorenz J., Jogansen U. (1986). Dose-time correlation in the irradiation of the lung of piglets of evaluating a model of human radiogenic pneumopathy. Med Radiol. (Mosk). 31:36-40. (English Abstract) (Russian)

Hersh E., Funk C., Petersen E., Mosier D. (1990). Biological activity of diethyldithiocarbamate (Ditiocarb, Imuthiol) in an animal model of retrovirus-induced immunodeficiency disease and in clinical trials in patients with HIV infection. The Ditiocarb Study Group. Dev Biol Stand 72:355-63.

Hershko C., Gordeuk V., Thuma P., Theanacho E., Spira D., Hider R., Peto T., Brittenham G. (1992). The antimalarial effect of iron chelators: studies in animal models and in humans with mild falciparum malaria. J Inorg Biochem 47(3-4):267-77.

Herzig J.W., Gerber W., Salzmann R. (1987). Heart failure and Ca + activation of the cardiac contractile system: hereditary cardiomyopathy in hamsters (BIO 14.6), isoprenaline overload and the effect of APP 201-533. Basic Res Cardiol. 82:326-40.

Herzog H., Rösch F., Stöcklin G., Lueders C., Qaim S.M., Feinendegen L.E. (1993). Measurement of Yttrium-86 radiopharmaceuticals with PET and radiation dose calculation of analogous Yttrium-90 radiotherapeutics. J Nucl Med. 34(12):2222-6.

Hesselton R.M., Yang W.C., Medveczky P., Sullivan J.L. (1988): Pathogenesis of Herpes virus sylvilagus infection in cottontail rabbits. Am J Pathol. 133(3):639-47.

Hettleman B.D., Sabina R.L., Drezner M.K., Holmes E.W., Swain T.L. (1983). Defective adenosine triphosphate synthesis. An explanation for skeletal muscle dyfunction in phosphate-deficient mice. J Clin Invest. 72:582-9.

Heupler F.A. Jr., Ferrario C.M., Averill D.B., Batt-Silverman C. (1985). Initial coronary air embolus in the differential diagnosis of coronary artery spasm. Am J Cardiol. 55:657-61.

Heymer B., Spanel R., Haferkamp O. (1982). Experimental models of arthritis. Curr Top Pathol. 71:123-52.

Hicks R.J., Kassiou M., Peter E., Katsifis A.G., Garra M., Power J., Najdovski L., Lambrecht R.M. (1995). Iodine-123 N-methyl-4-iododexetimide: a new radioligand for single-photon emission tomographic imaging of myocardial muscarinic receptors. Eur J Nucl Med. 22:339-45.

Higgins A.J., Lees P., Sedgwick A.D. (1987). Development of equine models of inflammation. The Ciba-Geigy Prize for Research in Animal Health. Vet Res. 120:517-22.

Hilberg T., Bugge A., Beylich K., Ingum J., Bjorneboe A., Morland J. (1993). An animal model of postmortem amitriptyline redistribution. J Forensic Sci 38(1):81-90.

Hilbig H., Winkelmann E. (1986). The microphthalmic 944 strain of mice as a model for ontogenesis studies of the visual system. Volumetric and Golgi studies on the lateral geniculate body in the pars dorsalis. J Hirnforsch. 27:471-84. (English Abstract). (German)

Hill J.H., Plant R.L., Harris D.M., Grossweiner L.I., Rok B., Setter A.J. (1986). The nude mouse xenograft system: a model for photodetection and photodynamic therapy in head and neck squamous cell carcinoma. Am J Otolaryngol. 7:17-27.

Hill J.L., Yu D.T. (1987). Development of an experimental animal model for reactive arthritis induced by Yersinia enterocolitica infection. Infect Immun. 55:721-6.

Hinder R.A. (1986). Peptic ulceration--what can be expected from animal models. Scand J Gastroenterol. 125:195-202.

Hinrichs S., Fontes J., Bills N., Schneider P. (1991). Transgenic models of human cancer. Princess Takamatsu Symp 22:259-74.

Hinshaw L. (1989). Development of animal models for application to clinical trials in septic shock. Prog Clin Biol Res 308:835-46.

Hinshaw L.B., Brackett D.J., Archer L.T., Beller B.K., Wilson M.F. (1983). Detection of the 'hyperdynamic state' of sepsis in the baboon during lethal E coli infusion. J Trauma. 23:361-5.

Hirai A., Kumagai A. (1982). Animal model for gout. Jikken Dobutsu. 31:143-51.(Japanese)

Hirano T., Iwasaki K., Yamane Y. (1988): Osteonecrosis of the femoral head of growing, spontaneously hypertensive rats. Acta Orthop Scand. 59(5):530-5.

Hirayama R., Takagi Y., Nihei Z., Hirokawa K., Mishima Y. (1987). Establishment of new animal model of the periotoneal metastasis. Nippon Geka Gakkai Zasshi. 88:1047.

Hirose S., Shirai T.(1985). Single gene mutation models of systemic lupus erythematosus. Seikagaku. 57:593-8. (Japanese)

Hirschberg M., Hofferberth B. (1988): New model of cerebral thrombosis in dogs. Stroke 19(6):741-6.

Hjorth R.N., Bonde G.M., Piner E., Hartzell R.W., Rorke L.B., Rubin B.A. (1984). Experimental neuritis induced by a mixture of neural antigens and influenza vaccines. A possible model for Guillain-Barre syndrome. J Neuroimmunol. 6:1-8.

Hlinak Z., Krejci, I. (1990). Long-term behavioural consequences of sodium nitrite hypoxia: an animal model. Act Nerv Super (Praha) 32(1):48-9.

Ho F.C., Fu K.H. (1987). A new model of AA-amyloidosis induced by oral pistane in BALB/c mice. Br J Exp Pathol. 68:413-20.

Hoedemaeker P., Aten J., Hogendoorn P., Kawasaki K., van L. E., de H., Fleuren G. (1991). Pathogenesis of glomerulonephritis: experimental models revisited. Adv Nephrol Necker Hosp 20:73-90.

Hof H., Kuhn B. (1984). Antibiotic therapy in the compromised host--presented a model for listeriosis in the mouse. II. Effect of tetracycline. Immun Infekt. 11:61-4. (English Abstract).

Hofflin J.M., Conley F.K., Remington J.S. (1987). Murine model of intracerebral toxoplasmosis. J Infect Dis. 155:550-7.

Hoffman G.S., Ellsworth C.A., Wells E.E., Franck W.A., Mackie R.W. (1983). Spinal arachnoiditis. What is the clinical spectrum? II. Arachnoiditis induced by Pantopaque/autologous blood in dogs, a possible model for human disease. Spine. 8:541-51.

Hofmann A.F. (1984). Animal models of calcium cholelithiasis. Hepatology. 4:209S-211S.

Holaday J.W., Pasternak G.W., Faden E.I. (1982). Naloxone or TRH fails to. improve neurologic deficits in gerbil models of stroke. Life Sci..31:385-92.

Holden C. (1986). A pivotal year for lab animal welfare. Tighter regulations, higher costs, and refined methodologies likely lead to decreased animal use. Science 232:147-50.

Holland J. (1988). Animal models of alopecia. Clin Dermatol 6(4):159-62.

Hollander C.F. (1984). The place of animal models in gerontological research. Eur J clin Invest. 14:i-ii.

Hollander C.F., Mos J. (1986): The old animal as a model in research on brain aging and Alzheimer's disease/senile dementia of the Alzheimer type. Prog Brain Res. 70:337-43.

Hollander D.H., Gonder J.D. (1985). Indigenous intravaginal pentatrichmonads. vitiate the usefulness of squirrel monkeys (Saimiri sciureus)} as models for trichomoniasis in men. Genitourin Med. 61:212.

Hollyfield J.G., Anderson R.E., LaVail M.M. (Ed.) (1993). Retinal degeneration: clinical and laboratory applications. International Symposium on Retinal Degenerations, 1992, Sardinia, Italy. New York: Plenum Press. 365 P.

Holm J., Hansson G. (1990). Cellular and immunologic features of carotid artery disease in man and experimental animal models. Eur J Vasc Surg 4(1):49-55.

Holzbach R.T. (1984). Animal models of cholesterol gallstone disease. Hepatology. 4(5 Suppl):191S-198S.

Homburger F., Bernfeld P. (1985). Preferred animal model in tobacco-inhalation studies. JNCI. 75:393.

Home Office (1992). The use of animal in research, development and testing. Parlamentary Office of Sience and Technology. September, 92p.

Homma Y. (1981). Experimental models of lung diseases pulmonary fibrosis (idiopathic interstitial pneumonia). Kyobu Shikkan Gakkai Zasshi. 19:813-9. (English Abstract). (Japanese)

Honjo S., Narita T., Kobayashi R., Hiyaoka A., Fujimoto K., Takasaka M. et al. (1990). Experimental infection of African green monkeys and cynomolgus monkeys with a SIVAGM strain isolated from a healthy African green monkey. J Med Primatol 19(1):9-20.

Hood Jr. W.B. (1983). Future directions for nonclinical evaluation. Circulation 68(Suppl I):I98-I104.

Hook R.R. Jr., Berkelhammer J., Oxenhandler R.W. (1982). Melanoma: Sinclair swine melanoma. Am J Pathol. 108:130-3.

Hope G., Dawson W., Engel H., Ulshafer R., Kessler M., Sherwood M. (1992). A primate model for age related macular drusen. Br J Ophthalmol 76(1):11-6.

Horchner F., Zillmann U., Metzner M., Schonefeld A., Mehlitz. (1985). West African dogs as a model for research on trypanotolerance. Trop Med Parasitol. 36:257-8.

Horellou P., Marlier L., Privat A., Darchen F., Scherman D., Henry J., Mallet J. (1990). Exogeneous expression of L-dopa and dopamine in various cell lines following transfer of rat and human tyrosine hydroxylase cDNA: grafting in an animal model of Parkinson's disease. Prog Brain Res 82:23-32.

Horio T., Miyauchi H., Asada Y. (1991). The hairless guinea pig as an experimental animal for photodermatology. Photodermatol Photoimmunol Photomed 8(2):69-72.

Horiuchi K., Yomoda I., Ohta H., Endo K., Yokoyama A. (1991). Search for polynuclear pentavalent technetium complex of dimercaptosuccinic acid [Tc(V)-DMS] tumour localization mechanism. I. Medullary thyroid carcinoma animal model. Eur J Nucl Med 18(10):796-800.

Horton C.E.Jr., Davisson M.T., Jacobs J.B., Bernstein G.T., Retik A.B., Mandell J. (1988): Congenital progressive hydronephrosis in mice: a new recessive mutation. J Urol. 140(5 Pt 2):1310-5.

Hosenpud J.D., Hart M.V., Morton M.J., Hohiwer A.R., Resko J.A. (1983). Progesterone-induced hyperventilation in the guinea pig. Respir Physiol. 52:259-64.

Hosoda Y., Yoshimura Y., Higaki S. (1981). A new breed of mouse showing multiple osteochondral lesions--two mouse. Ryumachi. 21(Suppl):157-64.

Hosokawa Y. (1991). Mucosal lesions of the stomach in liver cirrhosis with a special reference to phospholipid metabolism. Gastroenterol Jpn 26(3):329-35.

Hossmann K.A. (1991). Animal models of cerebral ischemia. 1. Review of literature. Cerebrovasc Dis. 1(Suppl 1):2-15.

Hossmann K.A., Mies G., Paschen W. et al. (1985). Multiparametric imaging of blood flow and metabolism after middle cerebral artery occlusion in cats. J Cereb Blood Flow Metab. 5:97-107.

Hoste H., Fort G. (1992). Experimental infections with Nematodirus spathiger in rabbits. J Helminthol 66(3):227-30.

Houchens D.P., Ovejera A.A., Riblet S.M., Slagel D.E. (1983). Human brain tumor xenografts in nude mice as a chemotherapy model. Eur J Cancer Clin Oncol. 19:799-805.

Houff S.A., London w.T., Zu Rhein G.M., Padgett B.L., Walker D.L., Sever J.L. (1983). New world primates as a model of viral-induced astrocytomas. Prog Clin Biol Res. 105:223-6.

Hough A.J. Jr., Hubbard W.C., Oates J.A. (1983). VX2 carcinoma, pulmonary metastases, and neutrophilic leukocytosis. Possible animal model of tumor-associated granulocytosis. Am J Pathol. 112:231-7.

Houghton J.A., Houghton P.J., Webber B.L. (1982). Growth and characterization of childhood rhabdomyosarcomas as xenografts. JNCI. 68:437-43.

Howard C.F. Jr. (1984). Diabetes mellitus: relationships of non-human primates and other animal models to human forms of diabetes. Adv Vet Sci Comp Med. 28:115-49.

Howard J.L., Pollard G.T. (1983). Are primate models of neuropsychiatric disorders useful to the pharmaceutical industry? Prog Clin Biol Res. 131:307-2

Howe A., Webster W. (1990). Exposure of the pregnant rat to warfarin and vitamin K1: an animal model of intraventricular hemorrhage in the fetus. Teratology 42(4):413-20.

Howett M., Kreider J., Cockley K. (1990). Human xenografts. A model system for human papillomavirus infection. Intervirology 31(2-4):109-15.

Howie A., Kizaki T., Beaman M., Morland C., Birtwistle R., Adu D. et al. (1989). Different types of segmental sclerosing glomerular lesions in six experimental models of proteinuria. J Pathol 157(2):141-51.

Hozawa K. (1988). [Experimental model for otitis media with effusion induced by the type III hypersensitivity reaction]. Nippon Jibiinkoka Gakkai Kaiho 91(2):197-203.

Hsiung G., Chan V. (1989). Evaluation of new antiviral agents: II. The use of animal models. Antiviral Res 12(5-6):239-58.

Huang T. (1984). Animal models used to study the therapeutic effect and mechanism of Chinese herbal drugs in the treatment of psoriasis. Chung Hsi I Chieh Ho Tsa Chih. 4:428-9. (English Abstract). (Chinese)

Huang Y., Richardson J., Tong A., Zhang B., Stone M., Vitetta E. (1993). Disseminated growth of a human multiple myeloma cell line in mice with severe combined immunodeficiency disease. Cancer Res 53(6):1392-6.

Hubbard G.B., Shimazu T., Yukioka T., Langlinais P.C., Mason A.D., Pruitt B.A. jr. (1988): Smoke inhalation injury in sheep. Am J Pathol. 133(3):660-3.

Hudson S., Dix R., Streilein J. (1991). Induction of encephalitis in SJL mice by intranasal infection with herpes simplex virus type 1: a possible model of herpes simplex encephalitis in humans. J Infect Dis 163(4):720-7.

Hultman J., Forsberg J.O., Hansson H.E., Ronquist G. (1982). A paracorporeal rat heart model for ischemic and reperfusion studies. Ups J Med Sci. 87:235-42.

Humber D., Hetherington C., Atlaw T., Eriso F. (1989). Leishmania aethiopica: infections in laboratory animals. Exp Parasitol 68(2):155-9.

Humphrey C.D., Montag D.M., Pittman F.E. (1985). Experimental infection of hamsters with Campylobacter jejuni. J Infect Dis. 151:485-93.

Humphrey S.J., McCall R.B. (1982). A rat model for predicting orthostatic hypotension during acute and chronic antihypertensive drug therapy. J Pharmacol Methods. 7:25-34.

Hunag D.F., Shen T.Y. (1993). A versatile total synthesis of epibatidine and analogs. Tetrahedon Letters 34(28):4477-80.

Hunneyball I.M., Crossiey M.J., Spowage M. (1986). Antigen-induced arthritis in mice. Br J Clin Pract. 43:13-20.

Hunter A.J., Caulfield M.P., Kimberlin R.H. (1986). Learning ability of mice infected with different strains of scrapie. Physiol Behav.36:1089-92.

Hurn I.L., Fisher J.C., Rudolph R., Utley J.F. (1983). A method for producing chronic radiation injury in rodent skin. Invest Radiol.18:552-3.

Hurtrel B., Chakrabarti L., Hurtrel M., Maire M., Dormont D., Montagnier L. (1991). Early SIV encephalopathy. J Med Primatol 20(4):159-66.

Hutchings D., Dow-Edwards D. (1991). Animal models of opiate, cocaine, and cannabis use. Clin Perinatol 18(1):1-22.

Hutchings D.E., Zmitrovich A., Church S., Malowany D. (1993). Methadone during pregnancy: the search for a valid animal model. Ann Ist Super Sanita. 29(3):439-44.

Huxtable C.R., Dorling P.R. (1982). Animal model of human disease. Mannosidosis. Swainsonine-induced mannosidosis. Am J Pathol.107:124-6.

Hwang D.R., Eckelman W.C., Mathias C.J., Petrillo E.W.Jr., Lloyd J., Welch M.J. (1991). Positron-labeled angiotensin-converting enzyme (ACE) inhibitor: Fluorine-18-fluorocaptopril. Probing the ACE activity in vivo by positron emission tomography. J Nucl Med. 32:1730-7.

Iakovleva L.A., Timanovskaia V.V., Indzhiia L.V., Lapin B.A., Voevodin A.F. (1987): Modelling of malignant lymphoma in rabbits using primate oncogenic viruses. Preliminary report. Biull Eksp Biol Med. 103:336-8. (English Abstract). (Russian)

Iakovleva O.N., Rycheva T.A., Petrovskaia V.G. (1982). Comparative study of Salmonella typhimurium strains of various origins in murine models of enteral and intranasal infection. Zh Mikrobiol Epidemiol Immunobiol. 9:53-7. (English Abstract). (Russian)

Iancu T.C. (1993). Animal models in liver research: iron overload. Adv Vet Sci Comp Med. 37:379-401.

Iancu T.C., Shiloh H. (1988): Experimental iron overload. Ultrastructural studies. Ann N Y Acad Sci. 526:164-78.

Ibarra-Rubio M., Cruz C., Tapia E., Pena JC., Pedraza-Chaverri J. (1990). Serum angiotensin converting enzyme activity and plasma renin activity in experimental models of rats. Clin Exp Pharmacol Physiol 17(6):391-9.

Ido T. et al. (1978). Labeled 2-deoxy-D-glucose analogs. ^{18}F-labeled 2-deoxy-2-fluoro-D-glucose, 2-deoxy-2-fluoro-D-mannose and ^{14}C-2-deoxy-2-fluoro-D-glucose. J Label Compounds Radiopharm. 14:175-84.

Iesaka Y., Aonuma K., Gosselin A.J., Pinakatt T., Stanford W., Benson J., Sampsell R., Roganski J.J., Lister J.W. (1983). Susceptibility of infarcted canine hearts to digitalis-toxic ventricular tachycardia. J Am Coll Cardiol. 2:45-51.

Ignatovski B., Borcic V. (1981). Acute experimental (endogenous) hepatic coma and the clinical syndrome of acute hepatocellular injury]. Acta Chir Iugosl. 28:193-201. (English Abstract). (Scrotian)

Ikeda H., Koga Y., Kuwano K., Nakayama H., Ueno T., Yoshida N. et al. (1993). Cyclic flow variations in a conscious dog model of coronary artery stenosis and endothelial injury correlate with acute ischemic heart disease syndromes in humans. J Am Coll Cardiol 21(4):1008-17.

Ikeda K., Matsumoto T., Fukumoto S., Kurokawa K., Ueyama Y., Fujishize K., Tamaoki N., Saito T., Ohtake K., Ogata E. (1988): A hypercalcemic nude rat model that completely mimics human syndrome of humoral hypercalcemia of malignancy. Calcif Tissue Int. 43(2):97-102.

Ilgren E.B. (1993). Mesotheliomas of animals: a comprehensive, tabular compendium of the world's literature. Boca Raton, Fla.: CRC Press. 356 P.

Illavia S.J., Webb H.E., Pathak S. (1982). Demyelination induced in mice by a virulent Semliki Forest virus. I. Virology and effects on optic nerve. Neuropathol Appl Neurobiol. 8:35-42.

Imai A., Morishita K., Kurihara Y. (1984). Indigenous microfloras and resistance to bacterial infection in mice with experimentally induced diabetes: a possible animal model for opportunistic infection. Can J Microbiol. 30:186-91.

Imataka K., Kitahara Y., Naito S., Fujii J. (1993). A new model for infective endocarditis of the mitral valve in rabbits. Am Heart J 125(5 Pt 1):1353-7.

Imperato-McGinley J., Binienda Z., Arthur A., Mininberg D.T., Vaughan E.D., Quimby F.W. (1985) The development of a male pseudohermaphroditic rat using an inhibitor of the enzyme 5 alpha-reductase. Endocrinology. 116:807-12.

Infantino A., Fabris C., Basso D., Del F. G., Munaretto S., Plebani M., Panozzo M., Meggiato T., Fassina A., Lise M., et al. (1992). Acute reflux pancreatitis in rats: a comparison between two experimental models. Gastroenterol Jpn 27(5):657-61.

Ingalls T.H. (1982). Mutations in the hamster. Arch Environ Health. 37:61.

Innis R.B., Al-Tikriti M.S., Zoghbi S.S., Baldwin R.M., Sybirska E.H., Laruelle M.A., Malison R.T., Seibyl J.P., Zimmermann R.C., Johnson E.W., Smith E.O., Charney D.S., Heninger G.R., Woods S.W., Hoffer P.B. (1991). SPECT imaging of the bezodiazepine receptor: Feasibility of in vitro potency measurements from stepwise displacement curves. J Nucl Med. 32:1754-61.

Inoue T., Aikawa K., Tezuka H., Kada T., Shultz L.D. (1986). Effect of DNA-damaging agents on isolated spleen cells and lung fibroblasts from the mouse mutant "wasted," a putative animal model for ataxia-telangiectasia. Cancer Res. 46:3979-82.

Inoue Y. (1986). Animals with hereditary brain diseases and neurological research. Hokkaido Igaku Zasshi. 61:165-7. (Japanese)

Irving G. 3. (1991). A perspective on the selection of experimental models. Neurosci Biobehav Rev 15(1):15-20.

Isaacs J.T. (1987). Development and characteristics of the available animal model systems for the study of prostatic cancer. Prog Clin Biol Res, 239:513-76.

Isaji M., Momose Y., Naito J. (1989). Enhancement of inflammatory reactions in a non-immunological air pouch model in rats. Br J Exp Pathol 70(6):705-16.

Ishii K., Kita T., Kume N., Nagano Y., Kawai C. (1988): Uptake or acetylated LDL by peritoneal macrophages obtained from normal and Watanabe heritable hyperlipidemic rabbits, an animal model for familial hypercholesterolemia. Biochim Biophys Acta. 14;962 (3):387-9.

Ishizuki S., Kanda N., Kaneta S., Fujihira E. (1984). Progressive foot swelling in BUF rats. A new animal model for screening of anti-inflammatory and anti-rheumatic drugs. Arch Int Pharmacodyn Ther. 271:303-14.

Ismaiel M., Greenman J., Morgan K., Glover M., Rees A., Scully C. (1989). Periodontitis in sheep: a model for human periodontal disease. J Periodontol 60(5):279-84.

Ismailov E.M. (1982). Pulmonary circulation and right ventricular function in an experimental model of acute altitude-induced pulmonary edema. Biull Eksp Biol Med. 94:18-20. (English Abstract). (Russian)

Ito N., Shirai T. (1986). Cancer development and animal models. Nippon Rinsho. 44:311-7.

Itoh M., Hiramine C., Hojo K. (1991). A new murine model of autoimmune orchitis induced by immunization with viable syngeneic testicular germ cells alone. I. Immunological and histological studies. Clin Exp Immunol 83(1):137-42.

Iumatov E.A., Pevtsova E.I., Mezentseva L.N. (1988): Physiologically adequate experimental model of aggression and emotional stress. Zh Vyssh Nerv Deiat. 38(2):350-4 (English Abstract). (Russian).

Ivanov A.I., Khitrov N.K. (1983). Heart function and the mechanisms of its regulation in modelling adaptation to hypoxia by 2,4-dinitrophenol administration. Kardiologiia. 23:94-8. (English Abstract). (Russian)

Ivanova I.A., Bobkov IuG. (1984). Comparative study of several preparations in different models of cerebral hypoxia. Biull Eksp Biol Med. 98:567-70. (English Abstract). (Russian)

Iverson W.O., Fetterman G.H., Jacobson E.R., Olsen J.H., Senior D.F., Schobert E.E. (1982). Polycystic kidney and liver disease in Springbok: I. Morphology of lesions. Kidney Int. 22:146-55.

Ivic M., Strahinjic S., Teodosic S., Stefanovic V. (1988): Disorders of calcium and phosphate metabolism regulation in an experimental model of acute uremia. Sr Arli Celok Lek. 116(4):371-82. (English Abstract).

Iwase M. (1991). A new animal model of non-insulin-dependent diabetes mellitus with hypertension: neonatal streptozotocin treatment in spontaneously hypertensive rats. Fukuoka Igaku Zasshi 82(7):415-27.

Izotov V.K., Chunikbin S.P. (1982). Modeling a persistent infection by tick-borne encephalitis virus strains in a cell culture of the clawed toad. Zh Mikrobiol Epidemiol Immunobiol. 10:56-9. (English Abstract).

Jabs D.A., Prendergast R.A. (1994). Murine models of Sjogren's syndrome. Adv Exp Med Biol. 350:623-30.

Jackson A., Crossman A.R. (1984). Experimental choreoathetosis produced by injection of a gamma-aminobutyric acid antagonist into the lentiform nucleus in the monkey. Neurosci Lett. 46:41-5.

Jackson C., Hutson, N., Steward, S., & McDonald, T. (1990). Megakaryocytopoiesis in man and laboratory animals. Conclusions derived from comparative studies and recently discovered animal models with megakaryocyte anomalies. Prog Clin Biol Res, 356:11-23.

Jackson D.M., Eady R.P. (1986). Monkeys infected with Ascaris suum (a new in vivo model of airway disease): protective effect of nedocromil sodium and sodium cromoglycate against bronchial antigen challenge. Eur J Respir Dis. 147:202-5.

Jacobs R.L., Lux G.K., Speilvogel R.L., Eichberg J.W., Gleiser C.A.(1984). Nasal polyposis in a chimpanzee. J Allergy Clin Immunol.74:61-3.

Jaeger P., Jones W., Kashgarian M., Baron R., Clemens T.L., Segre G.V., Hayslett J.P. (1987). Animal model of primary hyperparathyroidism.. Am J Physiol. 252 (Pt 1):E790-8.

Jahrling P.B., Smith S., Hesse R.A., Rhoderick J.B. (1982). Pathogenesis of Lassa virus infection in guinea pigs. Infect Immun. 37:771-8.

Jansen B., Tryphonas L., Wong J., Thorner P., Maxie M.G., Valli V.E., Baumal R., Barrur P.K. (1986). Mode of inheritance of Samoyed hereditary glomerulopathy: an animal model for hereditary nephritis in humans. J Lab Clin Med. 107:551-5.

Jansen P.L., Oude-Elferink R.P. (1993). Hereditary conjugated hyperbilirubinemia in Wistar rats: a model for the study of ATP-dependent hepatocanalicular organic anion transport. Adv Vet Sci Comp Med. 37:175-95.

Jantos C., Altmannsberger M., Weidner W., Schiefer H. (1990). Acute and chronic bacterial prostatitis due to E. coli. Description of an animal model. Urol Res 18(3):207-11.

Jasper J.M., Nelkin D. (1992). The animal rights crusade. New York: The Free Press Macmillan.

Jaspers S.R., Tischler M.E. (1984). Atrophy and growth failure of rat hindlimb muscles in tail-cast suspension. J Appl Pysiol. 57:1472-9.

Jastreboff P., Brennan J., Sasaki C. (1988). An animal model for tinnitus. Laryngoscope 98(3):280-6.

Jastreboff P.J., Sasaki C.T. (1994). An animal model of tinnitus: a decade of development. Am J Otol. 15:19-27.

Jellinek H. (1982). A new model for arteriosclerosis. An electron- microscopic study of the lesions induced by i.v. administered fat. Atherosclerosis. 43:7-18.

Jenden D.J., Russell R.W., Booth R.A., Lauretz S.D., Knusel B.J., Roch M. (1987). A model of hypocholinergic syndrome produced by a false choline analog, N-aminodeanol. J Neural Transm [Suppl] 24:325-9.

Jensen D.M., Machicado G.A., Tapia J.L., Kauffman G., Franco P., Beilin D. (1983). A reproducible canine model of esophageal varices. Gastroenterology. 84:573-9.

Jensen H., Hau J. (1990). A murine model for the study of the impact of Aspergillus fumigatus inoculation on the foeto-placental unit. Mycopathologia 112(1):11-8.

Jermy A., Fisher C., Vincent A., Willcox N., Newsom-Davis J. (1989). Experimental autoimmune myasthenia gravis induced in mice without adjuvant: genetic susceptibility and adoptive transfer of weakness. J Autoimmun 2(5):675-88.

Jeynes B. (1988). Treatment of experimentally induced cerebral atherothromboembolism in an animal model with streptokinase and taurochenodeoxycholate. Artery 15(5):259-71.

Jiang X. (1989). [A model of daunorubicin-induced nephrotic syndrome in the rat]. Chung Hua I Hsueh Tsa Chih 69(5):288-90.

Jiao S., Matsuzawa Y., Matsubara K., Kubo M., Tokunaga K., Odaka H., Ikeda H., Matsuo T., Tarui S. (1991). Abnormalities of plasma lipoproteins in a new genetically obese rat with non-insulin-dependent diabetes mellitus (Wistar fatty rat). Int J Obes 15(7):487-95.

Jimenez S.A., Christner P. (1994). Animal models of systemic sclerosis. Clin Dermatol. 12(3):425-36.

Jing H.D. (1984). An atherosclerosis model using the Japanese quail. Chung Hua Hsin Hsueh Kuan Ping Tsa Chih. 12:222-4. (Chinese)

Jinnah H., Gage F., Friedmann T. (1990). Animal models of Lesch-Nyhan syndrome. Brain Res Bull 25(3):467-75.

Job C.K. (1993). Animal models for early leprosy. Indian J Lepr. 65(1):29-37.

Jobe P., Mishra P., Ludvig N., Dailey J. (1991). Scope and contribution of genetic models to an understanding of the epilepsies. Crit Rev Neurobiol 6(3):183-220.

Johansson A., Svensson O., Blomgren G., Eliasson G., Nord C. (1991). Anaerobic osteomyelitis. A new experimental rabbit model. Clin Orthop (265):297-301.

Johnson E.L., Turkington T.G., Iaszczak R.J., Gilland D.R., Vaidyanathan G., Greer K.L., Coleman R.E., Zalutsky M.R. (1995). Quantitation of [211]At in small volumes for evaluation of targeted radioimmunotherapy in animal models. Nucl Med Biol. 22:45-54.

Johnson K.J., Glovsky M., Schrier D. (1984). Pulmonary granulomatous vasculitis. Pulmonary granulomatous vasculitis induced in rats by treatment with glucan. Am J Pathol. 114:515-6.

Johnson P., Hirsch V. (1991). Pathogenesis of AIDS: the non-human primate model. AIDS 5 Suppl 2:S43-8.

Johnson W.J., Muirhead K.A., Meumier P.C., Voha B.J., Schmitt T.C., Wimartino M.J., Hanna N. (1986). Macrophage activation in rat models of inflammation and arthritis. Systemic activation precedes arthritis induction and progression. Arthritis Rheum. 29:1122-30.

Johnstone P.A. (1987). The search for animal models of leprosy. Int J Lepr Other Mycobact Dis. 55:535-47.

Jokinen M.P., Clarkson T.B., Prichard R.W. (1985). Animal models in atherosclerosis research. Exp. Mol Pathol. 42:1-28.

Jolly R.D., Shimada A., Dalefield P.R., Slack P.M. (1987). Mannosidosis: ocular lesions in the bovine model. Curr Eye Res. 6:1073-8.

Jonas A.M. (1984). The mouse in biomedical research. Physiologist.27:330-46.

Jones J.B., Lange R.D. (1983). Cyclic Hematopoiesis: animal models. Exp Hematol. 11:571-80.

Jones M., Abbitt B. (1993). Animal model of human disease. Bovine beta-mannosidosis. Am J Pathol 142(3):957-60.

Jones T.C. (1982). Animal models of inherited metabolic disease - an overview. Prog. Clin Biol Res. 94:5-7.

Jordan G.W., Cohen S.H. (1987). Encephalomyocarditis virus-induced diabetes mellitus in mice: model of viral pathogenesis. Rev Infect Dis. 9:917-24.

Jordan V.C. (1987). Laboratory models of breast cancer to aid the elucidation of antiestrogen action. J Lab Clin Med. 109:267-77.

Jordan W.P. Jr. (1982). The guinea pig as a model for predicting photoallergic contact dermatitis. Contact Dermatitis. 8:109-16.

Jori G., Reddi E., Rubaltelli F. (1990). Bronze baby syndrome: an animal model. Pediatr Res 27(1):22-5.

Juniewicz P., Fetrow N., Marinelli J., Wolf M., Young E., Lamb J., Isaacs J. (1991). Evaluation of Win 49,596, a novel steroidal androgen receptor antagonist, in animal models of prostate cancer. Prostate 18(2):105-15.

Jurgelski W. (1983). An alternative animal model for perinatal carcinogenesis. Biol Res. Pregnancy Perinatol. 4:3-16.

Just M., Tripier D., Seiffge D. (1991). Antithrombotic effects of recombinant hirudin in different animal models. Haemostasis 21 Suppl 1:80-7.

Kadaba R., Simpson C. (1990). Disparate effect of tamoxifen in rats with experimentally induced endometriosis. Endocrinology 126(6):3263-7.

Kahraman M., Prieur D. (1990). Chediak-Higashi syndrome in the cat: prenatal diagnosis by evaluation of amniotic fluid cells. Am J Med Genet 36(3):321-7.

Kaijima M., Tanaka T., Daita G., Ohgami S., Yonemasu Y. (1981). A new model of epilepsy--a small epileptic focus by microinjection of kainic acid into the unilateral hippocampus in cats. No To Shinkei. 33:ll33-40. (English Abstract). (Japanese)

Kaiserlian D., Savino W., Uriel J., Hassid J., Dardenne M., Bach J.F. (1986). The wasted mutant mouse II. Immunological abnormalities in a mouse described as a model of ataxia-telangiectasia. Clin Exp Immunol. 63:562-9.

Kajdacsy-Balla A., Howeedy A., Bagasra O. (1987). Syphilis in the Syrian hamster. A model of human venereal and congenital syphilis. Am J Pathol.126:599-601.

Kakoma I., James MA., Whiteley H., Montelegre F., Buese M. et al. (1992). Platelet kinetics and other hematological profiles in experimental Plasmodium falciparum infection: a comparative study between Saimiri and Aotus monkeys. Kisaengchunghak Chapchi 30(3):177-82.

Kakulas B.A., Howell J.M., Roses A.D. (Ed.) (1992). Duchenne muscular dystrophy: animal models and genetic manipulation. New York: Raven Press. 308 P.

Kal H.B., Van Berkel A.H., Zurcher C., Smink T., Van Bekkum D.W. (1986). A rat lung cancer model based on intrapulmonary implantation of tumour material. Radiother Oncol. 6:231-8.

Kallman R.F., Brown J.M., Denekamp J., Hill R.P., Kummermehr J. (1985). The use of rodent tumors in experimental cancer therapy. Conclusions and recommendations from an international workshop. Cancer Res. 45:6541-5.

Kallos P., Kallos L. (1984). Experimental asthma in guinea pigs revisited. Int Arch Allergy Appl Immunol. 73:77-85.

Kalush F., Rimon E., Mozes E. (1992). Neonatal lupus erythematosus in offspring of mothers with experimental systemic lupus erythematosus. Am J Reprod Immunol 28(3-4):264-8.

Kameyama T., Nabeshima T., Kozawa T. (1986). Step-down-type passive avoidance-and escape-learning method. Suitability for experimental amnesia models. J Pharmacol Methods. 16:39-52.

Kaminishi M., Sadatsuki H., Johjima Y., Oohara T., Kondo Y. (1987): A new model for production of chronic gastric ulcer by duodenogastric reflux in rats. Gastroenterology. 92:1913-8.

Kane J.L., Woodland R.M., Elder M.G., Dargougar S. (1985). Chlamydial pelvic infection in cats: a model for the study of human pelvic inflammatory disease. Genitourin Med. 61:311-8.

Kaneko D., Nakamura N., Ogawa T. (1985). Cerebral infarction in rats using homologous blood emboli: development of a new experimental model. Stroke. 16:76-84.

Kaneko J.J. (1987). Animal models of inherited hematologic disease. Clin Chim Acta. 165:1-19.

Kaneshima H., Baum C., Chen B., Namikawa R., Outzen H., Rabin L. et al. (1990). Today's SCID-hu mouse. Nature 348(6301):561-2.

Kanfer J.N., Stephens M.C., Singh H., Legler G. (1982). The Gaucher mouse. Prog Clin Biol Res. 95:627-44.

Kanno T., Nakamura T., Jain V.K., Sugimoto T. (1987). An experimental model of communicating hydrocephalus in C57 black mouse. Acta Neurochir (Wien). 86:111-4.

Kanwar S.S., Samra H., Ganguly N.K., Mahajan R.C. (1986): Comparative evaluation of Giardia lamblia infection in mouse and rat. Indian J Med Res. 84:577-81.

Kao M., Ludwig H., Gosztonyi G. (1984). Adaptation of Borna disease virus to the mouse. J Gen Viol. 65 (Pt 10):1845-9.

Kapp U., Wolf J., von K. C., Tawadros S., Rottgen A., Engert A., Fonatsch C., Stein H., Diehl V. (1992). Preliminary report: growth of Hodgkin's lymphoma derived cells in immune compromised mice. Ann Oncol 3 Suppl 4:21-3.

Kapuscinski A. (1987): Cerebral blood flow in the experimental model of the clinical death of rats. Neuropatol Pol. 25(3):287-98. (English Abstract). (Polish)

Karapetian A.E., Isaakian Z.S., Lalaian A.A. (1987): Role of tissue antigen in modeling balantidiasis in the adult white rat. Med Parazitol (Mosk).

Karasawa T., Shikata T. (1981). Animal model of non-A, non-B hepatitis infection. Nippon Rinsho. 39:3190-200. (Japanese)

Karita M., Kouchiyama T., Okita K., Nakazawa T. (1991). New small animal model for human gastric Helicobacter pylori infection: success in both nude and euthymic mice. Am J Gastroenterol 86(11):1596-603.

Karol M.H. (1994). Animal models of occupational asthma. Eur Respir J. 7(3):555-68.

Karpiak S., Tagliavia A., Wakade C. (1989). Animal models for the study of drugs in ischemic stroke. Annu Rev Pharmacol Toxicol 29:403-14.

Karrer F.M., Rhenman B., Buckley A.R., Steinbronn K.K., Putnam C.W. (1984). A reproducible large animal model of acute hepatic failure. Curr Surg. 4:464-7.

Karvonen R.L., Fernandez-Madrid F., Maughan R.L., Palmer K.C., Fernandez-Madrid I. (1987). An animal model of pulmonary radiation fibrosis with biochemical, physiologic, immunologic, and morphologic observations. Radiat Res. 111:68-80.

Kase F. (1981). Experimental models of human congenital coagulation defects. Probl Gematol Pereliv Krovi. 26:41-4. (Russian)

Kasik J.W., Leuschen M.P., Case M.J., Nelson R.M. Jr. (1985). Limitations of premature rabbit model of IVH. J Neurosurg. 63:816-7.

Kaspareit-Rittinghausen J., Deerberg F., Rapp K., Wcislo A. (1990). Renal hypertension in rats with hereditary polycystic kidney disease. Z Versuchstierkd 33(5):201-4.

Kassiou M., Scheffel U., Ravert H.T., Mathews W.B., Musachio J.L., Lambrecht R.M., Dannals R.F. (1995). [^{11}C]-A-69024: A potent and selective non-benzazepine radiotracer for in vivo studies of dopamine D_1 receptors. Nucl Med Biol. 22:221-6. Also see abstract A05. World Wide Web (WWW) Point to HTTP://GABRIOLA.PET.MED.UBC.CA/WTTC95.HTML

Kataoka K., Sasaki T., Sezumi H., Kato M., Yamane Y. (1988): A rat model of chronic pancreatic insufficiency induced by injection of zein-oleic acid-linoleic acid solution into the pancreatic duct. Nippon Shokakibyo Gakkai Zasshi. 85 (7):1431. (Japanese)

Kato S. (1985). Behavioral changes in Rhesus monkeys induced by repeated administration of ephedrine. Seishin Shinkeigaku Zasahi. 87:583-94. (English Abstract). (Japanese)

Katz R.J. (1982). Animal model of depression: pharmacological sensitivity of a hedonic deficit. Pharmacol Biochem Behav. 16:965-8.

Katz R.J., Sibel M. (1982). Animal model of depression: tests of three structurally and pharmacologically novel antidepressant compounds. Pharmacol Biochem Behav. 16:973-7.

Kaufman H.H., Pruessner J.L., Bernstein D.P., Borit A., Ostron P.T., Cahall D.L. (1985). A rabbit model of intracerebral hematoma. Acta Neuropathol. (Berl). 65:318-21.

Kaufman P.L., Bito L.Z., DeRousseau C.J. (1982). The development of presbyopia in primates. Trans Ophthalmol Soc UK. 102 (Pt 3):323-6.

Kaufman R.C., Amankwah K.S., Dunaway G., Maroun L., Arbuthnot J., Roddick J.W. Jr. (1981). An animal model of gestational diabetes. Am J Obstet Gynecol. 141:479-82.

Kaufmann C., Weinberger D., Stevens J., Asher D., Kleinman J., Sulima M., Gibbs C. J., Gajdusek D. (1988). Intracerebral inoculation of experimental animals with brain tissue from patients with schizophrenia. Failure to observe consistent or specific behavioral and neuropathological effects. Arch Gen Psychiatry 45(7):648-52.

Kawai S., Aikawa M., Kano S., Suzuki M. (1993). A primate model for severe human malaria with cerebral involvement: Plasmodium coatneyi-infected Macaca fuscata. Am J Trop Med Hyg 48(5):630-6.

Kawamata J. (1984). Experimental animal information file: WHHL (Watanabe heritable hyperlipidemic rabbit). Gan To Kagaku Ryoho. 11:1895-7.

Kawamata J., Matsushita H. (1987): Overview of the state of the art in development and utilization of animal models in Japan. Prog Clin Biol Res. 229:11-25.

Kawamata J., Melby E.C. (Ed.) (1985). Animal models: assessing the scope of their use in biomedical research. New York: Alan R. Liss, Inc.

Kawamura S., Yasui N., Shirasawa M., Fukasawa H. (1991). Rat middle cerebral artery occlusion using an intraluminal thread technique. Acta Neurochir (Wien) 109(3-4):126-32.

Kazmierczak S., Lott J., Caldwell J. (1988). Acute intestinal infarction or obstruction: search for better laboratory tests in an animal model. Clin Chem 34(2):281-8.

Keane T., Rosner G., Gingrich J., Poulton S., Walther P. (1991). The therapeutic impact of dipyridamole: chemopotentiation of the cytotoxic combination 5-fluorouracil/cisplatin in an animal model of human bladder cancer. J Urol 146(5):1418-24.

Keehn J.D. (1986). Animal Models for Psychiatry. Methuen Inc, New York. 237 pp.

Keenam C.M., Hendricks L.D., Lightner L., Webster H.K., Johnson A.J. (1984). Visceral leishmaniasis in the German shepherd dog. Infection, clinical disease, and clinical pathology. Vet Pathol. 21:74-9.

Keisler L.W., Walker S.E. (1987). Suppression of reproductive function in autoimmune NZB/W mice: effective doses of four contraceptive steroids.Am J Reprod Immunol Microbiol.14:115-21.

Kekomaki M., Wehle M., Walker R.D. (1985). The growing rabbit with a solitary, partially-obstructed kidney. Analysis of an experimental model with reference to the renal concentrating ability. J Urol. 133:870-2.

Kellerhals B., Zogg R. (1991). Tinnitus-induced weight loss in rats. An animal model for tinnitus research. ORL J Otorhinolaryngol Relat Spec 53(6):331-4.

Kenmochi T., Asano T., Nakagori T., Arita S., Isono K. (1989). [Studies on rat infectious pancreatitis models by subcapsular injection of dog's bile and appendix contents]. Nippon Shokakibyo Gakkai Zasshi 86(12):2840.

Ker C., Wu S. (1992). A simple animal model for inducing and releasing surgical jaundice in rats. Kao Hsiung I Hsueh Ko Hsueh Tsa Chih 8(10):520-4.

Kerbel R.S., Man M.S., Dexter P. (1984). A model of human cancer metastasis: extensive spontaneous and artificial metastasis of a human pigmented melanoma and derived variant sublines in nude mice. JNCI. 72:93-108.

Kern E. (1991). Value of animal models to evaluate agents with potential activity against human cytomegalovirus. Transplant Proc 23 (3 Suppl 3):152-5, discussion 155.

Kersh R., Handren J., Hergrueter C., May J. J. (1989). Microvascular surgical experimental thrombosis model: rationale and design. Plast Reconstr Surg 83(5):866-72; discussion 873-4.

Kerwar S., Oromsky A. (1989). Methotrexate in rheumatoid arthritis: studies with animal models. Adv Enzyme Regul 29:247-65.

Kerwar S.S., Oromsky A.L. (1986). Studies on type II collagen induced arthritis. Br J Clin Pract. 43:32-40.

Kerwin R.W., Pilowsky L.S. (1995). Traditional receptor theory and its application to neuroreceptor measurements in fuctional imaging. Eur J Nucl Med. 22:699-710.

Kesecioglu J., Telci L., Denkel T., Tutuncu A., Esen F., Akpir K., Lachmann B. (1992). Comparison of different modes of artificial ventilation with extracorporeal CO2 elimination on gas exchange in an animal model of acute respiratory failure. Adv Exp Med Biol 317:893-9.

Kesel M.L., Ellis R.P. (1988): A reversible-tie technique of the rabbit gut for bacterial colonization and toxin production. Lab Anim Sci. 38(5):621-3.

Keshavarzian A., Doria M., Sedghi S., Kanofsky J., Hecht D., Holmes E. et al. (1992). Mitomycin C-induced colitis in rats: a new animal model of acute colonic inflammation implicating reactive oxygen species. J Lab Clin Med 120(5):778-91.

Keshavarzian A., Rizk G., Urban G., Willson C. (1990). Ethanol-induced esophageal motor disorder: development of an animal model. Alcohol Clin Exp Res 14(1):76-81.

Kessler M.J., Howard C.F. Jr., London W.T. (1985). Gestational diabetes mellitus and impaired glucose tolerance in an aged Macaca mulatta. J Med Primatol. 14:237-44.

Ketyi I. (1981). Suckling mouse model of urinary tract infections caused by Escherichia coli. Acta Microbiol Acad Sci Hung. 28:393-9.

Key M.E., Bernhard M.I., Hoyer L.C., Foon K.A., Oldham R.K., Hanna M.G. Jr. (1983). Guinea pig line 10 hepatocarcinoma model for monoclonal antibody serotherapy: in vivo localization of a monoclonal antibody in normal and malignant tissues. J Immunol. 130:1451-7.

Khan S.R., Hackett R.L. (1985). Calcium oxalate urolithiasis in the rat: is it a model for human stone disease? A review of recent literature. Scan Electron Microsc. (Pt. 2):759-74.

Khanmirzoev F., Kulikovskaia I., Dadasheva N., Rabinovich S. (1990). [The modelling of the multiple drug resistance of the malarial parasites. 1. The combined resistance of Plasmodium berghei to chloroquine and fansidar] Modelirovanie mnozhestvennoi lekarstvennoi ustoichivosti maliariinykh parazitov. Soobshchenie 1. Sochetannaia ustoichivost' Plasmodium berghei k khlorokhinu i fansidaru. Med Parazitol (Mosk) (5):60-3.

Khatib R., Chason J.L., Lerner A.M. (1982). A mouse model of transmural myocardial necrosis due to coxsackievirus B4: observations over 12 months. Intervirology. 18:197-202.

Khodtsev A.S. (1986). Models of autoimmune diseases of the retina. Fiziol Cheloveka. 12:100-9. (Russian)

Khodzhagel'diev T. (1984). Formation of nicotine addiction in mongrel white rats. Biull Eksp Biol Med. 98:576-8. (English Abstract).

Khomenko A.G., Golyshevskaia V.I. (1981). Model of destructive tuberculosis in guinea pigs. Biull Eksp Biol Med. 92:627-9. (English Abstract). (Russian)

Kiel R., Smith F., Chason J., Khatib R., Reyes MP. (1989). Coxsackievirus B3 myocarditis in C3H/HeJ mice: description of an inbred model and the effect of exercise on virulence. Eur J Epidemiol 5(3):348-50.

Kilbourn M.R. (1990). Fluorine-18 Labeling of Radiopharmaceuticals. Nuclear Science Series, Washington, D.C.: National Academic Press. 149p.

Kilbourn M.R., Carey J.E., Koeppe R.E., Haka M.S. et al. (1989). Biodistribution, dosimetry, metabolism and monkey PET studies of [^{18}F]GBR13119. Imaging the dopamine uptake system in vivo. Nucl 16:569-76.

Kilpatrick L., Polin R., Douglas S., Corkey B. (1989). Hepatic metabolic alterations in rats treated with low-dose endotoxin and aspirin: an animal model of Reye's syndrome. Metabolism 38:73-7.

Kilpatrick-Smith L., Hale D., Douglas S. (1989). Progress in Reye syndrome: epidemiology, biochemical mechanisms and animal models. Dig Dis 7(3):135-46.

Kim Y.S., Kim Y. (1981). A new animal model for fetal macrosomia in diabetic pregnancy. Exp Mol Pathol. 35:388-93.

Kimata K. (1982). Cartilage matrix deficiency: a new genetic disorder in the mouse and related subjects . Seikagaku.54:162-8. (Japanese)

Kimura R.S. (1982). Animal models of endolymphatic hydrops. Am J Otolaryngol. 3:447-51.

Kindt T., Hirsch V., Johnson P., Sawasdikosol S. (1992). Animal models for acquired immunodeficiency syndrome. Adv Immunol 52:425-74.

King F.A., Yarbrough C.J. (1985). Medical and behavioral benefits from primate research. Physiologist. 28:75-87.

King N.W. (1986). Simian models of acquired immunodeficiency syndrome (AIDS): a review. Vet Pathol. 23:345-53.

Kingdon H.S., Hassell T.M. (1981). Hemophilic dog model for evaluating therapeutic effectiveness of plasma protein fractions. Blood. 58:868-72.

Kinnamon K.E., Davidson D.E. Jr., Rane D.S. (1985). Screening procedure using chicks infected with the sporozoites of Plasmodium gallinaceum in an antimalarial drug development programme. Bull WHO. 63:119-23.

Kirn A., Gut J.P., Bingen A., Steffan A.M. (1983). Murine hepatitis induced by frog virus 3: a model for studying the effect of sinusoidal cell damage on the liver. Hepatology. 3:105-11.

Kisker C.T. (1987): The animal models for hemorrhage and thrombosis in the neonate. Thromb Haemost. 57:118-22.

Kiss J., Schlumpf M., Balazs R. (1989). Selective retardation of the development of the basal forebrain cholinergic and pontine catecholaminergic nuclei in the brain of trisomy 16 mouse, an animal model of Down's syndrome. Brain Res Dev Brain Res 50(2):251-64.

Kita T., Nagano Y., Yokoda M., Ishii K. Kume N., Ooshima A., Yoshida H., Kawai C. (1987). Probucol prevents the progression of atherosclerosis in Watanabe heritable hyperlipidemic rabbit, an animal model for familial hypercholesterolemia. Proc Natl Acad Sci USA. 84:5928-31.

Kitahara M., Katakura R., Suzuki J., Sasaki T. (1987). Experimental combination chemotherapy of ACNU and 5-FU against cultured glioma model (spheroid) and subcutaneous rat glioma. Int J Cancer. 15;(40):557-63.

Klamer T.W., Donegan W.L., Max M.H. (1983). Breast tumor incidence in rats after partial mammary resection. Arch Surg. 118:933-5.

Klausen B. (1991). Microbiological and immunological aspects of experimental periodontal disease in rats: a review article. J Periodontol 62(1):59-73.

Klein E., Marangos P.J., Montgomery P., Bacher J., Uhde T.W. (1987): Adenosine receptor alterations in nervous pointer dogs. Clin Neuropharmacol. 10(5):462-9.

Klein H.H., Nebendahl K., Lindert S., Schrader J. et al. (1986). A modified regionally ischemic porcine heart preparation with eligible residual blood flows. Basic Res Cardiol. 81:384-93.

Klemm W., Bratton G., Hudson L., Sherry C., Dziezyc J. (1993). A possible feline model for human blepharospasm. Neurol Res 15(1):41-5.

Kleven M.S., Anthony E.W., Woolverton W.L. (1990). Pharmacological characterization of the discriminative stimulus effects of cocaine in Rhesus monkeys. J Pharm Exp Ther. 254:312-7.

Klimenko P.A., Ryzhova I.A., Orlov V.N., Grishin V.L., Kulaev D.V. (1986). Experimental renal failure and utero-placental circulatory insufficiency. Akush Ginekol (Mosk). 10:39-41. (English Abstract). (Russian)

Kline J. Jr., Reid K.H. (1985). The acute periventricular injury syndrome: a possible animal model for psychotic disease. Psychopharmacology (Berlin). 87:292-7.

Kloting I., Hahn H.J. (1981). Breeding of spontaneously diabetic sand rats (Psammomys obesus) under laboratory conditions. Z Versuchstierkd.23:84-90. (German)

Kluth D., Lambrecht W., Reich P., Buhrer C. (1991). SD-mice--an animal model for complex anorectal malformations. Eur J Pediatr Surg 1(3):183-8.

Kluwe W.M., Abdo K.M., Huff J. (1984). Chronic kidney disease and organic chemical exposures: evaluations of causal relationships in humans and experimental animal. Fundam Appl Toxicol. 4:889-901.

Knights K.M., Gourlay G.K., Hall P.D., Adams J.F., Cousins M.J. (1987). Halothane hepatitis in an animal model: time course of hepatic damage.Br J Exp Pathol. 68:613-24.

Knobler R.L., Rodriguez M., Lampert P.W., Oldstone M.B. (1983). Virologic models of chronic relapsing demyelinating disease. Acta Neuropathol [Suppl] (Berl). 9:31-7.

Knochel J.P. (1982). Models of hypophosphaetamia and phosphate depletion. Adv Exp Med Biol. 151:191-8.

Kobat K., Buterbaugh G.G., Eccles C.U. (1985). Methylazoxymethanol as a development model of neurotoxicity. Neurobehav Toxicol Teratol.7:519-25.

Kocsis B., Fedina L., Pasztor E. (1990). Comparison of methods eliciting cerebral ischaemic pressor response in the cat. Neurol Res 12(1):49-53.

Kodama M., Matsumoto Y., Fujiwara M., Masani F., Izumi T., Shibata A. (1990). A novel experimental model of giant cell myocarditis induced in rats by immunization with cardiac myosin fraction. Clin Immunol Immunopathol 57(2):250-62.

Kodama S., Igisu H., Siegel D A., Suzuki K. (1982). Glycosyleceramide synthesis in the developing spinal cord and kidney of the twitcher mouse, an enzymatically authentic model of human Krabbe disease. J Neurochem. 39:1314-8.

Kodama T., Kestler H. 3., Burns D., Ringler D., King N., Daniel M., Desrosiers R. (1990). Non-human primate lenti viruses: models for human infection. Dev Biol Stand 72:267-71.

Kohashi O., Aihara K., Ozawa A., Kotani S., Azuma I. (1982). New model of a synthetic adjuvant, N-acetylmuramyl-L-alanyl-D-isoglutamine- induced arthritis: clinical and histologic studies in athymic nude and euthymic rats. Lab Invest. 47:27-36.

Kohler B., Richter U., Mochmann H. (1988): Animal experiments with Campylobacter coli using suckling pigs. Arch Exp Veterinarmed. 42(2):238-53 (English Abstract). (German)

Kohler J., Silverman NA, Levitsky S., Pavel D.G., Eckner F.A. (1984). A model of cyanotic heart disease: functional, pathological, and metabolic sequelae in the immature canine heart. J Surg Res. 37:309-13.

Kohn D.F., Chinookoswong N., Chou S.M (1984). Animal model of human disease. Congenital hydrochephalus. Am J Pathol. 114:184-5.

Kohno S., Munoz J.A., Williams T.M., Teuscher C., Bernard C.C., Tung K.S. (1983). Immunopathology of murine experimental allergic orchitis. J Immunol. 130:2675-82.

Kohno S., Sasayama K., Doutsu Y., Yamashita K., Shibuya N., Miyazaki T., Koga H., Nakazato H., Nagasawa M., Suyama N. (1986). Experimental Pseudomonas pneumonia model in normal mice. Kansenshogaku Zasshi.60:1165-71. (English Abstract). (Japanese)

Kohrman K., Kirkland J., Danneman P. (1989). Response of various animal species to experimental infection with different strains of Staphylococcus aureus. Rev Infect Dis 11 Suppl 1:S231-6; discussion S236-7.

Koike S., Horie H., Sato Y., Ise I., Taya C., Nomura T., Yoshioka I., Yonekawa H., Nomoto A. (1993). Polio virus-sensitive transgenic mice as a new animal model. Dev Biol Stand 78:101-7.

Koizumi F. (1980). Animal model of rheumatism. Ryumachi. 20:371-82. (Japanese)

Kokubu M., Amatsu M. (1985). Experimental otitis media with effusion induced by electron beam irradiation to pharyngeal orifice of auditory tube in guinea pig. Auris Nasus Larynx. 1:S159-60.

Kolbasa K.P., Lancaster C., Olafsson A.S., Gilbertson S.K., Robert A. (1988): Indomethacin-induced gastric antral ulcers in hamsters. Gastroenterology. 95(4):932-44.

Kolomiets N.D., Votiakov V.I. (1987). Pathogenesis of amyotrophic leukospongiosis reproduced in guinea pigs by retrobulbar infection. Vopr Virusol.32:480-7. (English Abstract). (Russian)

Komai M., Shirakawa H., Kimura S. (1988): Newly developed model for vitamin K deficiency in germ free mice. Int J Vitam Nutr Res. 58(1):55-9.

Komeichi H., Katsuta Y., Aramaki T., Okumura H. (1991). A new experimental animal model of portal hypertension. Intrahepatic portal obstruction by injecting DEAE-cross-linked dextran microspheres into the portal vein in the rabbit. Nippon Ika Daigaku Zasshi 58(3):273-84.

Konishi K., Satoh S., Ida S., Takishima T. (1984). A rabbit model for hypersensitivity pneumonitis. Tohoku J Exp Med. 142:381-9.

Konishi Y., Mii Y., Maruyama H., Masuhara K. (1984). Malignant fibrous histiocytoma. Am J Pathol. 115:469-72.

Kono Y. (1986). Pulmonary lesions in MRL/1 mice-arteritis, phlebitis, pneumonitis. Ryumachi. 26:77-83. (English Abstract). (Japanese)

Kooistra K.L., Rodriguez M., Powis G., Yaksh T.L., Harty G.J., Hilton J.F., Lows E.R. Jr. (1986). Development of experimental models for meningeal neoplasia using intrathecal injection of 9L gliosarcoma and Walker 256 carcinosarcoma in the rat. Cancer Res. 46:317-23.

Kopchok G., White R., Tabbara M., Cavaye D., Cormier F., Peng S. (1993). A canine iliac artery occlusion model. J Invest Surg 6(1):65-70.

Kopp S., Mejersjo C., Clemenson E. (1983). Induction of osteoarthrosis in the guinea pig knee by papain. Oral Surg. 55:259-66.

Koppang N. (1993). The significance of animal models for human ceroid-lipofuscinosis. J Inherit Metab Dis. 16(2):272-3.

Kore A. (1990). Species differences: the applicability of data from one animal model to another. Vet Hum Toxicol 32(5):473-5.

Kornacewicz-Jach Z. (1985). Hemodynamics in coronary embolism in dogs. Ann Acad Med Stetin. 31:155-68. (English Abstract) (Polish)

Korneev A., Sheveleva G. (1991). [The use of the perfused rat heart as a model for selecting anti-hypoxic compounds] Nekotorye aspekty ispol'zovaniia perfuziruemogo serdtsa krysy kak modeli dlia otbora antigipoksicheskikh soedinenii. Farmakol Toksikol 54(3):67-70.

Kornetsky C., Wheeling H.S. (1982). An animal model for opiate induced euphoria and analgesia. Ther Umsch. 39:617-23.

Kornguth S.E., Bersu E.T., Auerbach R., Sobkowicz H.M., Schutta H.S., Scott G.L. (1986). Trisomy 16 mice: neural, morphological, immunological studies. Ann NY Acad Sci. 477:160-78.

Kort W.J., Weijma I.M., Westbroek D.L. (1987). Is the 7,12-dimethylbenza-anthracene-induced rat mammary tumor model suitable as a preclinical model to study mammary tumor malignancy? Cancer Invest. 5:443-7.

Kosnikova I.V., Ovchinnikov I.V. (1987). Methods for reproducing acute experimental ischemia of the extremities in rats. Pathol Fiziol Eksp Ter. 4:74-5. (Russian)

Kostowski W., Dyr W., PuciLowski O. (1990). Activity of diltiazem and nifedipine in some animal models of depression. Pol J Pharmacol Pharm 42(2):121-7.

Koto M., Miwa M., Shimizu A., Tsuji K. Okamoto M., Adachi J. (1987). Inherited hydrocephalus in Csk: Wistar-Imamichi rats; Hyd strain: a new disease model for hydrocephalus. Jikken Dobutsu. 36:157-62.

Kottgen E., Beiswenger M., James L.F., Bauer C. (1988): In vivo induction of gliadin-mediated enterocyte damage in rats by the mannosidase inhibitor, swainsonine: a possible animal model for celiac disease. Gastroenterology. 95(1):100-6.

Kotwica Z., Persson L., Hardemark H., Pahlman S. (1989). [Nerve tissue protein S 100 level in the cerebrospinal fluid as an indicator of the extent of brain damage in cerebral ischemic stroke. Experimental study of a rat model of stroke] BiaLko S-100 w pLynie mozgowo-rdzeniowym jako wskaznik wielkosci uszkodzenia tkanki nerwowej w udarze niedokrwiennym mozgu. Praca doswiadczalna na modelu udaru u szczura. Neurol Neurochir Pol 23(3):203-7.

Kotz D. (1995). Scanning the animal world. J Nucl Med. 36:16N-36N.

Koufman J., Branch M., Ryu J. (1988). A comparison of the carbon dioxide and neodymium: YAG lasers in a canine model of acquired sub-glottic stenosis. J Otolaryngol 17(5):223-6.

Kountouras J., Billing B.H., Scheuer P.J. (1984). Prolonged bile duct obstruction: a new experimental model for cirrhosis in the rat. Br J Exp Pathol. 65:305-11.

Kovalenko F., Razakov S., Khakberdiev P., Aminzhanov M., Zbarskii A., Ballad N. (1990). [Experimental imaginal Echinococcus multilocularis infestation of golden hamsters] Eksperimental'nyi imaginal'nyi mnogokamernyi ekhinokokkoz zolotistykh khomiakov. Med Parazitol (Mosk) (6):41-3.

Kovalenko F.P., Dzhabarova V.I., Rudakov V.A., Krotov A.I., Shadrin B.P. (1986). Methods of reproducing a model of larval multilocular echinococcosis with a primary lesion of the liver or the lungs. Med Parazitol (Mosk). 5:71-4. (English Abstract). (Russian)

Kovalenko V.S., Evartau E.E., Bershadskii B.G. (1984). Behavioral manifestations of the abstinence syndrome in the rat. Zh Vyssh Nerv Deiat. 34:581-3. (Russian)

Kraemer G.W., Ebert M.H., Lake C.R., McKinney W.T. (1983). Amphetamine challenge: effects in previously isolated rhesus monkeys and implications for animal models of schizophrenia. Prog Clin Biol Res. 131:199-218.

Krauss J., Mayo-Bond L., Rogers C., Weber K., Todd R. 3., Wilson J. (1991). An in vivo animal model of gene therapy for leukocyte adhesion deficiency. J Clin Invest 88(4):1412-7.

Kreider J.W., Bartlett G.L. (1981). The Shope papilloma-carcinoma complex of rabbits: a model system of neoplastic progression and spontaneous regression. Adv Cancer Res. 35:81-110.

Krendal F.P., Kudrin A.N. (1982). Characteristics of the development of model psychosis in rats in intracerebral administration of lysergic acid diethylamide. Farmakol Toksikol. 45:16-9. (English Abstract).

Kristensen K., Nørbygaard E. (Eds.) (1987). Safety and efficacy of radiopharmaceuticals. In: Cox P.H. (Ed.) Series on Developments in Nuclear Medicine. Vol 14. Dordrecht: Martinus Nijhoff Publishers. 371 pp.

Kroes R., Beems R.B., Bosland M.C., Bunnik G.S., Simkeldam E.J. (1986). Nutritional factors in lung, colon, and prostate carcinogenesis in animal models. Fed Proc. 45:136-41.

Kronauge J.F., Noska M.A., Davison A. et al. (1992). Interspecies variation in biodistribution of technetium (2-carbomethoxy-2-isocyanopropane)$_6^+$. J Nucl Med. 33:1357-65.

Kronauge J.F., Noska M.A., Davison A., Holman B.L., Jones A.G. (1992). Interspecies variation in biodistribution of technetium (2-carbomethoxy-2-isocyanoporpane)$_6^+$. J Nucl Med. 33:1357-65.

Krug H., Mahowald M., Clark C. (1989). Progressive ankylosis (ank/ank) in mice: an animal model of spondyloarthropathy. III. Proliferative spleen cell response to T cell mitogens. Clin Exp Immunol 78(1):97-101.

Krybus A.N. (1984). Experimental neurosis in developing rats. Zh Vyssh Nerv Deiat. 34:151-5. (English Abstract). (Russian)

Kryshen V.P., Smirnova T.V., Ardelian V.N. (1984). Experimental simulation of liver abscess in the rabbit. Patol Fiziol Eksp Ter. 2:68-9. (Russian)

Kryzhanovskii G., Karpova M., Abramova E., Abrosimov I. (1992). [The antiepileptic effects of sodium valproate and the calcium antagonist riodipine when used jointly in a model of focal penicillin-induced epileptic activity] Antiepilepticheskie effekty val'proata natriia i antagonista kal'tsiia riodipina pri ikh sochetannom primenenii na modeli fokal'noi penitsillin-indutsirovannoi epileticheskoi aktivnosti. Biull Eksp Biol Med 114(10):369-70.

Kryzhanovskii G.N., Lobasiuk B.A., Mokhovikov A.N., Bartsevich L.B., Mosketi K.V. (1987). Modelling psychosis in cats by creating a generator of pathologically enhanced excitation in one of the septal nuclei. Biull Eksp Biol Med. 104:405-8 (English Abstract). (Russian)

Kryzhanovskii G.N., Makul'kin R.F.,Shandra A.A., Godlevskii L.S., Rozhkov V.S. (1987): Modelling of the parkinsonian syndrome by the administration of kainic acid into the caudate nucleus. Biull Eksp Biol Med. 103:650-3 (English Abstract). (Russian)

Kubota K., Som P., Brill AB., Sacker D., Meinken G., Srivastava S., Atkins H. (1989). Comparative dual-tracer studies of carbon-14 tryptophan and iodine-131 HIPDM in animal models of pancreatic diseases. J Nucl Med 30(11):1848-55.

Kubota K., Som P., Oster Z.H., Brill A.B., Goodman M.M., Knapp Jr. F.E. et al. (1988). Detection of cardiomyopathy in an animal model using quantitative autoradiography. J Nucl Med. 29:1697-703.

Kubota R., Kubota K., Yamada S., Tada M., Ido T., Tamahashi N. (1995). Microautoradiographic study for the differentiation of intratumoral macrophages, granulation tissues and cancer cells by the dynamics of fluorine-18 fluorodeoxyglucose uptake. J Nucl Med.35:104-12.

Kudo M., Aoyama A., Ichimori S., Fukunaga N. (1982). An animal model of cerebral infarction. Homologous blood clot emboli in rats. Stroke. 13:505-8.

Kudo Y., Shiosaka S., Matsuda M., Tohyama M. (1989). An attempt to cause the selective loss of the cholinergic neurons in the basal forebrain of the rat: a new animal model of Alzheimer's disease. Neurosci Lett 102(2-3):125-30.

Kuehn M.R., Bradley A., Robertson E.J., Evans M.J. (1987). A potential animal model for Lesch-Nyhan syndrome through introduction of HPRT mutations into mice. Nature. 326:295-8.

Kukain R.A., Nagaeva L.I., Lozha V.P. (1983). Chronic lympholeukemia in cattle as an experimental model for finding the oncogen. Vopr Onkol.29:73-8. (Russian)

Kukla L.J,, Abramson E.C., McCuire W.P., Shevrin D.H., Lad T., Kukreja SC. (1984). Cis-platinum treatment for malignancy-associated humoral hypercalcemia in an athymic mouse model. Calcif Tissue Int. 36:559-62.

Kumano K., Kogure K., Tanaka T., Sakai T. (1986). A new method of inducing experimental chronic renal failure by cryosurgery. Kidney Int. 30:433-6.

Kumar S., Sigmon D., Miller T., Carpenter B., Khan S., Malhotra R., Scheid C., Menon M. (1991). A new model of nephrolithiasis involving tubular dysfunction/injury. J Urol 146:1384-9.

Kuriyama K., Ichikawa K. (1982). An experimental asthma model in unanesthetized rat, and the difference in effect of disodium cromoglycate between passive cutaneous anaphylaxis model and asthma model in rat. Pharmacobiodyn. 5:751-9.

Kurokawa Y., Hashi K., Okuyama T., Sasaki S. (1989). An experimental model of cerebral venous hypertension in the rat. Neurol Med Chir (Tokyo) 29(3):175-80.

Kurz K.D., Johnson J.A., Fowler W.L. Jr., Siripaisarnpipat S., Payne C.G. (1981). Absence of an antihypertensive effect of 12 hour infusions of an angiotensin antagonist in chronic renal hypertensive rabbits. Clin Exp Hypertens. 3:1195-205.

Kusche J., Menningen R., Leisten L., Krakamp B. (1988). Large bowel tumor promotion by diamine oxidase inhibition: animal model and clinical aspects. Adv Exp Med Biol 250:745-52.

Kuwabara S., Andoh S., Uno J., Matsumoto S., Ishikawa S. (1988): Experimental model of brainstem infarction. Neurol Med Chir (Tokyo). 28(3):223-9. (English Abstract). (Japanese)

Kuzan F., Patton D., Allen S., Kuo C. (1989). A proposed mouse model for acute epididymitis provoked by genital serovar E, Chlamydia trachomatis. Biol Reprod 40(1):165-72.

Kuznetsov V. (1991). [Effect of adaptation to continuous stress on the contractile function and electric stability of the heart] Vliianie adaptatsii i nepreryvnomu stressornomu vozdeistviiu na sokratitel'nuiu funktsiiu i elektricheskuiu stabil'nost' serdtsa. Kardiologiia 31(6):85-6.

Kuzon W.M. Jr., Walker P.M., Mickle D.A., Harris K.A., Pynn B.R., McKee N.H. (1986). An isolated skeletal muscle model suitable for acute ischemia studies. J Surg Res. 41:24-32.

Kyogoku M. (1982). Disease model for refractory diseases. Gan To Kagaku Ryoho. 9:1863-70.

Laas R., Igloffstein J. (1983). Cerebral infarction due to carotid occlusion and carbon monoxide exposure. I. Pathophysiological and neuropathologicla investigations. J Neurol Neurosurg Psychiatry. 46:756-67.

Labrid C. (1988): Experimental models in cerebral ischemia: application to the study of duxil. Rev Med Interne. 9(1):21-6. (French)

Lacey D.J. (1984). Hippocampal dendritic abnormalities in a rat model of phenylketonuria. Ann Neurol. 16:577-80.

Lachmann B. (1989). Animal models and clinical pilot studies of surfactant replacement in adult respiratory distress syndrome. Eur Respir J Suppl 3:98s-103s.

Ladds P.W., Daniels P.W. (1982). Animal model of human disease. Squamous cell carcinoma. Ovine squamous cell carcinoma. Am J Pathol. 107:122-3.

Lafreniere R., Rosenberg S.A. (1986). A novel approach to the generation and identification of experimental hepatic mestastases in a murine model. JNCI. 76:309-22.

Lahti A., Maibach H.I. (1984). An animal model for nonimmunologic contact urticaria. Toxicol Appl pharmacol. 76:219-24.

Lal H., Emmett-Oglesby M.W. (1983). Behavioral analogues of anxiety. Animal models. Neuropharmacology. 22:1423-41.

Lambrecht R.M. and Eckelman W.C. (Eds) (1983).: Animal Models in Radiotracer Design. Springer-Verlag, New York. 260 pp.

Lambrecht R.M., Eckelman W.C., Rescigno A. (1983). Animal models in biomedical research and radiotracer design. In: Lambrecht R.M., Eckelman W.C. (Eds). Animal Models in Radiotracer Design. Heidelberg: Springer Verlag. pp 1-34.

Lambrecht R.M., Hara T., Gallagher B.M., Wolf A.P., Ansari A., Atkins A. (1978). Cyclotron isotopes and radiopharmaceuticals. XXVIII. Potassium-38 for myocardial perfusion studies. Int J Appl Rad Isotopes 29:667-71.

Lambrecht R.M., Rescigno A. (Ed.) (1983). Tracer Kinetics and Physiologic Modelling - Theory To Practice. In: Lecture Notes in Biomathematics (S. Levin), Springer Verlag, Heidelberg:502

Lambrecht R.M., Wolf A.P. (1973). The cyclotron and short-lived halogen isotopes for radiopharmaceutical applications. Radiopharmaceuticals and Labeled Compounds, IAEA, Vienna, Vol I, pp 275-90.

Lambrecht R.M., Woodhouse N., Phillips R., Wolczak D.F. et al. (1988). Investigational study of iodine-124 with a positron camera. Amer J Physiologic Imaging 3:197-200.

Lamm M.E., Emancipator S.N., Gallo G.R. (1984). Relevance of an experimental model to clinical IgA nephropathy. Contrib Nephrol. 40:32-6.

Lamperth, L., Dalakas, MC., Dagani, F., Anderson, J., Ferrari, R. (1991). Abnormal skeletal and cardiac muscle mitochondria induced by zidovudine (AZT) in human muscle in vitro and in an animal model. Lab Invest, 65 (6):742-51.

Landa Garcia II., Arias Diaz J., Torres Garcia A., Jover Navalon J.M., Gomez Cutierrez M., Calleja Kempin J. et al. (1988): Experimental model of chronic portal hypertension. Rev Esp Enferm Apar Dig. 73(2):131-7. (English Abstract). (Spanish)

Landau I., Chabaud A. (1994). Plasmodium species infecting Thamnomys rutilans: a zoological study. Adv Parasitol. 33:49-90.

Lander E.b., Hewitt C.W., Black K.S., Martin D.C. (1986). Evaluation of the rat renal allograft model in comparison to man: a physiological perspective. J Urol. 136:710-4.

Landymore R.W., Kinley L.E., Cameron C.A. (1985). Intimal hyperplasia in autogenous vein grafts used for arterial bypass: a canine model. Cardiovasc Res. 19:589-92.

Lang C.H., Bagby G.J., Bornside G.H., Vail L.J., Spitzer J.J. (1983). Sustained hypermetabolic sepsis in rats: characterization of the model. J Surg Res. 35:201-10.

Lang J.A., Sinclair N.L., Burson J.M., Sigmund C.D. (1994). Transgenic animals as tools in hypertension research. Proc Soc Exp Biol Med. 205(2):106-18.

Langford M.P., Yin-Murphy M., Barber J.C., Heard H.K., Stanton G.J. (1986). Conjunctivitis in rabbits caused by enterovirus type 70 (EV70). Invest Ophthalmol Vis Sci. 27:915-20.

Langhorne J. (1994). The immune response to the blood stages of Plasmodium in animal models. Immunol Lett. 41(2-3):99-102.

Lankford M., Roscoe A., Pennington S., Myers R. (1991). Drinking of high concentrations of ethanol versus palatable fluids in alcohol-preferring (P) rats: valid animal model of alcoholism. Alcohol 8(4):293-9.

Lannfelt L., Folkesson R., Mohammed A.H., Winblad B., Hellgren D., Duff K., Hardy J. (1993). Alzheimer's disease: molecular genetics and transgenic animal models. Behav Brain Res. 57(2):207-13.

Lapidot T., Pflumio F., Dick J.E. (1993). Modeling human hematopoiesis in immunodeficient mice. Lab Anim Sci. 43(2):147-50.

Lapin B.A., Shevtsova Z.V., Krylova R.I., Korzaia L.I. (1988). Viral hepatitis A in lower Old World monkeys (possibility of use as a model for vaccine testing). Biull Eksp Biol Med. 105:17-9 (Eng. Abstr.) (Russian)

Larkin D., Easty D. (1990). Experimental Acanthamoeba keratitis: I. Preliminary findings. Br J Ophthalmol 74(9):551-5.

Larson S.M., Pentlow K.S., Volkow N.D., Wolf A.P., Lambrecht R.M., Finn R.D., Graham M.C. et al. (1992). PET scanning of ^{124}I-3F8 as a novel method of tumor dosimetry during treatment planning for radioimmunotherapy in a child with neuroblastoma. J Nucl Med. 33:2020-3.

Lassman H. (1983). Chronic relapsing experimental allergic encephalomyelitis its value as an experimental model for multiple sclerosis. J Neurol. 229:207-20.

Lathe R., Mullins J.J. (1993). Transgenic animals as models for human disease - report of an EC Study Group. Transgenic Res. 2(5):286-99.

Lauricella M.A., Riarte A., Lazzari J.O., Barousse A.P., Segura E.L. (1986): Chagas' disease in dogs experimentally infected with Trypanosoma cruzi. Medicina (B Aires). 46:195-200 (English Abstract). (Spanish)

Laver N., Robison W. J., Pfeffer B. (1993). Novel procedures for isolating intact retinal vascular beds from diabetic humans and animal models. Invest Ophthalmol Vis Sci 34(6):2097-104.

Laviola G. (1993). Mouse models of emotional postpartum disorders. Ann Ist Super Sanita. 29(1):153-62.

Lawler J.E., Cox R.H., Sanders B.J., Mitchell V.P (1988): The borderline hypertensive rat: a model for studying the mechanisms of environmentally induced hypertension. Health Psychol. 7(2):137-47.

Le Douarin N.M. (1987): Chimeras of the spinal cord between quail and chicken. A new experimental model for studying demyelinating diseases. Pathol Biol (Paris). 35:325-31 (English Abstract). (French)

Le Gal La Salle G., Cavalheira E.A., Feldblum S., Maresova D. (1983). Experimental models of epilepsy. Their predictive value. Therapie. 38:123-33. (English Abstract). (French)

Le Magnen J., Marfaing-Jallat P. (1984). Further study of induced behavioral dependence on ethanol in rats. Alcohol. 1:269-73.

Le May D.R., Neal S., Neal S., Zelenock G.B., D'Alecy L.G. (1987). Paraplegia in the rat induced by aortic cross-clamping: model characterization and glucose exacerbation of neurologic deficit. J Vasc Surg. 6:383-90.

Le Q., Cortez S., Nguyen H., Shah S., Baricos W. (1992). Glomerular neutral metalloproteinase: characterization and activity in animal models of human glomerular disease. Matrix Sup 1:415-6.

Leader R.W., Hegreberg G.A., Padgett G.A., Wagner B.M. (1983). Comparative pathology of connective tissue diseases. Monogr Pathol. 24:150-62.

Lecci A., Borsini F., Volterra G., Meli A. (1990). Pharmacological validation of a novel animal model of anticipatory anxiety in mice. Psychopharmacology (Berl) 101(2):255-61.

Ledent C., Parmentier M., Vassart G., Dumont J.E. (1994). Models of thyroid goiter and tumors in transgenic mice. Mol Cell Endocrinol. 100(1-2):167-9.

LeDuc J.W., Lemon S.M., Keenan C.M., Graham R.R., Marchwicki-R.H., Binn L.N. (1983). Experimental infection of the New World owl monkey (Aotus trivirgatus) with hepatitis. A virus. Infect Immun. 40:766-72.

Lee A., Fox J., Otto G., Murphy J. (1990). A small animal model of human Helicobacter pylori active chronic gastritis. Gastroenterology 99(5):1315-23.

Lee J., Kim T., Chiocca E., Medhkour A., Martuza RL. (1990). Growth of human schwannomas in the subrenal capsule of the nude mouse. Neurosurgery 26(4):598-605.

Lee M.I., Oakes G.K., Lam R., Hobel C.J. (1982). The rabbit: a suitable model for investigation of vascular responsiveness during pregnancy. Clin Exp Hypertens [B]. 1:429-39.

Lee T.D., Zhao T., Chi Z., Wong H., Shen M., Rodey G. (1983). Cortisone-induced immunotolerance to nematode infection in CBA/Ca mice. II. A model for human chronic trichuriasis. Immunology. 48:571-7.

Lees P., Higgins A.J., Sedgwick A.D., May S.A. (1987). Applications of equine models of acute inflammation. The Ciba-Geigy Prize for Research in Animal Health. Vet Rec. 120:522-9.

Lehman T.J., Mahnovski V. (1988): Animal models of vasculitis. Lessons we can learn to improve our understanding of Kawasaki disease. Rheum Dis Clin North Am. 14(2):479-87.

Lehman T.J., Warren R., Giett D., Mahnouski V., Prescott M. (1988): Variable expression of Lactobacillus casei cell wall-induced coronary arteritis: an animal model of Kawasaki's disease in selected inbred mouse strains. Clin Immunol Immunopathol. 48(1):108-18.

Leib D.A, Hart C.A, McCarthy K. (1988): Alpha herpes virus saimiri in rabbits: a model for human encephalitis? J Gen Virol. 69(Pt 7):1609-15.

Leibovici J., Wolman M. (1984) Animal models for tumor progression. Anticancer Res. 4:165-8.

Leiby D.A., el Naggar H.M., Schad G.A. (1987). Thirty generations of Ancylostoma duodenale in laboratory-reared beagles. J Parasito. 73:844-8.

Leiter E.H., Prochazka M., Coleman D.L. (1987). The non-obese diabetic (NOD) mouse. Am J Pathol. 128:380-3.

Leng M.L. (1982). Jumping chickens: relevance to hazards in humans. Science. 215:1421-2.

Leon J., Kamino H., Steinberg J., Pellicer A. (1988). H-ras activation in benign and self-regressing skin tumors (keratoacanthomas) in both humans and an animal model system. Mol Cell Biol 8(2):786-93.

Leonard B.E. (1984). The olfactory bulbectomized rat as a model of depression. Pol J Pharmacol Pharm. 36:561-9.

Leonard J.M., Abramczuk J.W., Pezen D.S., Rutledge R., Belcher J.H., Hakim F. et al. (1988): Development of disease and virus recovery in transgenic mice containing HIV proviral DNA. Science. 23; 242(4886):1665-70.

Lerch M.M., Adler G. (1994). Experimental animal models of acute pancreatitis. Int J Pancreatol. 15(3):159-70.

Lerer B., Stanley M., Altman H., Kcegan M. (1986). An animal model of electro-convulsive-therapy-induced amnesia. Possible neurochemical correlates. Ann NY Acad Sci. 462:91-8.

Lerner A.B., Shiolara T., Boissy R.E., Jacobson K.A., Lamoreud M.L., Moellmann G.E. (1986). A mouse model for vitiligo. J Invest Dermatol. 87:299-304.

Lesser T., Ebner E., Zwiener U. (1989). [The hemodynamics of the lung circulation of minipigs after experimentally-caused Sedlarik's pulmonary embolism. I. Sedlarik's pulmonary embolism model in comparison to existing embolism models] Zur Hämodynamik des Lungenkreislaufes des Minischweins nach experimentell ausgelöster Lungenembolie nach Sedlarik. I. Das Lungenemboliemodell nach Sedlarik im Vergleich zu bisherigen Emboliemodellen. Z Exp Chir Transplant Künstliche Organe 22(6):342-6.

Letvin N.L, Daniel M.D, Sehgal P.K, Desrosiers R.C, Hunt R.D, Waldron L.M, Mackey J.J., Schmidt D.K., Chalifoux L.V., King N.W. (1985). Induction of AIDS-like disease in macaque monkeys with T-cell tropic retrovirus STLV-III. Science. 230:71-3.

Letvin N.L., Eaton K.A., Aldrich W.R., Sehgal P.K., Blake B.J., Schlossman S.F., King N.W., Hunt R.D. (1983) Acquired immunodeficiency syndrome in a colony of macaque monkeys. Proc Natl Acad Sci USA. 80:2718-22.

Letvin N.L., Hunt R.D., Finberg R. (1984). Animal models of AIDS. Semin Oncol. 11:18-28.

Letvin N.L., King N.W. (1991). Naturally Occurring Animal Models of the Aquired Immune Deficiency Syndrome (AIDS). Amer J Physiologic Imaging 6:1-15.

Levin E. (1992). Nicotinic systems and cognitive function. Psychopharmacology 108:417-21.

Levine N., Queen L., Chalom A.A., Daniels L.J. (1982). Animal model of intracutaneous melanoma. J Invest Dermatol. 78:191-3.

Lewis A.J., Kirchner T., Dervinis A., Rosenthale M.E. (1982). Ascaris-induced allergic asthma in the conscious dog: a model for the pharmacologic modulation of immediate type hypersensitivity. J Pharmacol Methods. 7:35-46.

Lewis S., Erickson R., Barnett L., Venta P., Tashian R. (1988). N-ethyl-N-nitrosourea-induced null mutation at the mouse Car-2 locus: an animal model for human carbonic anhydrase II deficiency syndrome. Proc Natl Acad Sci U S A 85(6):1962-6.

Lewis S.A., Lyon I.C., Elliott R.B. (1985). Outcome of pregnancy in the rat with mild hyperphenylalaninaemia and hypertyrosinaemia: implications for the management of "human maternal PKU". J Inherited Metab Dis. 8:113-7.

Leyten R., Vroemen J.P., Blanckaert N., Heirwegh K.P. (1986). The congenic normal R/APfd-j/j rat strains: a new animal model of hereditary non-haemolytic unconjugated hyperbilirubinaemia due to defective bilirubin conjugation. Lab Anim. 20:335-42.

Li T.K., Lumeng L. (1984). Alcohol preference and voluntary alcohol intakes of inbred rat strains and the National Institutes of Health heterogeneous stock of rats. Alcoholism (NY). 8:485-6.

Li T.K., Lumeng L., McBride W.J., Murphy J.M. (1987). Rodent lines selected for factors effecting alcohol consumption. Alcohol (Suppl) 1: 91-6.

Li W., Qian H. (1993). [Human ovarian epithelial adenocarcinoma with peritoneal metastasis and ascites established in murine models]. Chung Hua Fu Chan Ko Tsa Chih 28(1):38-40, 61.

Li Y., Togashi Y., Sato S., Emoto T., Kang JH., Takeichi N., Kobayashi H., Kojima Y., Une Y., Uchino J. (1991). Spontaneous hepatic copper accumulation in Long-Evans Cinnamon rats with hereditary hepatitis. A model of Wilson's disease. J Clin Invest 87(5):1858-61.

Li Z. (1992). [Experimental infection with hepatitis E virus in rhesus monkeys]. Chung Hua I Hsueh Tsa Chih 72(11):658-60, 701-2.

Lieber C.S., DeCarli L.M. (1988): Journal of Medical Primatology Volume 3, 1974: An experimental model of alcohol feeding and liver injury in the baboon. Nutr Rev. 46(7):263-4.

Likar I.N., Robinson R.W. (1985). Atherosclerosis: cattle as a model for study in man. Monogr Atheroscler. 12:1-175.

Like A.A., Anthony M., Guberski D.L., Rossini A.A. (1982). Spontaneous autoimmune diabetes mellitus in the BB rat. Diabetes. 31(Suppl 1 Pt 2):7-13.

Lillehei K.O., Chandler W.F., Knake J.E. (1984). Real time ultrasound characteristics of the acute intracerebral hemorrhage as studied in the canine model. Neurosurgery. 14:48-51.

Lillrank S., Oja S., Saransaari P., Seppala T. (1991). Animal models of amphetamine psychosis: neurotransmitter release from rat brain slices. Int J Neurosci 60(1-2):1-15.

Limb G., Brown K., Wolstencroft R., Ellis B., Dumonde D. (1989). The production of arthritis in the guinea-pig by intra-articular reaction between lymphokines and inflammatory leucocytes. Br J Exp Pathol 70(4):443-56.

Lin J., Cheng J., Tzeng C., Yeh M., Meng C. (1991). An animal model for colon cancer metastatic cell line with enhanced metastasizing ability. Establishment and characterization. Dis Colon Rectum 34(6):458-63.

Lindsay T.F. (1994). The in vivo gracilis muscle model of skeletal muscle ischemia. J Invest Surg. 7(1):17-26.

Lindsberg P., Frerichs K., Burris J., Hallenbeck J., Feuerstein G. (1991). Cortical microcirculation in a new model of focal laser-induced secondary brain damage. J Cereb Blood Flow Metab 11(1):88-98.

Lindsey W., Masterson T., Spotnitz W., Wilhelm M., Morgan R. (1990). Seroma prevention using fibrin glue in a rat mastectomy model. Arch Surg 125(3):305-7.

Lindsley M., Patick A., Prayoonwiwat N., Rodriguez M. (1992). Coexpression of class I major histocompatibility antigen and viral RNA in central nervous system of mice infected with Theiler's virus: a model for multiple sclerosis [see comments]. Mayo Clin Proc 67(9):829-38.

Linhart W., Spendel S., Weber G., Zadravec S. (1990). Septic arthritis - an experimental animal model useful in free oxygen radical research. Z Versuchstierkd 33(2):65-71.

Linsky C.B., Diamond M.P., Cunningham T., Constantine B., DeCherney A.H., diZerega G.S. (1987): Adhesion reduction in the rabbit uterine horn model using an absorbable barrier, TC-7. J Reprod Med. 32:17-20.

Linville D.G., Williams S., Raskiewicz J.L., Arneric S.P. (1993). Nicotinic antagonists modulate basal forebrain (BF) control of cortical cerebral blood flow in anesthetized rats. J Pharmacol Exp Ther. 267:440-61.

Lips J., Jongsma H., Eskes T. (1988). Alloxan-induced diabetes mellitus in pregnant sheep and chronic fetal catheterization. Lab Anim 22(1):16-22.

Lipson A., Webster W., Brown-Woodman P., Osborn R. (1989). Moebius syndrome: animal model - human correlations and evidence for a brainstem vascular etiology. Teratology 40:339-50.

Lister R. (1990). Ethologically-based animal models of anxiety disorders. Pharmacol Ther 46(3):321-40.

Little R.R., Parker K.M., England J.P., Goldstein D.E. (1982). Glycosylated hemoglobin in Mystromys albicaudatus: a diabetic animal model. Lab Anim Sci. 32:44-7.

Liu A., Katzenellenbogen J.A., VanBrocklin H.F., Mathias C.J., Welch M.J. (1991). 20-[18F]fluoromibolerone, a positron-emitting radiotracer for androgen receptors: Synthesis and tissue distribution studies. J Nucl Med. 32:81-8.

Liu L.X., Zhang X.Y., Song H.Y., Niu H.Z., Li Z.J. (1985). Studies on the hamster colitis model. Wei Sheng Wu Hsueh Pao. 25:60-5. (English Abstract). (Chinese)

Liu Q. (1992). [Establishing orthotopic transplanted models of human pancreatic cancer in nude mice and study on their biological properties]. Chung Hua Chung Liu Tsa Chih 14(6):403-6.

Lloyd D.H., Noble W.C. (1982). Dermatophilus congolensis as a model pathogen in mice for the investigation of factors influencing skin infection. Br Vet J. 138:51-60.

Loc'h C., Bourguignon M., Maziere B., Stulzaft O., Ottavani M., Hantraye P., Chabriat H., Raynaud C., Syrota A., Maziere M. (1991). 123I-Iodolisuride, un nouvel agent pour l'étude des récepteurs dopaminergiques D2 par tomographie d'émission monophotonique (SPECT). J Med Nucl Biophy. 15(4):420-7.

Logothetis J., Karacostas D., Karoutas G., Artemis N., Mansouri A., Milonas I. (1983). A new model of subarachnoid hemorrhage in experimental animals with the purpose to examine cerebral vasospasm. Exp Neurol. 81:257-78.

London E.D., Scheffel U., Kimes A.S., Kellar K.J. (1995). In vivo labeling of nicotinic cholinergic receptors in brain using [H-3]epibatidine. Eur J Pharmacology 278:R1-R2.

Long Z., Sun C.S., White E.M., Horowitz B., Sito A.F. (1993). Hepatitis B viral clearance studies using duck virus model. Dev Biol Stand. 81:163-8.

Longnecker D.S. (1981). Animal model of human disease. Carcinoma of the pancreas in azaserine-treated rats. Am J Pathol. 105:94-6.

Longnecker D.S., Wiebkin P., Schaeffer B.K., Roebuck B.D. (1984). Experimental carcinogenesis in the pancreas. Int Rev Exp Pathol. 26:177-229.

Loo Y.H., Rabe A., Potempska A., Wang P., Fersko R., Wisniewski H.M. (1983-1984). Experimental maternal phenylketonuria: an examination of two animal models. Dev Neurosci. 6:227-34.

Loor F., Jachez B., Montecino-Rodriguez E., Klein A.S., Kuntz L., Pflumio F., Fonteneau P. et al. (1988). Radiation therapy of spontaneous autoimmunity: a review of mouse models. Int J Radiat Biol. 53: 119-36.

Lord E.M., Burkhardt G. (1984). Assessment of in situ host immunity to syngeneic tumors utilizing the multicellular spheroid model. Cell Immunol. 85:340-50.

Lorente C.A., Tassinari M.S., Keith D.A. (1981). The effects of phenytoin on rat development: an animal model system for fetal hydantoin syndrome. Teratology. 24:169-80.

Lorentz W.B. Jr., Shihabi Z.K., Weidner N. (1987). Galactosemic nephropathy in the rat. Clin Physiol Biochem. 5:261-7.

Lorenzo A.V. (1985). The preterm rabbit: a model for the study of acute and chronic effects of premature birth. Pediatr Res. 19:201-5.

Loscher W., Schmidt D. (1988): Which animal models should be used in the search for new antiepileptic drugs? A proposal based on experimental and clinical considerations. Epilepsy Res. 2(3):145-81.

Lothrop C.D. Jr., Caulson P.A., Nolan H.L., Cole B., Jones J.B., Sanders W.L. (1987). Cyclic hormonogenesis in gray collie dogs: interactions of hematopoietic and endocrine systems. Endocrinology. 120:1027-32.

Louis E.D., Williamson P.D., Darcey T.M. (1987): Experimental models of chronic focal epilepsy: a critical review of four models. Yale J Biol Med. 60:255-72.

Lovenberg W. (1987): Animal models for hypertension research. Prog Clin Biol Res. 229:225-40.

Lovik M. (1987). Experimental murine leprosy and its relevance for the study of resistance to mycobacterial infections in man. Int J Lepr Other Mycobact Dis. 55:689-701.

Low P.A., Schmelzer J.S., Ward K.K., Yao J.K. (1986). Experimental chronic hypoxic neuropathy: relevance to diabetic neuropathy. Am J Physiol. 250:E94-9.

Lu S.Q. (1986). Giardia lamblia infection in the gerbil (Meriones unguiculatus): an animal model. Chung Hua I Hsueh Tsa Chih. 66:157-8,189. (English Abstract). (Chinese)

Lubbesmeyer H., Basadre J., Mollmann M., Traber L., Maguire J., Herndon DN., Traber D. (1989). Hydroxyethyl starch and lung lymph flow in an ovine model of endotoxemia. Prog Clin Biol Res 308:815-9.

Lucas C., Cheriex E., van d. V. F., Habets J., van d. N. T., Penn O., Wellens H. (1992). Imipramine induced heart failure in the dog: a model to study the effect of cardiac assist devices. Cardiovasc Res 26(8):804-9.

Lucey E.C. (1983). Experimental emphysema. Clin Chest Med. 4:389-403.

Lun A., Dominick B., Gross J. (1990). An animal model of perinatal hypoxic brain damage: behavioural aspects. Biomed Biochim Acta 49(10):1021-6.

Lun A., Gruetzmann H., Wustmann C., Szuesz L., Dominick B., Horvath G., Fischer HD., Nagy I., Gross J. (1989). Effect of pyritinol on the dopaminergic system and behavioural outcome in an animal model of mild chronic postnatal hypoxia. Biomed Biochim Acta 48(2-3):S237-42.

Lund D.D., Schmid P.G., Roskoski R. Jr. (1983). Neurochemical indices of autonomic innervation of heart in different experimental models of heart failure. Adv Exp Med Biol. 161:179-98.

Lundell A., Bergqvist D., Leide S., Lindblad B., Ljungberg J. (1991). The effect of a thromboxane receptor antagonist on acute ePTFE arterial graft thrombogenicity - an experimental study in sheep. Eur J Vasc Surg 5(3):321-6.

Luscombe G., Jenner P., Marsden C.D. (1986). 5-HT-mediated myoclonus in the guinea pig as a model of brainstem 5-HT and tryptamine receptor action. Adv Neurol. 43:529-43.

Lusso P., Markham P., DeRocco S., Gallo R. (1990). In vitro susceptibility of T lymphocytes from chimpanzees (Pan troglodytes) to human herpesvirus 6 (HHV-6): a potential animal model to study the interaction between HHV-6 and human immunodeficiency virus type 1 in vivo. J Virol 64(6):2751-8.

Luyten G., Mooy C., De J. P., Hoogeveen A., Luider T. (1993). A chicken embryo model to study the growth of human uveal melanoma. Biochem Biophys Res Commun 192(1):22-9.

Lyden P.D., Selig J., Martin R.P., Yoshida s., Bailey M., Rothrock J.F., Alksne J.A. (1985). A new model of focal cerebral ischemia: validation and utility. Bull Clin Neurosci. 50:69-75.

Ma J.W., (1982). Exploration on Radix trichosanthis on the model of anaphylactic shock in mice. Chung Yao Tung Pao. 7:33-5. (Chinese)

Machado e. S. J., de O. R., Rodrigues e. S. R., Maldonado J., Rey L. (1991). [Wild rodents as experimental models of schistosomiasis mansoni: Akodon arviculoides (Rodentia: Cricetidae)] Roedores silvestres como modelos experimentais da esquistossomose mansonica: Akodon arviculoides (Rodentia: Cricetidae). Rev Inst Med Trop Sao Paulo 33(4):257-61.

Maciver I., Silverman S., Brown M., O'Reilly T. (1991). Rat model of chronic lung infections caused by non-typable Haemophilus influenzae. J Med Microbiol 35(3):139-47.

Mackinnon S.E., Dellon A.L., Hudson A.R., Hunter D.A. (1984). Chronic nerve compression--an experimental model in the rat. Ann Plast Surg. 13: 112-20.

Macklis R., Kaplan W., Ferrara J., Atcher R., Hines J., Burakoff S., Coleman C. (1989). Alpha particle radio-immunotherapy: animal models and clinical prospects. Int J Radiat Oncol Biol Phys 16(6):1377-87.

MacLellan D.G., Shulkes A., Hardy K.J. (1986). Profile of gastric stress following acute cervical cord injury: an animal model. Aust NZ J Surg. 56:499-504.

MacLeod I.A., Bow C.R., Joffe S.N. (1982). A quantifiable bleeding gastric ulcer in dogs for assessing the neodymium Yag laser. Endoscopy. 14:9-10.

Madel J.T. (1985). Animal models of osteomyelitis. Am J Med. 78:213-7.

Magid N.M., Young M.S., Wallerson D.C., Goldweit R.S., Carter J.N., Devereux R.B., Borer J.S. (1988): Hypertrophic and functional response to experimental chronic aortic regurgitation. J Mol Cell Cardiol. 20(3):239-46.

Maguire H.C. Jr., Kaidbey K. (1982). Experimental photoallergic contact dermatitis: a mouse model. J Invest Dermatol. 79:147-52.

Mahajan D.K. (1988): Polycystic ovarian disease: animal models. Endocrinol Metab Clin North Am. 17(4):705-32.

Mahowald M.L., Krug H., Taurog J. (1988): Progressive ankylosis in mice. An animal model of spondylarthropathy. I. Clinical and radiographic findings. Arthritis Rheum. 31(11):1390-9.

Maiboroda A.D. (1983). Inbred mice and their viruses as a model in virology. Vestn Akad Med Nauk SSSR. 9:68-71. (English Abstract)

Maier S.F. (1984). Learned helplessness and animal models of depression. Prog Neuropsychopharmacol Biol Psychiatry. 8:435-46.

Mailman R.B., Lewis M.H., Kilts C.D. (1981). Animal models related to developmental disorders: theoretical and pharmacological analyses. Appl Res Ment Retard. 2:1-12.

Mak J., Choong M., Lam P., Suresh K. (1990). Experimental infection of the leaf-monkeys, Presbytis cristata and Presbytis melalophos with subperiodic Brugia malayi. Acta Trop (Basel) 47(4):223-6.

Makino H., Theng LZ., Kumagai I., Takatori K., Ota Z., Yoshifusa H. (1990). [Progressive glomerular sclerosis and renal failure in rat with 7/8 nephrectomy model]. Nippon Jinzo Gakkai Shi 32(2):127-36.

Malemud C.J. (1993). Markers of osteoarthritis and cartilage research in animal models [published erratum appears in Curr Opin Rheumatol 1993; 5(5):667]. Curr Opin Rheumatol. 5(4):494-502.

Malemud C.J., Goldberg V.M., Moskowitz R.W. (1986). Pathological, biochemical and experimental therapeutic studies in meniscectomy models of osteoarthritis in the rabbit-its relationship to human joint pathology. Br J Clin Pract. 43:21-31.

Mall G., Mattfeldt T., Hasslacher C., Mann J. (1986). Morphological reaction patterns in experimental cardiac hypertrophy - a quantitative stereological study. Basic Res Cardio. 1:193-201.

Malo C., Morin C.L. (1986). Establishment of an animal model of ovalbumin sensitised mouse to study protein induced enteropathy. Gut. 27:1298-305.

Malov Ius., Solodovniko V.I. (1982). Arthus phenomenon in the wall of the stomach as a model for studying peptic ulcer. Patol Fiziol Eksp Ter. 95:28-30. (Russian)

Maltais L.J., Lane P.W., Beamer W.G. (1984). Anorexia, a recessive mutation causing starvation in preweaning mice. J Hered. 75:468-72.

Mamedov L.A., Nikolaev A.V., Iunuskhodzhaev E., Zakharov V.V., Semenova N.A. (1988): A method for creating an experimental model of abscess. Arkh Patol. 50(8):82-4. (English Abstract). (Russian)

Mandell J., Koch W.K., Nidess R., PreMinger G.M., McFarland E. (1983). congential polycystic kidney disease. Genetically transmitted infantile polycystic kidney disease in C57BL/6J mice. Am J Pathol. 113:112-4.

Manenti A., Botticelli A., Buttazzi A., Gibertini G. (1992). Acute pulmonary edema after over-infusion of crystalloids versus plasma: histological observations in the rat. Pathologica 84(1091):331-4. Also: Pathologica 84(1091):325-9.

Mankin H. (1990). Experimental models in sarcomas. Curr Opin Oncol 2(3):500-4.

Manley B., Chong E., Walton C., Economides A., Cobbe S. (1989). An animal model for the chronic study of ventricular repolarisation and refractory period. Cardiovasc Res 23(1):16-20.

Manna V., Bem J., Marks R. (1982). An animal model for chronic ulceration. Br J Dermatol. 106:169-81.

Mano M.T., Potter B.J., Belling G.B., Chavadej J., Hatzel B.S. (1987). Fetal brain development in response to iodine deficiency in a primate model (Callithrix jacchus jacchus). J Neurol Sci. 79:287-300.

Mano M.T., Potter B.J., Belling G.B., Hetzel B.S. (1985). Low-iodine diet for the production of severe I deficiency in marmosets (Callithrix jacchus jacchus)}. Br J Nutr. 54:367-72.

Mantyjarvi R.A., Jagerroos H.J., Seppa A. (1987). An animal model of allergic alveolitis. Eur J Respir Dis [Suppl], 154:111-9.

Manukhina E., Lapshin A., Meerson F. (1991). [Effect of adaptation to periodic hypoxia on post-infarction fall of blood pressure and hyperactivation of the endothelium] Vliianie adaptatsii k periodicheskoi gipoksii na postinfarktnoe padenie davleniia i giperaktivatsiiu endoteliia. Fiziol Zh 37(3):98-105.

Marantidi A., Dzhikidze E., Krylova R., Stipkovich L. (1991). [Use of monkeys for modeling human Mycoplasma infection] Ispol'zovanie obez'ian dlia modelirovaniia mikoplazmozov cheloveka. Vestn Akad Med Nauk SSSR (6):51-5.

Marantidi A.N., Dzhikidze E.K., Krylova R.I., Sztipkovics L. (1987): Experimental Mycoplasma infection of the urogenital tract in monkeys. Zh Mikrobiol Epidemiol Immunobiol. 1:87-90 (English Abstract). (Russian)

March W.F., Gherezghiher T., Koss M., Nordquist R. (1984). Ultrastructural and pharmacologic studies on laser-induced glaucoma in primates and rabbits. Lasers Surg Med. 4:329-35.

Marczynski T., Urbancic M. (1988). Animal models of chronic anxiety and "fearlessness". Brain Res Bull 21(3):483-90.

Marder V., Shortell C., Fitzpatrick P., Kim C., Oxley D. (1992). An animal model of fibrinolytic bleeding based on the rebleed phenomenon: application to a study of vulnerability of hemostatic plugs of different age. Thromb Res 67(1):31-40.

Mardh P.A., Holst E., Moller B.R. (1984). The grivet monkey as a model for study of vaginitis. Challenge with anaerobic curved rods and Gardnerella vaginalis. Scand J Urol Nephrol [Suppl]. 86:201-5.

Marennikova S.S., Matsevich G.R., Chekunova E.V., Nikulina V.G., Rozina E.E. (1986). Development and practical use of new experimental models of the various forms of herpetic infection. Vopr Virasol. 31:59-65. (English Abstract). (Russian)

Marescaux C., Micheletti G., Vergnes M., Depaulis A., Rumbach L., Warter J.M. 1984. A model of chronic spontaneous petit mal-like seizures in the rat: comparison with pentylenetetrazol-induced seizures. Epilepsia. 25:326-31.

Marg E. (1982). Prentice-Memorial Lecture: Is the animal model for stimulus deprivation amblyopia in children valid or useful? Am J Optom Physiol. 59:451-64.

Markgraf C., Kraydieh S., Prado R., Watson B., Dietrich W., Ginsberg M. (1993). Comparative histopathologic consequences of photothrombotic occlusion of the distal middle cerebral artery in Sprague Dawley and Wistar rats. Stroke 24(2):286-92; discussion 292-3.

Marks M.I., Ziegler E.G., Douglas H., Corbeil L.B. (1982). Lethal Haemophilus influenzae type b infection in mice. Infection. 10:261-6.

Marliss E.B. (1983). Workshop on the BB rat. Metabolism. 32 (7 Suppl 1):1-5.

Marni A., Grassi G., Romani F., Rigoni-Stern A. (1983). Advantages and disadvantages of an experimental model for the study of acute hepatic insufficiency. Arch Sci Med (Torino). 140:281-5. (English Abstract).

Marquardt J., Hermanns W., Schulz L.C., Leibald W. (1983). A persistent retrovirus infection of chickens as a possible model of human rheumatoid arthritis (RA). Zentralbl Veterinarmed [B]. 30:274-82.

Marquie G., Hadjiisky P., Arnaud O., Duhault J. (1991). Development of macroangiopathy in sand rats (Psammomys obesus), an animal model of non-insulin-dependent diabetes mellitus: effect of gliclazide. Am J Med 90(6A):55S-61S.

Marra C., Baker-Zander S., Hook E. 3., Lukehart S. (1991). An experimental model of early central nervous system syphilis. J Infect Dis 163(4):825-9.

Marriott C.J., Cadorette J.E., Lecomte R., Scasnar V., Rousseau J., van Lier J.E. (1994). High-resolution PET imaging and quantitation of pharmaceutical biodistributions in a small animal using avalanche photodiode detectors. J Nucl Med. 35:1390-7.

Marriott C.J., Cadorette J.E., Lecomte R., Scasnar V., Rousseau J., van Lier J.E. (1994). High resolution PET imaging and quantitation of pharmaceutical biodistributions in a small animal using avalanche photodiode detectors. J Nucl Med. 35:1390-7.

Marsh J.C., Shoemaker R.H., Suffness M. (1985). Stability of the in vivo P388 leukemia model in evaluation of antitumor activity of natural products. Cancer Treat Rep. 69:683-5.

Marshall C., Ishibe Y., Marshall B. (1988). A combined in vivo/in vitro small animal model for studying pulmonary responses. Methods Find Exp Clin Pharmacol 10(1):5-11.

Marshall R.J., Muir A.W., Winslow E. (1981). Development of a severe model of early coronary artery ligation-induced dysrhythmias in the anaesthetized rat. Br J Pharmacol. 73:951-9.

Martens A., van B. D., Hagenbeek A. (1990). Minimal residual disease in leukemia: studies in an animal model for acute myelocytic leukemia (BNML). Int J Cell Cloning 8(1):27-38.

Martin D.S., Balis M.E., Fisher B., Frei E., Freireich E.J., Heppner G.H., Holland J.F., Houghton J.A., Houghton P.J., Johnson R.K. (1986). Role of murine tumor models in cancer treatment research. Cancer Res. 46:2189-92.

Martin J., Edwards E., Johnson J., Henn F. (1990). Monoamine receptors in an animal model of affective disorder. J Neurochem 55(4):1142-8.

Martin L.N., Gormus B.J., Walf R.H., Walsh G.P., Meyers W.M., Binford C.H., Harboe M. (1984). Experimental leprosy in nonhuman primates. Adv Vet Sci Comp Med. 28:201-36.

Martin P., Irino M., Suzuki K., Lewis MH., Mailman R. (1991). The female brindled mouse as a model of Menkes' disease: the relationship of fur pattern to behavioral and neurochemical abnormalities. Dev Neurosci 13(3):121-9.

Martin Paredero V., Millas I., Casado S., Lopez Novoa J.M. (1984). Development and hemodynamic studies of a new model of experimental progressive hypertension due to restriction of the growth of the aorta in rats. Angiologia. 36:162-200. (Spanish)

Martin R.B., Butcher R.L., Sherwood L.L., Buckendahl P., Boyd R.D., Farris D., Sharkey N., Dannucci G. (1987): Effects of ovariectomy in beagle dogs. Bone. 8:23-31.

Martin S., Palmour R., Goldwater R., Gutkowsa J., Hughes C., Hamet P., Ervin FR. (1990). Characterization of a primate model of hypertension. The response of hypertensive and normotensive male vervets (Cercopithecus aethiops) to cold pressor stress, captopril administration, and acute bolus of atrial natriuretic factor. Am J Hypertens 3(1):27-32.

Martinell J., Whitney J.B. 3d., Popp R.A., Russell L.B., Anderson W.F. (1981). Three mouse models of human thalassemia. Proc Natl Acad Sci USA. 78:5056-60.

Martinez J.R., Bylund D.B., Mawhinney T., Camden J., Ray G. (1983). The chronically reserpinized rat as a model for cystic fibrosis: alterations in the mucous-secreting sublingual gland. Pediatr Res. 17:523-8.

Martinez J.R., Martinez A.M. (1988): The reserpine-treated rat as an experimental animal model for cystic fibrosis: abnormal Cl transport in pancreatic acinar cells. Pediatr Res. 24(4):427-32.

Martino G., DuPont BL., Wollmann R., Bongioanni P., Anastasi J., Quintans J., Arnason BG., Grimaldi L. (1993). The human-severe combined immunodeficiency myasthenic mouse model: a new approach for the study of myasthenia gravis. Ann Neurol 34(1):48-56.

Martorana P., Brand T., Gardi C., van E. P., de S. M., Calzoni P., Marcolongo P., Lungarella G. (1993). The pallid mouse. A model of genetic alpha 1-antitrypsin deficiency. Lab Invest 68(2):233-41.

Masoro E. (1992). The role of animal models in meeting the gerontologic challenge of the 21st century [see comments]. Gerontologist 32(5):627-33.

Masuda J., Tanaka K. (1984). A new model of cerebral arteriosclerosis induced by intimal injury using a silicone rubber cylinder in rabbits. Lab Invest. 51:475-84.

Mathias C.J., Welch M.J. (1983). ^{111}In-labeled platelets for the detection of vascular disorders in animal models. In: Lambrecht R.M., Eckelman W.C. (Eds). Animal models in radiotracer design. Heidelberg: Springer Verlag. pp 149-178.

Mathias C.M., Welch M.J., Raichle M.E. et al. (1990). Evaluation of a potential generator-produced PET tracer for cerebral perfusion imaging. Single-pass cerebral extraction measurement and imaging with radiolabeled Cu-PTSM. J Nucl Med. 31:351-9.

Matias J., Malloy V., Orentreich N. (1989). Animal models of androgen-dependent disorders of the pilosebaceous apparatus. 1. The androchronogenetic alopecia (AGA) mouse as a model for male-pattern baldness. Arch Dermatol Res 281(4):247-53.

Matsuda H., Kinuya K., Tsuji S., Terada H., Shiba K., Kojima K., Mori H., Sumiya H., Hisada K. (1990). [Preparation and assessment of an animal model of Alzheimer's disease]. Kaku Igaku 27(8):883-91.

Matsumori A., Kawai C. (1983). Animal models of cardiomyopathy. Int J Cardiol. 3:368-73.

Matsumori A., Kawai C., Crumpacker C.S., Abelmann W.H. (1987). Pathogenesis and preventive and therapeutic trials in an animal model of dilated cardiomyopathy induced by a virus. Jpn Circ J. 51:661-4.

Matsumoto T., Ezawa I., Morita K., Kawanobe Y., Ogata E. (1985). Effect of vitamin D metabolites on bone metabolism in a rat model of postmenopausal osteoporosis. J Nutr Sci Vitaminol (Tokyo). 31 (Suppl):S61-5.

Matsumoto T., Iida M., Nakamura S., Hizawa K., Kuroki F., Fujishima M. (1993). An animal model of longitudinal ulcers in the small intestine induced by intracolonically administered indomethacin in rats. Gastroenterol Jpn 28(1):10-7.

Matsumura K., Uno Y., Scheffel U., Wilson A.A., Dannals R.F., Wagner H.N.Jr. (1991). In vitro and in vivo characterization of 4-[^{125}I]Iododexetimide binding to muscarinic cholinergic receptors in the rat heart. J Nucl Med. 32:76-80.

Matsushita M., Tsuboyama T., Kasai R., Okumura H., Yamamuro T., Higuchi K., Kohno A., Yonezu T., Utani A. (1986). Age-related changes in bone mass in the senescence-accelerated mouse (SAM). SAM-R/3 and SAM-P/6 as new murine models for senile osteoporosis. Am J Pathol. 125:276-83.

Matsuura H., Kudo M., Ikeda Y., Isayama K., Nakazawa S. (1986). A model of brain abscess: septic homologous blood clot emboli in rats. J Neurosurg. 64:125-7.

Matti H. (1984). Animal models in antibacterial drug research. J. Antimicrob Chemoth. 14:101-2.

Maurer T. (1984). Experimental contact photoallergenicity: guinea pig models. Photodermatol. 1:221-31.

Mavroudis C., Ganzel B.L., Cox S.K., Palk H.C. Jr. (1987). Experimental aerobic-anaerobic thoracic empyema in the guinea pig. Ann Thorac Surg. 43:298-302.

Mavroudis C., Katzmark S., Howe W.R., Gray L.A. Jr. (1984). Creation of left-to-right shunts in the newborn pig: a new model. J Surg Res. 36:274-7.

Maximilien R., Poncy J., Monchaux G., Morin M., Masse R. (1992). Validity and limitations of animal experiments in assessing lung carcinogenicity of cadmium. IARC Sci Publ (118):415-24.

Mayzner-Zawadzka E. (1983). Malignant hyperthermia in the pig--studies on the pathogenesis of the syndrome. Pol Tyg Lek. 38:21-6.

Mazière B., Coenen H.H., Halldin C., Någren K., Pike V.W. (1992). PET radioligands for dopamine receptors and re-uptake sites: Chemistry and biochemistry. Nucl Med Biol. 19:497-512.

Mazière B., Mazière M. (1991). Positron emission tomography studies of brain receptors. Fundam Clin Pharmacol. 5:61-91.

Mazière M., Bottlaender M., Brouillet E., Varastet M., Schmid L., Fuseau C., Fournier D. (1992). In vivo modulation of the GABAergic neurotransmission by drugs acting at the benzodiazepine receptor visualized by positron emission tomography (PET) and electroencephalography (EEG), in normal and epileptic baboons. Funct Neurosurg. 31:1-12.

Mazoyer B.M., Heiss W.D., Comar D. (Eds.) (1993). PET studies on amino acid metabolism and protein synthesis. Dordrecht: Kluwer Academic Publishers.

McAfee J.C., Subramanian G. (1983). Experimental models and evaluation of animal data for renal radiodiagnostic agents. In: Lambrecht R.M., Eckelman W.C. (Eds). Animal models in radiotracer design. Heidelberg: Springer Verlag. pp 211-227.

McCall C.E., Taylor R.G., Cousart S.L., Woodruff R.D., Lewis J.C., O'Flaherty J.T. (1983). Pulmonary injury induced by phorbol myristate acetate following intravenous administration in rabbits. Acute respiratory distress followed by pulmonary interstitial pneumonitis and pulmonary fibrosis. Am J Pathol. 111:258-62.

McCaughran J.A. Jr., Edwards E., Friedman R., Schechter N. (1984). Myocardial cholinergic receptor sites and enzyme activity in the Dahl model of essential hypertension. Clin Exp Hypertens [A]. 6:811-26.

McClatchey M., Temple-Smith P., Southwick G. (1991). Animal models for epididymoepididymostomy. Development of an alternative microsurgical procedure for vasoepididymostomy. Br J Urol 68(5):524-30.

McClearn G. (1988). Animal models in alcohol research. Alcohol Clin Exp Res 12(5):573-6.

McClure H., Anderson D., Ansari A., Fultz P., Klumpp S., Schinazi R. (1990). Non-human primate models for evaluation of AIDS therapy. Ann N Y Acad Sci 616:287-98.

McClure H.M. (1984). Non-human primate models for human disease. Adv Vet Sci Comp Med. 28:257-304.

McCune J., Kaneshima H., Krowka J., Namikawa R., Outzen H., Peault B. et al. (1991). The SCID-hu mouse: a small animal model for HIV infection and pathogenesis. Annu Rev Immunol 9:399-429.

McCurdy R.E., Martinez R. (1981). The chronically reserpinized rat as a model for cystic fibrosis: alterations in pancreatic enzyme secretion and storage. Pediatr Res. 15:1308-13.

McDonald M.I., Lucone C.L., Durack D.T. (1984). An experimental model for pyogenic liver abscess. J Infect. 8:129-36.

McDonough K.H., Dunn R.B., Griggs D.M. (1984). Transmural changes in porcine and canine hearts after circumflex artery occlusion. Am J Physiol. 246 (4 PT.2):H601-7.

McGinn M.D., Chole R.A., Henry K.R. (1981). Cholesteatoma induction. Consequences of external auditory canal ligation in gerbils, cats, hamsters, guinea pigs, mice and rats. Acta Otolaryngol (Stockh). 97:297-304.

McGuire M.T., Brammer G.L., Raleigh M.J. (1983). Animal models: Are they useful in the study of psychiatric disorders? Prog Clin Biol Res. 131:313-28.

McKerrow J.H., Ritter D.M. (1993). Using SCID mice to study parasitic diseases. Lab Anim Sci. 43(2):136-8.

McLain D.E, Roe D.A. (1984). Fetal alcohol syndrome in the ferret (Mustela putorius). Teratology. 30:203-10.

McMahon S.B., Abel C. (1987). A model for the study of visceral pain states: chronic inflammation of the chronic decerebrate rat urinary bladder by irritant chemicals. Pain. 28:109-27.

McMartin D.N., Dodds W.J. (1982). Animal model of human disease: atrial thrombosis in aged Syrian hamsters. 107:277-9.

McNally P., Baker F., Mistry N., Walls J., Feehally J. (1990). Effect of nifedipine on renal haemodynamics in an animal model of cyclosporin A nephrotoxicity. Clin Sci 79(3):259-66.

McNeill J.R. (1980). Laboratory rat and mouse colonies: some implications for biomedical research. Lucas Heights, Australia. ISBN-No. 0 642 59684 0. 38pp.

McVicker J.H., Lava N.S., Mittag T.W., Ringel S.P. (1982). D-penicillamine-induced neuromuscular disease in guinea pigs. Exp Neurol. 76 (l):46-57.

Meacock S., Bodmer J., Billingham M. (1990). Experimental osteoarthritis in guinea-pigs. J Exp Pathol (Oxford) 71(2):279-93.

Meador V.P., Deyoe B.L. (1986). Experimentally induced Brucella abortus infection in pregnant goats. Am J Vet Res. 47:2337-42.

Medori R., Jenich H., Autilio-Gambetti L., Gambetti P. (1988). Experimental diabetic neuropathy: similar changes of slow axonal transport and axonal size in different animal models. J Neurosci 8(5):1814-21.

Meehan C.J., Davidson P.M., Young D.G., Foulis A.K. (1987): The partially diabetic pancreas: a histological study of a new animal model. Pancreas. 2:91-8.

Mefford I.N., Baker T.L., Boehme R., Foutz A.S., Ciaranello R.D., Barchas J.D., Dement W.C. (1983). Narcolepsy: biogenic amine deficits in an animal model. Science. 220:629-32.

Mehdizadeh S., Alaghband-Zadeh J., Gusterson B., Arlot M., Bradbeer JN., Loveridge N. (1989). Bone resorption and circulating PTH-like bioactivity in an animal model of hypercalcaemia of malignancy. Biochem Biophys Res Commun 161(3):1166-71.

Mehrotra R., Goyal P., Mehrotra S., Nath P. (1990). Animal models in Hepadna viruses. Indian J Pathol Microbiol 33(3):288-98.

Mehta A. (1989). Animal models of metabolism in newborn infants. Proc Nutr Soc 48(2):257-62.

Meissner G. (1981). The value of animal models for study of infection due to atypical mycobacteria. Rev Infect Dis. 3:953-9.

Mel'nishnov Iu., Sychev IuN. (1984). Experimental urolithiasis. Urol Nefrol (Mosk). 4:14-8.

Mela-Riker L., Alexander P., Bartos D., Bryant R.E., Connell R.S., Erwin L., Gilchrish B., Harrison M., Luallin D., Oh G. (1988): Chronic hyperdynamic sepsis in the rat: I. Characterization of the animal model. Circ Shock. 25(4):231-44.

Melby E.C. Jr. (1987): Overview of the state of the art in development and utilization of animal models in the U.S.A. Prog Clin Biol Res. 229:1-10.

Mella O., Bjerkvig R., Schem B., Dahl O. et al. (1990). A cerebral glioma model for experimental therapy and in vivo invasion studies in syngeneic BD IX rats. J Neurooncol 9(2):93-104.

Mello N.K., Bree M.P., Mendelson J.H. (1983). Comparison of buprenorphine and methadone effects on opiate self-administration in primates. J Pharmacol Exp Ther. 225:378-86.

Melton D. (1990). The use of gene targeting to develop animal models for human genetic diseases. Biochem Soc Trans 18(6):1035-9.

Mendlovic S., Brocke S., Shoenfeld Y., Ben-Bassat M., Meshorer A., Bakimer R., Mozes E. (1988). Induction of a systemic lupus erythematosus-like disease in mice by a common human anti-DNA idiotype. Proc Natl Acad Sci U S A 85(7):2260-4.

Meng C.L., Allbright J., Shklar G. (1981). Anaplastic carcinoma in the buccal pouches of hamsters as a model of oral cancer. J Dermatol Surg Oncol 7:1011-7.

Mennander A., Tiisala S., Halttunen J., Yilmaz S., Paavonen T., Hayry P. (1991). Chronic rejection in rat aortic allografts. An experimental model for transplant arteriosclerosis. Arterioscler Thromb 11(3):671-80.

Ment L.R., Stewart W.B., Duncan C.C., Lambrecht R. et al. (1983). Beagle puppy model of intra-ventricular hemorrhage. Effect of indomethacin on cerebral blood flow. J Neurosurg. 58:857-62.

Ment L.R., Stewart W.B., Duncan C.C., Lambrecht R.M. (1982). Beagle Puppy Model of Intraventricular Hemorrhage. J Neurosurg. 57:219-223.

Ment L.R., Stewart W.B., Duncan C.C., Pitt B.R. (1986). Beagle puppy model of perinatal cerebral insults by hypoxemia. J Neurosurg. 65:847-50.

Ment L.R., Stewart W.B., Duncan C.C., Scott D.T., Lambrecht R.M. (1983). Beagle Puppy Model of Intraventricular Hemorrhage: Effect of Indomethacin on Cerebral Blood Flow. J Neurosurg. 58:857-862.

Ment L.R., Stewart W.B., Duncan C.C., Scott D.T., Lambrecht R.M. (1984). Beagle Puppy Model of Intraventricular Hemorrhage: Effect of Indomethacin on Local Cerebral Glucose Utilization. J Neurosurg. 60:737-742.

Mercugliano M., Hyman S., Batshaw M. (1990). Behavioral deficits in rats with minimal cortical hypoplasia induced by methylazoxymethanol acetate. Pediatrics 85(3 Pt 2):432-6.

Merlino G. (1991). Transgenic animals in biomedical research. FASEB J 5(14):2996-3001.

Mertz A., Batsford S., Curschellas E., Kist M., Gondolf K. (1991). Cationic Yersinia antigen-induced chronic allergic arthritis in rats. A model for reactive arthritis in humans. J Clin Invest 88(2):632-42.

Meshcheriakova O.A. (1988): Behavior of rats of different strains in an Experimental model of emotional resonance. Zh Vyssh Nerv Deiat. 38(2):368-9. (Russian)

Messer A., Strominger N.L., Mazurkiewicz J.E. (1987). Histpthology of the late-onset motor neuron degeneration (Mnd) mutant in the mouse. J Neurogenet. 4:201-13.

Mestre M., Clairefond P., Mardiguan J., Trillou M., Le Fur G., Uzan A. (1985). Comparative effects of heparin and PK 10169, a low molecular weight fraction, in a canine model of arterial thrombosis. Thromb Res. 38:389-99.

Metcalf J.F., Michaelis B.A. (1984). Herpetic keratitis in inbred mice. Invest Ophtahlmol Vis Sci. 25:1222-5.

Metz J., Van der Westhuyzen J. (1987). The fruit bat as an experimental model of the neuropathy of cobalamin deficiency. Comp Biochem Physiol [A]. 88:171-7.

Meuleman D.G., Hobbelen P.M., van Dedem G., Moelker H.C. (1982). A novel anti-thrombotic heparinoid (Org 10172) devoid of bleeding inducing capacity: a survey of its pharmacological properties in experimental animal models. Thromb Res. 27:353-63.

Meyer O. (1981). Animal models in lupus. Rev Rhum Mal Osteoartic . 48:817-25.

Meyer W.J. 3d. (1986) Animal models of mineralocorticoid resistance. Adv Exp Med Biol. 196:197-211.

Michejda M., McCallough D. (1987). New animal model for the study of neural tube defects. Z Kinderchi. 42 (Suppl 1):32-5.

Michelson E.L. (1981). Canine models of ventricular tachyarrhythmia. Ann Intern Med. 95:648-9.

Michie H., Jahoda C., Oliver R., Johnson B. (1991). The DEBR rat: an animal model of human alopecia areata. Br J Dermatol 125(2):94-100.

Mildenberger M., Beach T., McGeer E., Ludgate C. (1990). An animal model of prophylactic cranial irradiation: histologic effects at acute, early and delayed stages. Int J Radiat Oncol Biol Phys 18(5):1051-60.

Milhaud G., Labat M.L., Litwin I., Moricard Y., Moutier R., Rimbaut C. et al. (1981). Osteopetro-rickets: a new congenital bone disorder. Metab Bone Dis Relat Res. 3:91-7.

Miller C., Alexander N., Sutjipto S., Lackner AA., Gettie A., Hendrickx A., Lowenstine L., Jennings M., Marx P. (1989). Genital mucosal transmission of simian immunodeficiency virus: animal model for heterosexual transmission of human immunodeficiency virus. J Virol 63(10):4277-84.

Miller C.J. (1994). Animal models of viral sexually transmitted diseases. Am J Reprod Immunol. 31(1):52-63.

Miller C.L., Lim R.C. (1986). Post-ischemia immunosuppression in a miniature swine model. Lab Anim Sci. 36:375-80.

Miller J., Bullock R., Graham DI., Chen M., Teasdale G. (1990). Ischemic brain damage in a model of acute subdural hematoma. Neurosurgery 27(3):433-9.

Miller J.E., Tschoepe R.L., Ziegler M.M. (1985). A new model of heterotopic rat heart transplantation with application for in vivo 31P nuclear magnetic resonance spectroscopy. Transplantation. 39:555-8.

Miller M.J., McNeill H., Mullane K.M., Caravella S.J., Clark D.A. (1988): SOD prevents damage and attenuates eicosanoid release in a rabbit model of necrotizing enterocolitis. Am J Physiol. 255(5 Pt 1):G556-65.

Miller T.E., Lecamwasam J.P., Ormrod D.J., Findon G., Cornish J. (1987). An animal model for chronic infection of the unobstructed urinary tract. Br J Exp Pathol. 68:575-83.

Millner R., Mann J., Pearson I., Pepper JR. (1991). Experimental model of left ventricular failure. Ann Thorac Surg 52(1):78-83.

Minana M.D., Portales M., Jorda A., Grisolia S. (1984). Lesch-Nyhan syndrome, caffeine model: increase of purine and pyrimidine enzymes in rat brain. J Neurochem. 43:1556-60.

Minato M., Houssin D., Morin J., Szekely A.M., Bismuth H. (1982). Surgically induced acute hepatic failure in the rat. Eur Surg Res. 14:185-91.

Mink S.N., Coalson J.J., Whitley L, Greville H, Jaduc C. (1984). Pulmonary function tests in the detection of small airway obstruction in a canine model of bronchiolitis obliterans. Am Rev Respir Dis. 130:1125-33.

Minne H.W., Pfeilschifter J., Scharla S., Mutschelknauss S., Schwarz A., Krempien B., Ziegler R. (1984) Inflammation-mediate osteopenia in the rat: a new animal model for pathological loss of bone mass. Endocrinology. 115:50-4.

Minor R.R., Wootton J.A., Prockop D.J., Patterson D.F. (1987): Genetic diseases of connective tissues in animals. Curr Probl Dermatol. 17:199-215.

Mintun M.A., Dennis D.R., Welch M.J., Mathias C.J., Schuster D.P. (1987). Measurement of pulmonary vascular permeability with PET and gallium-68 transferrin. J Nucl Med. 28:1704-16.

Mir G.N., Alioto R.L. (1982). A semichronic diarrheal model. J Pharmacol Methods. 7:115-20.

Mironova T.K., Pasternak N.I., Khristich A.I. (1984). Natural reproduction of all stages of a generalized meningococcal infection in mice. Zh Mikrobiol Epidemiol Immunobiol. 6:31-5. (English Abstract). (Russian)

Misawa M., Kawamura T., Takenouchi K. (1989). A new bronchial asthma model using calcium ionophore A23187 in guinea pigs. Jpn J Pharmacol 51(3):446-9.

Mitchell I., Turk J. (1989). An experimental animal model of granulomatous bowel disease. Gut 30(10):1371-8.

Mitchell J., Ling WD, Bohr D.F. (1984). Deoxycorticosterone acetate hypertension in the sheep. J Hypertens. 2:473-8.

Mitro A., Marsala J., Jalc P., Pomfy M., Marossy A., Daxnerova Z., Sebokova. (1983). Method of the development of irreversible, complete cerebral ischemia in dog. Neuropatol Pol. 21:315-21.

Miyajima M., Tsuji S., Matsushita H. (1984). The present status of animal models for human diseases in Japan (1983). Jikken Dobutsu. 33:369-97. (Japanese)

Miyake T., Taguchi O, Ikeda H., Sato Y., Takeuchi S., Nishizuka Y. (1988). Acute oocyte loss in experimental autoimmune oophoritis as a possible model of premature ovarian failure. Am J Obstet Gynecol. 158 186-92.

Miyamoto Y., Yama S., Watanabe Y., Nikkawa T., Niida T., Kazuno Y., Takeda U., Sasaki H., Kawaoto H., Takemura T. (1987). Clinical laboratory studies on patients with Kawasaki disease (MCLS) and on the pathohistologic model of mice infected with Streptococcus sanguis. Kansenshogaku Zasshi. 61:510-22 (English Abstract.). (Japanese)

Miyata T., Torisu M., Toh H., Goya T. (1993). Prolonged lung edema formation during the generalized Shwartzman reaction in rabbits - can it be a model for septic lung disease? Circ Shock 39(1):44-51.

Miyawaki S., Mitsuoka S., Sakiyama T., Kitagawa T. (1982). Sphingomyelinosis, a new mutation in the mouse: a model of Niemann-Pick disease in humans. J Hered. 73:257-63.

Mock D.M., Mock N.I., Weintraub S. (1988): Abnormal organic aciduria in biotin deficiency: the rat is similar to the human. J Lab Clin Med. 112 (2):240-7.

Modig J., Borg T. (1986). Biochemical markers in a porcine model of adult respiratory distress syndrome induced by endotoxemia. Resuscitation. 14:225-36.

Modlin R.L., Ormerod L.D., Walsh G.P., Rea T.H., Meyers W.M., Binford C.H., Martin L.N., Walf R.H., Gormus B.J. (1986). In situ characterization of T lymphocyte subpopulations in leprosy in the mangabey monkey. Clin Exp Immunol. 65:260-4.

Moe G.W., Stopps T.P., Howard R.J., Armstrong P.W. (1988): Early recovery from heart failure: insights into the pathogenesis of experimental chronic pacing-induced heart failure. J Lab Clin Med. 112(4):426-32.

Moessinger A.C., Bassi G.A., Ballantyne G., Collins M.H., James L.S., Blanca W.A. (1983). Experimental production of pulmonary hypoplasia following amniocentesis and oligohydramnios. Early Hum Dev.8:343-50.

Mohn G., van K. H., Zeilmaker MJ. (1992). Gastrointestinal carcinogenesis: experimental models. Eur J Cancer Prev 1 Suppl 3:37-43.

Mohr U., Dungworth D.L., Capen C.C. (Ed.) (1992). Pathobiology of the aging rat. Washington D.C.: International Live Sciences Institute.

Mohr U., Reznik G. (1982). Three hamster species as models in cancer research. IARC Sci Publ. 34:437-42.

Mohr W., Kirkpatrick C.J. (1983). The relevance of animal experiments to human arthritis and the effect of drug therapy on experimentally induced arthritis in animals. Z Rheumatol. 42:159-70.

Moise K. J., Hesketh D., Belfort M., Saade G., Van d. V. I., Hudson K., Rodkey L. (1992). Ultrasound-guided blood sampling of rabbit fetuses. Lab Anim Sci 42(4):398-401.

Moller B.R., Freundt E.A. (1983). Monkey animal model for study of mycoplasmal infections of the urogenital tract. Sex Transm Dis. 10 (4 Suppl):359-62.

Molnar L., Hegedus K., Fekete I. (1988): A new model for inducing transient cerebral ischemia and subsequent reperfusion in rabbits without craniectomy. Stroke. 19(10):1262-6.

Momomura S., Bradley A.B., Grossman W. (1984). Left ventricular diastolic pressure-segment length relations and end-diastolic distensibility in dogs with coronary stenoses. An angina physiology model. Circ Res.55:203-14.

Monaco W., Wormington C. (1990). The rhesus monkey as an animal model for age-related maculopathy. Optom Vis Sci 67(7):532-7.

Mondino B.J., Caster A.I., Dethlefs B. (1987). A rabbit model of staphylococcal blepharitis. Arch Ophthalmol. 105:409-12.

Monk M., Handyside A., Hardy K., Whittingham D. (1987). Pre-implantation diagnosis of deficiency of hypoxanthine phosphoribosyl transferase in a mouse model for Lesch-Nyhan syndrome. Lancet. 2:423-5.

Montano L.M., Selman M., Paramo I., Vargas M.H. (1987). Acute allergic bronchoconstriction in the guinea-pig: advantages of intratracheal immunization. Arch Invest Med (Mex) 18:37-50.

Montgomery J., Mamer O., Colle E. (1991). Metabolism of deuterium-labeled nonanoic acids in the riboflavin-deficient rat model of multiple acyl-CoA dehydrogenase deficiency. Biol Mass Spectrom 20(4):179-85.

Moon K., Wester R., Maibach H. (1990). Diseased skin models in the hairless guinea pig: in vivo percutaneous absorption. Dermatologica 180(1):8-12.

Moore J.V. (1983). Growth sites for experimental tumours: tail vs. flank. Br J Radiol. 56:433-4.

Mordent J. (1986). Man versus beast: Pharmacokinetic scaling in mammals. J Pharm Sciences 75:1028-40.

Morita M. (1989). [Animal model of motion sickness in rats]. Nippon Jibiinkoka Gakkai Kaiho 92(9):1424-35.

Moriwaki K. (1987): Genetic significance of laboratory mice in biomedical research. Prog Clin Biol Res. 229:53-72.

Moroni F., Lombardi G., Moneti G., Cortesini C. (1983). The release and neosynthesis of glutamic acid are increased in experimental models of hepatic encephalopathy. J Neurochem. 40:850-4.

Morreale V., Herman B., Der-Minassian V., Palkovits M., Klubes P., Perry D. et al. (1993). A brain-tumor model utilizing stereotactic implantation of a permanent cannula. J Neurosurg 78(6):959-65.

Morrow J., Awad J., Kato T., Takahashi K., Badr K., Roberts L. 2., Burk R. (1992). Formation of novel non-cyclooxygenase-derived prostanoids (F2-isoprostanes) in carbon tetrachloride hepatotoxicity. An animal model of lipid peroxidation. J Clin Invest 90(6):2502-7.

Moser K.M., Maurer J., Jassy L., Kremsdorf R., Konopka R., Shure D. et al. (1982). Sensitivity, specificity, and risk of diagnostic procedures in a canine model of Streptococcus pneumoniae pneumonia. Am Rev Respir Dis. 25:436-42.

Moses B., Chan D., Hruban R., Forastiere A., Richtsmeier W. (1993). Comparison of intra-arterial and intravenous infusion of cisplatin for head and neck squamous cell carcinoma in a modified rat model. Arch Otolaryngol Head Neck Surg 119(6):612-7.

Moshakis V., Carter R.L. (1984). Neoplastic invasion of the arterial wall and its modification by surgery: an experimental model. Br J Surg. 71:119-22.

Mosier D., Gulizia R., Baird S., Wilson D., Spector D., Spector S. (1991). Human immunodeficiency virus infection of human-PBL-SCID mice. Science 251(4995):791-4.

Mosier D.E., Gulizia R.J., Baird S.M., Wilson D.B. (1988): Transfer of a functional human immune system to mice with severe combined immunodeficiency. Nature. 15;335(6187):256-9.

Moskowitz D., Schneider A., Lane P., Schmitz P., Gillespie K. (1992). Effect of epidermal growth factor in the rat 5/6 renal ablation model. J Am Soc Nephrol 3(5):1113-8.

Moss G.S., Gould S.A., Rosen A.L., Sehgal L.R., Sehgal H.L. (1986). Animal model for nephrotoxicity of haemoglobin tetramer. Lancet. 1:1219.

Mossakowski M.J. (1981). Experimental modelling of hepatogenic encephalopathy. Neuropatol Pol. 19:261-76.

Mostwin J., Karim O., van K. G., Brooks E. (1991). The guinea pig as a model of gradual urethral obstruction. J Urol 145(4):854-8.

Mountz J.D., Gause W.C. (1993). Murine models of autoimmune disease and Sjogren's syndrome. Curr Opin Rheumatol. 5(5):557-69.

Mourya D.T., Padbidri V.S., Dhanda V. (1983). Mosquito inoculation technique for the diagnosis of Q fever employing an animal model . Indian J Med Res. 78:201-4.

Mousa S., Cooney J., Stevens S. (1992). Kinetics of technetium-99m-Sestamibi and thallium-201 in a transient ischemic myocardium animal model: insight into the 'redistribution' phenomenon. Cardiology 81(2-3):157-63.

Mousa S.A. (1991). Animal Models in Radiotracer Design of a ^{99m}Tc-Labelled Myocardial Perfusion Agent. Amer J Physiologic Imaging 6:16-25

Moyana T., Lalonde J. (1990). Carrageenan-induced intestinal injury in the rat - a model for inflammatory bowel disease. Ann Clin Lab Sci 20(6):420-6.

Mrosovsky N., Melnyk R.B. (1982). Towards new animal models in obesity research. Int J Obes. 6:121-6.

Muchmore E., Moor-Jankowski J. (1983). Hepatitis research in chimpanzees: evaluations of clinical laboratory methodologies. J Med Primatol. 12:65-7.

Mue S. (1981). Animal model of lung diseases - bronchial asthma . Nippon Kyobu Shikkan Gakkai Zasshi. 19:802-6 (English Abstract) (Japanese)

Mueller-Sieburg C. (Ed.) (1992). Hematopoietic stem cells: animal models and human transplantation. Berlin; New York: Springer Verlag. 251 P.

Mufti S. (1990). An animal model of immune response associated with alcohol-related cancers. Prog Clin Biol Res 325:359-71.

Muhvich K., Myers R., Marzella L. (1988). Effect of hyperbaric oxygenation, combined with antimicrobial agents and surgery, in a rat model of intraabdominal infection. J Infect Dis 157(5):1058-61.

Mukoyama M., Yamazaki K., Kikuchi T., Tomita T. (1989). Neuropathology of gracile axonal dystrophy (GAD) mouse. An animal model of central distal axonopathy in primary sensory neurons. Acta Neuropathol (Berl) 79(3):294-9.

Mulholland G.K., Otto C.A., Jewett D.M., Kilbourn M.R. et al. (1992). Synthesis, rodent biodistribution, dosimetry, metabolism, and monkey images of carbon-11-labeled (+)-2α-tropanyl benzilate: A central muscarinic receptor imaging agent. J Nucl Med. 33:423-30.

Mullen K.D. (1987): Resurrection of the 90% hepatectomy rabbit model of acute liver failure. J Lab Clin Med. 110:128-9.

Mullenix P., Kernan W., Tassinari M., Schunior A., Waber D., Howes A., Tarbell NJ. (1990). An animal model to study toxicity of central nervous system therapy for childhood acute lymphoblastic leukemia: effects on behavior. Cancer Res 50(20):6461-5.

Muller A., Machnik F., Zimmermann T., Schubert H. (1988). Thioacetamide-induced cirrhosis-like liver lesions in rats--usefulness and reliability of this animal model. Exp Pathol 34(4):229-36.

Muller M., Heldstab A., Luginbuhl H. (1989). The woolly monkey (Lagothrix lagothricha): a possible model for human hypertension research. Schweiz Arch Tierheilkd 131(9):569-76.

Murata H. (1983). Experimental models of Kawasaki disease. Nippon Rinsho. 41:2075-9.

Murday A.J., Gershlick A.H., Syndercombe-Court Y.D., Ledingham S.J., Betts N.J., Lewis C.T., Mills P.G. (1983). Intimal hyperplasia in arterial autogenous vein grafts: a new animal model. Cardiovasc Res.17:446-51.

Murphy T., Dorfman G., Esparza A., Duwaji M., Smith W. (1992). Arteriosclerosis obliterans in a rabbit model. Invest Radiol 27(12):1059-63.

Murphy T.F., Dubori E.J., Clyde W.A. Jr. (1981). The cotton rat as an experimental model of human parainfluenza virus type 3 disease. Exp Lung Res. 2:97-109.

Murrison A.W. (1993). The contribution of neurophysiologic techniques to the investigation of diving related illness [see comments]. Undersea Hyperb Med. 20(4):347-73.

Musacchia X.J., Steffen J.K.M., Fell R.D. (1988): Disuse atrophy of skeletal muscle: animal models. Exerc Sport Sci Rev. 16:61-87.

Muscat R., Sampson D., Willner P. (1990). Dopaminergic mechanism of imipramine action in an animal model of depression. Biol Psychiatry 28(3):223-30.

Muscat R., Towell A., Willner P. (1988). Changes in dopamine autoreceptor sensitivity in an animal model of depression. Psychopharmacology (Berl) 94(4):545-50.

Mustard R., Fisher J., Hayman S., Matlow A., Mullen J., Odumeru J., Roomi M., Schouten B., Swanson H. (1989). Cardiopulmonary responses to Pseudomonas septicemia in swine: an improved model of the adult respiratory distress syndrome. Lab Anim Sci 39(1):37-43.

Myers S., Haley-Russell D., Bartula L., Nabzdyk W. (1990). Common bile ligation in the rabbit: an appropriate model for investigating the relationship of endogenous gallbladder prostanoid synthesis with evolving acute inflammation. Prostaglandins 40(2):165-85.

Myhrer T. (1993). Animal models of Alzheimer's disease: glutamatergic denervation as an alternative approach to cholinergic denervation. Neurosci Biobehav Rev 17(2):195-202.

Mylvaganam R., Sprinz P.G., Ahn Y.S., Harrington W.J. (1984). An animal model of alloimmune thrombocytopenia I. The role of the mononuclear phagocytic system (MPS). Clin Immunol Immunopathol. 31:163-70.

Nabozny G.H., David C.S. (1994). The immunogenetic basis of collagen induced arthritis in mice: an experimental model for the rational design of immunomodulatory treatments of rheumatoid arthritis. Adv Exp Med Biol. 347:55-63.

Nadeau A., Tancrede G., Rousseau-Migneron S. (1987): Acute diabetes mellitus does not impair survival rate in rats submitted to left coronary artery ligation. Can J Cardiol. 3:90-3.

Nadkarni G., Shimpi H., Noronha O. (1991). Biokinetics of [Tc-99m]-labelled liver-imaging agents in an animal model of liver cirrhosis. Indian J Gastroenterol 10(2):51-3.

Nagai H., Suda H., Kitagaki K., Goto S., Miura T., Koda A. (1990). Anti-allergic effects of ketanserin on animal models of allergic reactions. Arch Int Pharmacodyn Ther 307:172-82.

Nagano M., Takeda N., Dhalla N.S. (Ed.) (1994). The cardiomyopathic heart. New York, N.Y.: Raven Press. 464 P.

Nagata T., Ochikubo F., Yoshikawa Y., Yamanouchi K. (1990). Encephalitis induced by a canine distemper virus in squirrel monkeys. J Med Primatol 19(2):137-49.

Nagel E., Guthy E., Schattenfroh S., Pohlenz J., Pichlmayr R. (1988): Pathogenesis of Crohn's disease. Evaluation criteria for an animal model. Schweiz Med Wochenschr. 21;118(20):766-9.

Naitoh H., Nomura S., Kunimi Y., Yamaoka K. (1992). "Swimming-induced head twitching" in rats in the forced swimming test induced by overcrowding stress: a new marker in the animal model of depression? Keio J Med 41(4):221-4.

Nakagawa N., Ghishan FK. (1993). Transport of phosphate by plasma membranes of the jejunum and kidney of the mouse model of hypophosphatemic vitamin D-resistant rickets. Proc Soc Exp Biol Med 203(3):328-35.

Nakagawa Y. (1983). Animal models of cerebral ischemia. Hokkado Igaku Zasshi. 58:437-52.

Nakai M., Tomino T., Goto Y., Yamamoto J., Matsui Y., Togawa T., Ogino K. (1983). Quantitative evaluation of the pattern of shunt flow in the right ventricle and pulmonary artery of dogs with experimental ventricular septal defect. J Clin Invest. 72:779-88.

Nakai Y. (1982). Animal disease models of labyrinth diseases. Jikken Dobutsu. 31:61-8. (Japanese)

Nakajima Y., Goto N. (1983). Hydronephrosis in the inbred mouse strain DDD. Lab Anim. 17:143-7.

Nakamoto S., Terubagashi H., Akagi Y., Miyamoto Y., Tutumi M., Yokoi N., Itoi M. (1988): A rat experimental posterior subcapsular cataract model resembling human diabetic cataract. Nippon Ganka Gakkai Zasshi. 92(1):161-5. (English Abstract). (Japanese)

Nakamura H., Matsuo T. (1985). Animal models of abnormal bilirubin metabolism--Gunn rat and Corriedale sheep. Nippon Rinsho 43:1777-82. (Japanese)

Nakamura K., Murase N., Becich M., Furuya T., Todo S., Fung J. et al. (1993). Liver allograft rejection in sensitized recipients. Observations in a clinically relevant small animal model. Am J Pathol 142(5):1383-91.

Nakamura O., Hojo S., Takakura K., Nagashima K., Ishizaki R. Q (1982). Schmidt Ruppin-D-ASV-induced primary rat brain tumor model for therapeutic screening. No To Shinkei. 34:691-7. (English Abstract) (Japanese)

Nakamura T., Hara M., Kasuga T. (1989). Transplacental induction of peripheral nervous tumor in the Syrian golden hamster by N-nitroso-N-ethylurea. A new animal model for von Recklinghausen's neurofibromatosis. Am J Pathol 135(2):251-9.

Nakashima H., Asari S., Nishimoto A., Goldstein M. (1991). [The effect of chronic treatment of deprenyl in animal models of Parkinson's disease]. No To Shinkei 43(4):357-61.

Nakayama D.K., Harrison M.R., Berger M.S., Chinn D.H., Halks-Miller M., Edwards M.S.(1983). Experimental pulmonary hypoplasia due to oligohydramnios and its reversal by relieving thoracic compression. J Pediatr Surg. 18:347-53.

Namikawa R., Kaneshima H., Lieberman M., Weissman I.L. McCune J.M. (1988): Infection of the SCID-hu mouse by HIV-1. Science 23;242(4886):1684-6.

Nara P., Hatch W., Kessler J., Kelliher J., Carter S. (1989). The biology of human immunodeficiency virus-1 IIIB infection in the chimpanzee: in vivo and in vitro correlations. J Med Primatol 18(3-4):343-55.

Narfstrom K., Wrigstad A., Nilsson SE. (1989). The Briard dog: a new animal model of congenital stationary night blindness. Br J Ophthalmol 73(9):750-6.

Narukami H., Yoshioka K., Zhao J., Miike T. (1991). Experimental serotonin myopathy as an animal model of muscle degeneration and regeneration in muscular dystrophy. Acta Neuropathol (Berl) 81(5):510-6.

Naslund U., Haggmark S., Johansson G., Marklund S.L., Reiz S., Oberg A. (1986). Superoxide dismutase and catalase reduce infarct size in a porcine myocardial occlusion-reperfusion mode. J Mol Cell Cardiol.18:1077-84.

Natanson C. (1986). Gram-negative bacteremia produces both severe systolic and diastolic cardiac dysfunction in a canine model that stimulates human septic shock. J Clin Invest. 78:259-70.

Nath C., Gulati A., Dhawan K.N., Gupta G.P., (1988): Role of central histaminergic mechanism in behavioural depression (swimming despair) in mice. Life Sci. 42(24):2413-7.

Nathanielsz P.W. (Ed) (1985): Animal Models in Fetal Medicine, No. 1 (Monographs in Fetal Physiology). Perinatology, New York. 368 pp

National Center (1992) for Research Resources (U.S.). Regional primate research centers: a major national scientific resource for biomedical research. Bethesda, Md.: U.S. Dept. of Health and Human Services. 53 P.

Neal D. J., Dilworth J., Kaack M., Didier P., Roberts J. (1990). Experimental prostatitis in non-human primates: II. Ascending acute prostatitis. Prostate 17(3):233-9.

Nehis D.G. (1986). Experimental primate stroke model. Neurosurgery.18:388-9.

Neilson E.G., McCafferty E., Feldman A., Clayman M.D., Zakheim B., Korngold R. (1984). Spontaneous interstitial nephritis in kdkd mice. I. An experimental model of autoimmune renal disease. J Immunol. 133:2560-5.

Nemoto R., Mori H., Iwata K., Kato T., Harada M. (1981). A model of malignant urinary bladder tumor in rabbits. Tohoku J Exp Med. 134:257-63.

Neuwelt E.A., Johnson W.G., Blank N.K., Pagel M.A., Maslen-McClure C., McClure M.J., Wu P.M. (1985). Characterization of a new model of GM2-gangliosidosis (Sandhoff's disease) in Korat cats. J Clin Invest. 76:482-90.

Neven L., Khalil A., Pfaffinger D., Fless G., Jackson E., Scanu A. (1990). Rhesus monkey model of familial hypercholesterolemia: relation between plasma Lp[a] levels, apo[a] isoforms, and LDL-receptor function. J Lipid Res 31(4):633-43.

Newberne P.M., Nauss K.M. (1986). Dietary fat and colon cancer: variable results in animal models. Prog Clin Biol Res. 222:311-30.

Newbold R.R., Bullock B.C., McLachlam J.A. (1984) Diverticulosis and salpingitis isthmica nodosa (SIN) of the fallopian tube. Estrogen-induced diverticulosis and SIN of the mouse oviduct. Am J Pathol. 117:333-5.

Newbold R.R., Bullock B.C., McLachlan J.A. (1986). Adenocarcinoma of the rete testis. Diethylstilbestrol-induced lesions of the mouse rete testis. Am J Pathol. 125:625-8.

Nickel J., Grant S., Lam K., Olson M., Costerton J. (1991). Bacteriologically stressed animal model of new closed catheter drainage system with microbicidal outlet tube. Urology 38(3):280-9.

Nickel J., Olson M., Costerton J. (1991). Rat model of experimental bacterial prostatitis. Infection 19 Suppl 3:S126-30.

Nikkari S., Solakivi T., Jaakkola O. (1991). The hyperlipidemic hamster as an atherosclerosis model. Artery 18(6):285-90.

Nilsson R. (1982). The artificially ventilated preterm rabbit neonate as experimental model of hyaline membrane disease. Acta Anaesthesiol Scand. 26:89-103.

Ninan P.T., Insel T.M., Cohen R.M., Cook J.M., Skolnick P., Paul S.M. (1982). Benzodiazepine receptor-mediated experimental 'anxiety' in primates. Science. 218:1332-4.

Nivard J.L., Ward G.E., Stevens J.B., Maheswaran S.K. (1982). Model infection of the chicken embryo with Haemophilus somnus. Am J Vet Res. 43:1790-2.

Noble R.L. (1982). Prostate carcinoma of the Nb rat in relation to hormones. Int Rev Exp Pathol. 23:113-59.

Nomura T., Katsuki M., Yokoyama M., Tajima Y. (1987): Future perspectives in the development of new animal models. Prog Clin Biol Res. 229:337-53.

Nonaka I., Kikuchia, Suzuki T., Esaki K. (1986). Hereditary peroneal muscular atrophy in the mouse: an experimental model for congenital contractures (arthrogryposis). Exp Neurol. 91:571-9.

Nordeen S.K., Schaefer V.G., Edgell M.H., Hutchison C.A. 3rd, Schultz L.D., Swift M. (1984) Evaluations of wasted mouse fibroblasts and SV-40 transformed human fibroblasts as models of ataxia telangiectasia in vitro. Mutat Res. 140:219-22.

Noren G.R., Staley N.A., Einzig S., Mikell F.L., Asinger R.W. (1983). Alcohol-induced congestive cardiomyopathy: an animal model. Cardiovasc Res. 17:81-7.

Nose M., Kyogoku M. (1986). Lupus mice and arthritis. Ryumach.i 26:116-25.

Novak E.K., Sweet H.O., Prochazka M., Parentis M., Soble R., Raddington M., Cairo A., Swank R.T. (1988): Cocoa: a new mouse model for platelet storage pool deficiency. Br J Haematol. 69(3):371-8.

Nowaczynski M., Nowaczynski W., Mavoungou D., Lioy F., Wilkins G. Fung K., Boyo W. (1983). Aldosterone-binding globulin-induced hypertension in the rat. A new experimental model. Hypertension. 5(6 Pt 3):V163-71.

Nunn A., Linder K., Strauss H.W. (1995). Nitroimidazoles and imaging hypoxia. Eur J Nucl Med. 22:265-80.

Nunn A.D. (Ed.) (1992). Radiopharmaceuticals - Chemistry and Pharmacology. New York: Marcel Deker, Inc. 435 pp.

Nunoya T., Tajima M., Mizutani M., Umezawa H. (1985). A new mutant strain of Syrian hamster with myelin deficiency. Acta Neuropathol (Berl). 65:305-12.

Nuttall A., Smith H.J., Loveday B.E. (1985). A clinically relevant model of heart failure: effects of ticlopidine. Cardiovasc Res. 19:187-92.

O'Brien S.J., Nash W.G., Winkler C.A., Reeves R.M. (1982). Genetic anlaysis in the domestic cat as an animal model for inborn errors, cancer and evolution. Prog Clin Biol Res. 94:67-90.

O'Connor J.A., Scott R.L., Mellick P.W., Caldwell M.D. (1982). Perfused rat hindlimb wound model: lambda-carrageenan induced. Am J Physiol. 242:R570-6.

O'Rourke M.F., Avolio A.P., Nichols W.W. (1986). The kangaroo as a model for the study of hypertrophic cardiomyopathy in man. Cardiovasc Res. 20:398-402.

O'Connor M.K., Krom R.F., Carton E.G., Sanchez-Urdazpal L., Juni J.E., Ferguson D.M., Wiesner R.F. (1992). Ratio of hepatic arterial-to-portal venous blood flow - Validation of radionuclide techniques in an animal model. J Nucl Med. 33:239-45.

Obata H., Tao Y., Kido M., Nagata N., Tanaka I., Kuroiwa A. (1992). Guinea pig model of immunologic asthma induced by inhalation of trimellitic anhydride. Am Rev Respir Dis 146(6):1553-8.

Obelienius V., Vrana M., Kaderabek J., Blazek Z., Urbanova D. (1981). Experimental model of focal myocardial ischemia in the conscious dog. Cesk Fysiol. 30:431-6. (Czechoslovakian)

Office of Technology Assessment (1986). Alternatives to Animal Use in Research, Testing and Education. OTA, Washington.

Ogden J.A., Conlogue G.J. (1981). Spontaneous rickets in the wild arctic fox Alopex lagopus. Skeletal Radiol. 7:43-54.

Ogura A., Asano T., Matsuda J., Takano K., Nakagawa M., Fukui M. (1989). Characteristics of mutant mice (ICGN) with spontaneous renal lesions: a new model for human nephrotic syndrome. Lab Anim 23 (2):169-74.

Ohashi H., Ito Y., Tsuchiya J., Hino T., Nonomura O., Hayashi K., Sakata K. (1983). A rat's model of neurogenic stress gastric ulcer - studies on distribution of produced ulcers, and on effect of cimetidine and atropine. Nippon Shokakibyo Gakkai Zasshi. 80:147-55. (English Abstract) (Japanese)

Ohashi K., Kim J., Hara H., Aso R., Akimoto T., Nakama K. (1990). WBN/Kob rats. A new spontaneously occurring model of chronic pancreatitis. Int J Pancreatol 6(4):231-47.

Ohba K., Sawai T., Nobunaga T., Ishida N. (1985). Clinical and pathogenic studies on aged polyuria in the IVCS strain of mouse. Jikken Dobutsu. 34:123-30.

Ohnishi A., Inoue N., Yamamoto T., Murai Y., Hori H., Kogo M., Tanaka I., Akiyama T. (1985). Ethylene oxide induces central-peripheral distal axonal degeneration of the lumbar primary neurones in rats. Br J Ind Med. 42:373-9.

Ohnishi K. (1984). Transportal, secondary heptic alveolar echinococcosis of rats. J Parasitol. 70:987-8.

Ohno K., Ito U., Inaba Y. (1984). Regional cerebral blood flow and stroke index after left carotid artery ligation in the conscious gerbil. Brain Res. 297:151-7.

Ohnota H., Okada Y., Ushijima H., Kitamura T., Komuro K., Mizuochi T. (1990). 3'-Azido-3'-deoxythymidine prevents induction of murine acquired immunodeficiency syndrome in C57BL/10 mice infected with LP-BM5 murine leukemia viruses, a possible animal model for antiretroviral drug screening. Antimicrob Agents Chemother 34(4):605-9.

Ohta S., Tachikawa O., Makino Y., Tasaki Y., Hirobe M. (1990). Metabolism and brain accumulation of tetrahydroisoquinoline (TIQ) a possible parkinsonism inducing substance, in an animal model of a poor debrisoquine metabolizer. Life Sci 46(8):599-605.

Oite T., Shimizu F., Kihara I., Batsford S.R., Vogt A. (1983). An active model of immune complex glomerulonephritis in the rat employing cationized antigen. Am J. Pathol. 112:185-94.

Oka T., Nishimura H., Ueyama M., Kubota J., Kawamura K. (1993). Haemodynamic and neurohumoral changes in spontaneously hypertensive rats with aortocaval fistulae. Clin Sci (Colch) 84(5):531-5.

Okada T., Harada T., Bark D., Mayberg M. (1990). A rat femoral artery model for vasospasm. Neurosurgery 27(3):349-56.

Okayasu I., Hatakeyama S., Yamada M., Ohkusa T., Inagaki Y., Nakaya R. (1990). A novel method in the induction of reliable experimental acute and chronic ulcerative colitis in mice. Gastroenterology 98(3):694-702.

Okubo Y., Naruse T. (1988): Experimental nephritis models. Nippon Rinsho. 46(6):1434-9.

Okuyama S., Aihara H. (1984). The mode of action of analgesic drugs in adjuvant arthritic rats as an experimental model of chronic inflammatory pain: possible central analgesic action of acidic nonsteroidal anti-inflammatory drugs. Jpn J Pharmacol. 35:95-103.

Olivier B., Molewijk E., van Oorschot R., van der Poel G., Zethof T., van der Heyden J., Mos J. (1994). New animal models of anxiety. Eur Neuropsychopharmacol. 4(2):93-102.

Olsen E.G. (1985). An endocrine experimental model for myofibrillar disarray as found in hypertrophic cardiomyopathy. J Mol Cell Cardio. 2:35-40.

Olsen R.W., Wamsley J.K., Lee R.J., Lomax P. (1986). Benzodiazepine/barbiturate/GABA receptor-chloride ionophore complex in a genetic model for generalized epilepsy. Adv Neurol. 44:365-78.

Olson N.C., Brown T.T., Anderson D.L. (1985). Dexamethasone and indomethacin modify endotoxin-induced respiratory failure in pigs. J Appl Physiol. 58:274-84.

Olsson J., Gordon J., Pawlyk B., Roof D., Hayes A., Molday R., Mukai S., Cowley G., Berson E., Dryja T. (1992). Transgenic mice with a rhodopsin mutation (Pro23His): a mouse model of autosomal dominant retinitis pigmentosa. Neuron 9(5):815-30.

Omi N., Morikawa N., Ezawa I. (1992). The effect of spiny lobster shell powder on bone metabolism in ovariectomized osteoporotic model rats. J Nutr Sci Vitaminol (Tokyo) 38:555-63.

Omokawa S., Arai Y., Saito H., Furuya T., Sato T., Sato T. et al. (1991). A simple experimental model of total hepatectomy, hepatic ischemia and extrahepatic portal obstruction in rats using splenic transposition. Jpn J Surg 21(1):50-6.

Ondrula D., Nelson RL., Andrianopoulos G., Schwartz D., Abcarian H., Birnbaum A., Skosey J. (1993). Quantitative determination of pentane in exhaled air correlates with colonic inflammation in the rat colitis model. Dis Colon Rectum 36(5):457-62.

Opie L.H., Bruyneel K.J., Lubbe W.F.(1983). What has has the baboon to offer as model of experimental ischemia? Eur Hera J. 4 Suppl C:55-60.

Orlowaski J.P. (1986). Animal model of anaphylactic shock. Ann Emerg Med. 15:979-81.

Orme I.M. (1987): The dynamics of infection following BCG and Mycobacterium tuberculosis challenge in T-cell-deficient mice. Tubercle. 68(4):277-83.

Osborne W.R., Deeg H.J., Slichter S.J. (1986). A canine model of induced purine nucleoside phosphorylase deficiency. Clin Exp Immunol. 66:166-72.

Oser B.L. (1981). The rat as a model for human toxicological evaluation. J Toxicol Environ Health. 8:521-42.

Osieka R., Bamberg M., Pfeiffer R., Glatte P., Scherer E., Schmidt C.G. (1985). Effect of antineoplastic agents and ionizing radiation on a human testicular cancer heterograft. Strahlentherapie. 16:35-46. (English Abstract). (German)

Osipov V.V. (1988): An experiment at modelling alcoholism in minipigs. Farmakol Toksikol. 51(3):97-9. (English Abstract). (Russian)

Ossenkopp K.P. (1985). Animal models of motion sickness: are non-emetic species an appropriate choice? Physiologist. 28 (6 Suppl):S61-2.

Ossowska K., Schulze G., Wolfarth S., Coper H., Kaminska A., Hausmanowa-Petrusewicz I. (1992). Muscle stiffness and continuous electromyographic activity in old rats; an animal model for spasticity? Neuroscience 51(1):167-75.

Oster G., Kilburn K.H., Siegal F.P. (1983). Chemically induced congenital thymic dysgenesis in the rat: a model of the DiGeorge syndrome. Clin Immunol Immunopathol. 28:128-34.

Oster Z.H., Som P., W G.J., Weber D.A. (1991). Imaging of cocaine-induced global and regional myocardial ischemia. J Nucl Med. 32:1569-72.

Otsu T., Tsuno K., Nogami T., Esaki K., Higashi K., Saito Y., Yano T., Terasaki H., Morioka T. (1985). Veno-venous extacorporeal lung assist with a double lumen catheter in small dogs as an analogy of the human neonate. Kokyu To Junkan. 33:883-6. (Japanese)

Ott R.J., Tait D., Flower M.A., Babich J.W., Lambrecht R.M. (1992). Treatment planning for systemic radiotherapy of neural crest tumours using [124]I-mIBG positron emission tomography. Brit J Radiology 65:787-91.

Ottenweller J., Natelson B., Pitman D., Drastal S. (1989). Adrenocortical and behavioral responses to repeated stressors: toward an animal model of chronic stress and stress-related mental illness. Biol Psychiatry 26(8):829-41.

Otto U., Huland H. (1982). The clinical significance of NMRI NU/NU mice tumor model. Prog Clin Biol Res. 100:207-8.

Otto U., Huland H., Kloppel G., Baisch H. (1987): Xenogenic transplantation of human bladder- and renal-cell carcinoma into NMRI mice treated with cyclosporin A and into NMRI nu/nu mice. Introduction of a new experimental cancer model. Urol Int. 42:1-5.

Oubina J.R., Carballal G., Videla C.M., Cossio P.M. (1984). The guinea pig model for Argentine hemorrhagic fever. Am J Trop Med Hyg. 33:1251-7.

Overmier J.B., Burke P.D. (Ed.) (1992). Animal models of human pathology: a bibliography of a quarter century of behavioral research, 1967-1992. Washington, DC: American Psychological Association. 322 P.

Overstreet D., Double K., Schiller G. (1989). Antidepressant effects of rolipram in a genetic animal model of depression: cholinergic supersensitivity and weight gain. Pharmacol Biochem Behav 34(4):691-6.

Overstreet D.H. (1993). The Flinders sensitive line rats: a genetic animal model of depression. Neurosci Biobehav Rev. 17(1):51-68.

Overstreet D.H., Russell R.W., Crocker A.D., Gillin J.C., Janowsky D.S. (1988): Genetic and pharmacological models of cholinergic supersensitivity and affective disorders. Experientia 15;44(6):465-72.

Owen C.A. Jr., Ludwig J. (1982). Inherited copper toxicosis in Bedlington terriers: Wilson's disease (hepatolenticular degeneration). Am J Pathol. 106:432-4.

Owens M., Overstreet D., Knight D., Rezvani A., Ritchie J., Bissette G., Janowsky D., Nemeroff C. (1991). Alterations in the hypothalamic-pituitary-adrenal axis in a proposed animal model of depression with genetic muscarinic supersensitivity. Neuropsychopharmacology 4(2):87-93.

Owunwanne A., Al-Wafai I., Vallgren S., Sadek S., Abdel-Dayem H.M., Yacoub T. (1988). Comparison of Four Technetium-99m Radiopharmaceuticals for Detection and Localization of Gastrointestinal Bleeding in a Sheep Model. Amer J Physiologic Imaging 3:192-196.

Owunwanne A., Mahajan K.K., Abdel-Dayem H.M., Ericksson S.B., Sadek S., Yacoub T., Awdeh M. (1987). Development of an animal model using a closed system to study the sentisitivity of a radiopharmaceutical for the detection of gastrointestinal bleeding. Nuklearmedizin. 26:126-30.

Pacini D.L., Dubovi E.J., Clyde W.A. Jr. (1984). A new animal model for human respiratory tract disease due to adenovirus. J Infect Dis. 150:92:7.

Packchanian A., Emery R., Macdonald E.M., Rigdon R.N. (1982). Experimental leprosy with Mycobacterium lepraemurium in hairless mice (Mus musculus). Trans R Soc Trop Med Hyg. 76:183-6.

Padilla S., Veronesi B. (1988): Biochemical and morphological validation of a rodent model of organophosphorus-induced delayed neuropathy. Toxicol Ind Health. 4(3):361-71.

Page R.L., Garg P.K., Garg S., Archer G.E., Bruland Ø.S., Zalutsky M.R. (1994). PET imaging of osteosarcoma in dogs using a fluorine-18-labeled monoclonal antibody fab fragment. J Nucl Med. 35:1506-13.

Paigen B., Plump A.S., Rubin E.M. (1994). The mouse as a model for human cardiovascular disease and hyperlipidemia. Curr Opin Lipidol. 5(4):258-64.

Paller M.S., Murray B.M. (1985). Renal dysfunction in animal models of cyclosporine toxicity. Transplant Proc. 17 (4 Suppl 1):155-9.

Palmieri J.R., Connor D.H., Purnomo, Dennis D.T., Marwoto H. (1982). Experimental infection of Wuchereria bancrofti in the silvered leaf monkey Presbytis cristatus Eschscholtz, 56:243-5.

Palmieri J.R., Connor D.H., Purnomo, Dennis D.T., Marwoto H. (1983). Bancroftian filariasis. Wuchereria bancrofti infection in the silvered leaf monkey (Presbytis cristatus). Am J Pathol. 112:383-6.

Pamnani M., Huot S., Buggy J., Clough D., Naddy F. (1981). Demonstration of a humoral inhibitor of the Na+-K+pump in some models of experimental hypertension. Hypertension. 3 (6 Pt 2):II-96-101.

Panepinto L.M., Phillips R.W. (1986). The Yucatan miniature pig: characterization and utilization in biomedical research. Lab Anim Sci. 36:344-7.

Pang D., Sclobassi R.J., Horton J.A. (1986). Lysis of intraventricular blood clot with urokinase in a canine model: Part 1. Canine intraventricular blood cast model. Neurosurgery. 19:540-6; Part 2. Neurosurgery. 19:547-52; Part 3. Neurosurgery. 19:553-72.

Paniagua-Crespo E., Hasle D., Humphery-Smith I., Bellon C., Simitzis A. (1989). [Value of nu/nu mice in the production of experimental amoebic keratitis with Acanthamoeba] Interet de la souris nu/nu dans la realisation de la keratite experimentale a amibes libres du genre Acanthamoeba. C R Acad Sci III 309(11):499-503.

Papadimitriou J.M., Ashman R.B. (1986). The pathogenesis of acute systemic candidiasis in a susceptible inbred mouse strain. J. Pathol. 150:257-65.

Papp M., Willner P., Muscat R. (1991). An animal model of anhedonia: attenuation of sucrose consumption and place preference conditioning by chronic unpredictable mild stress. Psychopharmacology (Berl) 104(2):255-9.

Pappata S., Fiorelli M., Rommel T. et al. (1993). PET study of changes in local brain hemodynamics and oxygen metabolism after unilateral middle cerebral artery occlusion in baboons. J Cereb Blood Flow Metab 13:416-24.

Park C.M., Reid P.E., Owen D.A., Sanker J.M., Applegarth D.A. (1987). Morphological and histochemical changes in intestinal mucosa in the reserpine-treated rat model of cystic fibrosis. Exp Mol Pathol. 47:1-12.

Park N.H., Pavan-Langston D., Hettinger M.E., Geary P.A., August M.L., Albert D.M., Lin T.S., Prusoff W.H. (1982). Development of oral HSV-1 infection model in mice. Evaluation of efficacy of 5'-amino-5-iodo-2',5'- dideoxyuridine. Oral Surg. 53:256-62.

Park S., Selmanoff M. (1991). Dose-dependent suppression of postcastration luteinizing hormone secretion exerted by exogenous prolactin administration in male rats: a model for studying hyperprolactinemic hypogonadism. Neuroendocrinology 53(4):404-10.

Parker L.E., Netzloff. (1982). Decreased ornithine decarboxylase in the fetal hydantoin syndrome. Ann Clin Lab Sci. 12:216-22.

Parks D.A., Grogaard B., Granger D.N. (1982). Comparison of partial and complete arterial occlusion models for studying intestinal ischemia. Surgery. 92:896-901.

Paschal J., Holland G., Sison R., Berlin O., Bruckner D., Dugel P., Foos R. (1992). Mycobacterium fortuitum keratitis. Clinicopathologic correlates and corticosteroid effects in an animal model. Cornea 11(6):493-9.

Pasley J., White H., Barron A. (1990). Persistent chronic active cervicitis: a newly noted finding in an animal model of chlamydial genital disease [letter]. J Infect Dis 162(5):1219-20.

Pasqualini C.D. (1981). Comparative leukemia: of mice and men. Medicina (B Aires). 41 (Suppl):199-206.

Passaniti A., Adler S., Martin G. (1992). New models to define factors determining the growth and spread of human prostate cancer. Exp Gerontol 27(5-6):559-66.

Pasternak J.F., Groothuis D.R., Fischer J.M., Fischer D.P. (1983). Regional cerebral blood flow in the beagle puppy model of neonatal intraventricular hemorrhage: studies during systemic hypertension. Neurology (NY). 33:559-66.

Pataki A., Rordorf-Adam C. (1985). Polyarthritis in MRL 1pr/1pr mice. Rheumatol Int. 5:113-20.

Pate B.D., Snow B.J., Hewitt K.A., Morrison K.S., Ruth T.J., Calne D.B. (1991). The reproducibility of striatal uptake data obtained with positron emission tomography and fluorine-18-L-6-fluorodopa tracer in non-human primates. J Nucl Med. 32:1246-51.

Paterson P.Y. (1983). LT/EAE and the MS quest. Going to dogs and rats to study the patient. Cell Immunol. 82:55-74.

Patt J.T., Western G., Buck A., Fletcher S.R., Schubiger P.A. (1995). [^{11}C]-N-methyl and [^{18}F]-fluoroethylepibatidine ligands for the neuronal nicotinic receptor. Paper F02. World-Wide-Web (WWW). Point to HTTP: //GABRIOLA.PET.MED.UBC.CA/WTTC95.HTML

Pattengale P.K., Taylor C.R. (1983). Experimental models of lymphoproliferative disease. The mouse as a model for human non-Hodgkin's lymphomas and related leukemias. Am J Pathol. 113:237-65.

Patterson D.F., Haskins M.E., Jezyk P.F. (1982). Models of human genetic disease in domestic animals. Adv Hum Genet. 12:263-339.

Patterson E., Eller B.T., Lucchesi B.R. (1982). Ventricular fibrillation resulting from ischemia at a site remote from previous myocardial infarction. A conscious canine model of sudden coronary death. Am J Cardiol. 50:1414-23.

Patterson G.A., Todd T.R. (1982). A large animal model of pseudomonas pneumonia. J Surg Res. 33:214-9.

Patton D.L., Halbert S.A., Wang S.P. (1982). Experimental salpingitis in rabbits provoked by Chlamydia trachomatis. Fertil Steril. 37:691-700.

Paul L.C. (1993). Animal models of chronic heart and kidney allograft rejection. Transplant Proc. 25(2):2080-1.

Paule W., Bernick S., Strates B., Nimni M. (1992). Calcification of implanted vascular tissues associated with elastin in an experimental animal model. J Biomed Mater Res 26(9):1169-77.

Pawlowski K. (1983). An experimental model of inflammation. Postepy Hig Med Dosw. 37:519-35. (Polish)

Pazzaglia U., Zatti G., Gervaso P., Gatti A., Pio A. (1990). Experimental osteoporosis in the rat induced by a hypocalcic diet. Ital J Orthop Traumatol 16(2):257-65.

Pearce E.J., McLaren D.J. (1983). Schistosoma mansoni: in vivo and in vitro studies of immunity using the guinea pig model. Parasitology. 87 (Pt 3):465-79.

Pearl R., Baer E., Siegel L., Benson G., Rice S. (1992). Longitudinal distribution of pulmonary vascular resistance after endotoxin administration in sheep. Crit Care Med 20(1):119-25.

Pearson T.A., Dillman J., Malmros H., Sternby N. et al. (1983). Cholesterol-induced athero-sclerosis. Clonal characteristics of arterial lesions in the hybrid hare. Arteriosclerosis. 3:574-80.

Pedersen P., Biber B., Martinell S., Seeman T., Hasselgren P.O. (1984). Hemodynamic and hematologic changes in a standardized trauma-sepsis model in rats. Circ Shock. 14:13-23.

Pedley R., Dale R., Boden J., Begent R., Keep P., Green A. (1989). The effect of second antibody clearance on the distribution and dosimetry of radiolabelled anti-CEA antibody in a human colonic tumor xenograft model. Int J Cancer 43(4):713-8.

Peeters B., Van R. C., Van L. E., Coenen A. (1989). Anti-epileptic and behavioural actions of MK-801 in an animal model of spontaneous absence epilepsy [published erratum appears in Epilepsy Res 1989 Nov-Dec;4(3):234]. Epilepsy Res 3(2):178-81.

Pelfrene A.F. (1985). A search for a suitable animal model for bone tumors: a review. Drug Chem Toxicol. 8:83-99.

Pelletier J.P., Martel-Pelletier J., Howell D.S. (1983). Collagenolytic activity and collagen matrix breakdown of the articular cartilage in the Pond-Nuki dog model of osteoarthritis. Arthritis Rheum. 26:866-74.

Pemsingh R.S., MacPherson B.R., Scatt G.W. (1987). Mucous hypersecretion in the gallbladder epithelium of ground squirrels fed a lithogenic diet for the induction of cholesterol gallstones. Hepatology. 7:1267-71.

Pendleton D.B., Delano M.L., Sands H. et al. (1984). Pharmacological characterization of Tc-99m $(CN-t-butyl)_6^+$: A potential heart agent. J Nucl Med. 25:P15.

Penhale W.J., Ahmed S.A. (1982). Animal model of human disease. Lymphocytic thyroiditis. Autoimmune thyroiditis in rats induced by thymectomy and irradiation. Am J Pathol. 106:300-2.

Penn J., Thum L. (1989). The rat as an animal model for retinopathy of prematurity. Prog Clin Biol Res 314:623-42.

Penner J.D., Prieur D.J. (1987). A comparative study of the lesions in cultured fibroblasts of humans and four species of animals with Chediak-Higashi syndrome. Am J Med Genet, Oct; 28:445-54. Also: Am J Med Genet. 28:455-70.

Pentchev P.G. (1986). The cholesterol storage disorder of the mutant BALB/c mouse. A primary genetic lesion closely linked to defective esterification of exogenously derived cholesterol and its relationship to human type C Niemann-Pick disease. J Biol Chem. 261:2772-7.

Pentlow K.S., Graham M.C., Cheung N.K.U., Lambrecht R.M., Finn R., Larson S.M. (1991). Quantitative imaging of radiolabeled antibodies using iodine-124 and positron emission tomography. Medical Physics 18:357-66.

Pentlow K.S., Graham M.C., Lambrecht R.M., Larson S.M. et al. (1994). The use of positron emission tomographs for the quantitative imaging of iodine-124 in phantoms under clinical conditions. J Nucl Med. (submitted)

Pepeu G., Casamenti F., Pedata F., Cosi C., Pepeu I.M. (1986). Are the neurochemical and behavioral changes induced by lesions of the nucleus basalis in the rat a model of Alzheimer's disease? Prog Neuropsychopharmacol Biol Psychiatry. 10:541-51.

Pepeu G., Pepeu I., Casamenti F. (1990). The validity of animal models in the search for drugs for the aging brain. Drug Des Deliv 7(1):1-10.

Percy D.H., Barta J.R. (1993). Spontaneous and experimental infections in SCID and SCID/beige mice. Lab Anim Sci. 43(2):127-32.

Perese D., Ulman J., Viola J., Ewing S., Bankiewicz K. (1989). A 6-hydroxydopamine-induced selective parkinsonian rat model. Brain Res 494(2):285-93.

Perez-Saad H., Figueredo P., Urba-Holmgren R. (1984-85). Opiate abstinence head-shaking model in infant rats. Bol Estud Med Biol. 33:13-24.

Perpina M., Palau M., Cortijo J., Fornas E., Sanz C., Morcillo E. (1990). Relationship between non-specific airway hyperreactivity and antigen-induced contraction in an allergic animal model in vitro. Respiration 57(2):81-4.

Perry S., Dennie C.J., Coblentz C.L., Cleland S. (1994). Minimizing the risk of Q fever in the hospital setting. Can J Infect Control. 9(1):5-8.

Perryman L.E., McGuire T.C., Banks K.L. (1983). Animal model of human disease. Infantile X-linked agammaglobulinemia. Agammaglobulinemia in horses. Am J. Pathol. 111:125-7.

Peterson C., Vinayak S., Pazos A., Gale K. (1992). A rodent model of focally evoked self-sustaining status epilepticus. Eur J Pharmacol 221(1):151-5.

Peterson T. (1993). Pentoxifylline prevents fibrosis in an animal model and inhibits platelet-derived growth factor-driven proliferation of fibroblasts. Hepatology 17(3):486-93.

Petrovskaia V.G., Nastichkin I.A., Prozorovskii E.V. (1983). Dynamics of enterobacterial multiplication in a mouse model of intraperitoneal infection in the presence of iron cations as dependent on the availability and type of K antigens. Zh Mikrobiol Epidemiol Immunobiol. 9:53-60. (English Abstract). (Russian)

Pfeiffer C.J. (Ed) (1985): Animal Models for Intestinal Disease. CRC Press, Boca Raton,Fl. 320p.

Phelan J.P., Van lenten B.J., Fogelman A.M., Kean C., Haberland M.E., Edwards P.A. (1985). Notes on the breeding of the WHHL rabbit: an animal model of familial hypercholesterolemia. J Lipid Res. 26:776-8.

Philipp M., Aydintug M., Bohm R. J., Cogswell F., Dennis V., Lanners H., Lowrie R. J., Roberts E., Conway M., Karacorlu M., et al. (1993). Early and early disseminated phases of Lyme disease in the rhesus monkey: a model for infection in humans. Infect Immun 61(7):3047-59.

Phillips D.A., Fisher M., Smith T.W., Davis M.A. (1988): The safety and angiographic efficacy of tissue plasminogen activator in a cerebral embolization model. Ann Neurol. 23(4): 391-4.

Phillips J., Kelly R. J., Fonkalsrud E., Mirzayan A., Kim C. (1991). An improved model of experimental gastroschisis in fetal rabbits. J Pediatr Surg 26(7):784-7.

Phillips R. (1989). Circulatory shock in long and short pigs. Prog Clin Biol Res 299:265-75.

Phillips R.W., Panepinto L.M., Spangler R., Westmoreland N. (1982). Yucatan miniature swine as a model for the study of human diabetes mellitus. Diabetes. 31 (Suppl 1 Pt 2):30-6.

Phillips S.C. (1987). Can brain lesions occur in experimental animals by administration of ethanol or acetaldehyde? Acta Med Scand [Suppl]. 717:67-72.

Phillips T., Gurr K. (1989). A pre-conditioned arthritic hip model. J Arthroplasty 4(3):193-200.

Phillips T., Gurr K., Rao D. (1990). Hip implant evaluation in an arthritic animal model. Arch Orthop Trauma Surg 109(4):194-6.

Picha G., Goldstein J., Stohr E. (1990). Natural-Y Meme polyurethane versus smooth silicone: analysis of the soft-tissue interaction from 3 days to 1 year in the rat animal model. Plast Reconstr Surg 85(6):903-16.

Pickett R.D. (1987). Animal models for the evaluation of radiopharmaceuticals. In: Kristensen K., Norbygaard E. (Eds). Safety and Efficiency of Radiopharmaceuticals. Dordrecht: Martinus Nijhoff. pp 77-104.

Pierce C.S., Wicher K., Nakeeb S. (1983). Experimental Syphilis guinea pig model. Br J Vener Dis. 59:157-168.

Pifat D.Y., Smith J.F. (1987): Punta Toro virus infection of C57BL/6J mice: a model for phlebovirus-induced disease. Microb Pathog. 3(6):409-22.

Pignatiello M., Olson G., Kastin A., Ehrensing R., McLean J., Olson R. (1989). MIF-1 is active in a chronic stress animal model of depression. Pharmacol Biochem Behav 32(3):737-42.

Pillai N.R., Santhakumari G. (1984). Effects of nimbidin on acute and chronic gastro-duodenal ulcer models in experimental animals. Planta Med. 50:143-6.

Pincott J.R., Taffs L.F. (1982). Experimental scoliosis in primates: a neurological cause. J Bone Joint Surg [Br]. 64:503-7.

Pinder M., Leclerc A., Flockhart H., Egwang T. (1990). Macaca fascicularis, a non-permissive host for the human filarial parasite Loa loa. J Parasitol 76(3):373-6.

Pippin L.L. (1992). Animal models of ionizing radiation damage: technical report. Alexandria, V.A.: Defense Nuclear Agency. 51 P.

Pirovino M., Muller O., Zysset T., Honegger U. (1988): Amiodarone-induced hepatic phospholipidosis: correlation of morphological and biochemical findings in an animal model. Hepatology. 8(3):591-8.

Piwnica-Worms D. (1994). Making sense out of anti-sense: Challenges of imaging gene translation with radiolabeled oligonucleotides. J Nucl Med. 35:1064-6.

Pleskanovskaia S.A. (1986). Experimental models of cutaneous leishmaniasis in laboratory animals. Parazitologiia. 20:120-5. (English Abstract). (Russian)

Pogosianz H.E., Sokova O.I. (1982). Tumours of the Djungarian hamster. IARC Sci Publ. 34:451-5.

Poirier M., Beland F. (1992). DNA adduct measurements and tumor incidence during chronic carcinogen exposure in animal models: implications for DNA adduct-based human cancer risk assessment [see comments]. Chem Res Toxicol 5(6):749-55.

Poleshchuk V., Balaian M., Andzhaparidze A., Sobol' A., Dokin V., Guliaeva T., Titova I. (1990). [The modelling of hepatitis A and of enterally transmitted non-A, non-B hepatitis (hepatitis E) in Saguinus mystax tamarins] Modelirovanie gepatita A i enteral'no peredaiushchegosia gepatita ni A, ni B (gepatita E) na tamarinakh Saguinus mystax. Vopr Virusol 35(5):379-82.

Poleshchuk V.D., Novikova R.F. (1983). Parasitic diseases of laboratory animals as natural biological models. Vestn Akad Med Nauk SSSR. 9:72-5. (English Abstract). (Russian)

Pollack G.M., Shen D.D. (1985). A timed intravenous pentylenetetrazol infusion seizure model for quantitating the anticonvulsant effect of valproic acid in the rat. J Pharmacol Methods. 13:135-46.

Pollak K. (1989). [Preliminary results of comparative studies of cerebral hemiatrophy in humans and animals] Predvarite'lnye rezu'ltaty sravnite'lnogo issledovaniia gemiatrofii mozga u cheloveka i zhivotnykh. Zh Nevropatol Psikhiatr 89(10):127-9.

Pollard M. (1992). The Lobund-Wistar rat model of prostate cancer. J Cell Biochem Suppl 16H:84-8.

Pollard M., Luckert P.H. (1984). Animal models + treatment of prostate cancer. Prostate. 5:661-8.

Pollard M., Luckert P.H. (1987). Autochthonous prostate adenocarcinomas inLobund-Wistar rats: a model system. Prostate. 11:219-27.

Polotskii IuE., Tseneva GIa., Efremov V.E., Kleganov V.K. (1983). Modeling of pseudotuberculosis infection. Tr Inst Pastera. 60:91-103 (English Abstract). (Russian)

Ponzetto A., Forzani B., Smedile A., Hele C., Avanzini L., Novara R., Canese M.G., (1987). Acute and chronic delta infection in the woodchuck. Prog Clin Biol Res. 234:37-46.

Ponzetto A., Rapicetta M., Forzani B., Smedile A., Hele C., Morace G., di Rienzo A.M., Palladino P., Avanzini L., Gerin J.L. (1987) Hepatitis delta virus infection in Pekin ducks chronically infected by the duck hepatitis B virus. Prog Clin Biol Res. 234:47-9.

Pories S.E., Ramchurren N., Summerhayes I., Steele G. (1993). Animal models for colon carcinogenesis. Arch Surg. 128(6):647-53.

Port R., Sample J., Seybold K. (1991). Partial hippocampal pyramidal cell loss alters behavior in rats: implications for an animal model of schizophrenia. Brain Res Bull 26(6):993-6.

Porter D.G. (1992). Ethical Scores for Animal Experiments. Nature 356:101-102.

Portha B., Giroix M.H., Kergoat M., Bailbe D., Blondel O., Sarradas P. (1988): Animal models of non-insulin-dependent diabetes induced in the rat by experimental reduction of B cell mass. Journ Annu Diabetol Hotel Dieu. 33-46. (76 ref.) (French)

Portugal V., Garcia-Alonso I., Bilbao J., Barcelo P., Mugica P., Mendez J. (1993). [The hepatotrophic action of cyclosporin A in a model of hepatic ischemia in the rat] Estudio de la accion hepatotrofica de la ciclosporina A en un modelo de isquemia hepatica en la rata. Rev Esp Enferm Dig 83(4):255-9.

Posner M., Burt M., Stone M., Han B., Warren R., Vydelingum N., Brennan M. (1990). A model of reversible obstructive jaundice in the rat. J Surg Res 48 (3):204-10.

Potter G.K., Shen R.N., Chiao J.W. (1984). Nude mice as models for human leukemia studies. Am J Pathol. 114:360-6.

Pour P.M., Donnelly T., Stepan K. (1983). Modification of pancreatic carcinogenesis in the hamster model. 6. The effect of ductal ligation and excision. Am J Pathol. 113:365-72.

Power M., Olson M., Domingue P., Costerton J. (1990). A rat model of Staphylococcus aureus chronic osteomyelitis that provides a suitable system for studying the human infection. J Med Microbiol 33(3):189-98.

Powers J.D., Powers T.E., Varma K.J., Gabel A.A., Spurlock S.L. (1984). A health index to evaluate clinically a beta-hemolytic streptococcal infectious disease model in the horse. J Vet Pharmacol Ther. 7:213-7.

Pratt J.A., Rothwell J., Jenner P., Marsden C.D. (1986). p,p-DDT-induced myoclonus in the rat and its application as an animal model of 5-HT sensitive action myoclonus. Adv Neurol. 43:577-88.

Prause J.U., Elling F., Jensen O.A., Manthorpe R. (1986): The effect of bromhexine on the kidney lesions in NZB-NZW-F1 mice. Scand J Rheumatol [Suppl]. 61:286-90.

Pravenec M. (1986). Recombinant inbred strains - a model for the study of spontaneous hypertension in rats. Cesk Fysiol. 35:271-4. (Czechoslovakian)

Preac M. V., Patsouris E., Wilske B., Reinhardt S., Gross B., Mehraein P. (1990). Persistence of Borrelia burgdorferi and histopathological alterations in experimentally infected animals. A comparison with histopathological findings in human Lyme disease. Infection 18(6):332-41.

Preminger G.M., Koch W.E., Fried F.A., McFarland E., Murphy E.D., Mandell J. (1982). Murine congenital polycystic kidney disease: a model for studying development of cystic disease. J Urol. 127:556-60.

Pretolani M., Vargaftig B. (1993). From lung hypersensitivity to bronchial hyperreactivity. What can we learn from studies on animal models? Biochem Pharmacol 45(4):791-800.

Pretto E. (1991). Cardiac function after hepatic ischemia-anoxia and reperfusion injury: a new experimental model. Crit Care Med 19(9):1188-94.

Priborsky J., Muhlbachova E. (1990). Evaluation of in-vitro percutaneous absorption across human skin and in animal models. J Pharm Pharmacol 42(7):468-72.

Price D., Koo E., Sisodia S., Martin L., Koliatsos V., Muma N., Walker L., Cork L. (1990). Neuronal responses to injury and aging: lessons from animal models. Prog Brain Res 86:297-308.

Price D., Martin L., Clatterbuck R., Koliatsos V., Sisodia S., Walker L., Cork L. (1992). Neuronal degeneration in human diseases and animal models. J Neurobiol 23(9):1277-94.

Price D.L., Koliatsos V.E., Clatterbuck R.C. (1993). Cholinergic systems: human diseases, animal models, and prospects for therapy. Prog Brain Res. 98:51-60.

Price D.L., Sisodia S.S. (1994). Cellular and molecular biology of Alzheimer's disease and animal models. Annu Rev Med. 45:435-46.

Price J., Zhang R. (1990). Studies of human breast cancer metastasis using nude mice. Cancer Metastasis Rev 8(4):285-97.

Prieto G., Urba-Holmgren R., Holmgren B. (1991). Sleep and EEG disturbances in a rat neurological mutant (taiep) with immobility episodes: a model of narcolepsy-cataplexy. Electroencephalogr Clin Neurophysiol 79(2):141-7.

Prinzen F.W., Alewijnse R., Van der Vusse G.J., Kruger R.T. (1987). Coronary artery stenosis controlled by distal perfusion pressure: description of the servo-system and time-dependent changes in regional myocardial blood flow. Basic Res Cardiol. 82:375-87.

Pritchard D.G., Stuart F.A., Brewer J.I., Mahmood K.H. (1987): Experimental infection of badgers (Meles meles) with Mycobacterium bovis. Epidemiol Infect. 98:145-54.

Pritchard D.I., Eady R.P., Harper S.T., Jackson D.M., Orr T.S., Richards I.M., Trigg S., Wells E. (1983). Laboratory infection of primates with Ascaris suum to provide a model of allergic bronchoconstriction. Clin Exp Immunol. 54:469-76.

Pritzker K.P. (1994). Animal models for osteoarthritis: processes, problems and prospects. Ann Rheum Dis. 53(6):406-20.

Probert A.W. Jr., Schrier D.J., Gilbertson R.B. 1984. Effects of antiarthritic compounds on type II collgen-induced arthritis in rats. Arch Int Pharmacodyn Ther. 269:167-76.

Proceeding (1983) of the symposium on primate ethopharmacology. Ethopharmacology: Primate models of neuropsychiatric disorders. IX Congress of the International Primatological Society, Atlanta Georgia, August, 1972. Prog. Clin. Biol. Res. 131:1-334.

Proceedings (1982) of the International Symposium on Animal Models of Inherited Metabolic Disease. Animal models of inherited metabolic diseases. Bethesda, M.D., October 19-20, 1981. Prog. Clin. Biol. Res. 94:1-519.

Proceedings of the Sixth Charles River International Symposium on Laboratory Animals (1987). Animal models: assessing the scope of their use in biomedical research. Kyoto, Japan, October 8-9, 1985. Prog Clin Biol Res. (1987), 229:1-384.

Proietto J., Thorburn A.W. (1994). Animal models of obesity - theories of aetiology. Baillieres Clin Endocrinol Metab. 8(3):509-25.

Prop F.J., Weijer K., Spies J., Souw L., Peters K., Erich T. et al. (1986). Feline mammary carcinomas as a model for human breast cancer. I. Sensitivity of mammary tumor cells in culture to cytostatic drugs. A preliminary investigation of a predictive test. Anticancer Res. 6:989-94.

Provost P.J., Keller P.M., Banker F.S., Keech B.J., Klein H.J., Lowe R.S., Morton D.H., Phelps A.H., McAleer W.J., Ellis R.W. (1987). Successful infection of the common marmoset (Callithrix jacchus) with human varicella-zoster virus. J Virol. 61:2951-5.

Prusty S., Kemper T., Moss M.B., Hallander W. (1988). Occurrence of stroke in a non-human primate model of cerebrovascular disease. Stroke. 19:84-90.

Pruzansky M.E. (1987). A primate model for the evaluation of tendon adhesions. J Surg Res. 42:273-6.

Pryor G. (1990). Persisting neurotoxic consequences of solvent abuse: a developing animal model for toluene-induced neurotoxicity. NIDA Res Monogr 101:156-66.

Przedborski S., Jackson-Lewis V., Popilskis S., Kostic V., Levivier M., Fahn S., Cadet J. (1991). Unilateral MPTP-induced parkinsonism in monkeys. A quantitative autoradiographic study of dopamine D1 and D2 receptors and re-uptake sites. Neurochirurgie 37(6):377-82.

Pueschel S.M. (1985). Biological and behavioural assessments of young rhesus monkeys after intrauterine exposure to high phenylalanine concentrations. J Ment Defic Res. 29 (Pt. 3):247-56.

Puko V., Drozd I. (1990). [Condition of cell membranes in simulated motion sickness and use of alpha-tocopherol] Sostoianie kletochnykh membran pri modelirovanii bolezni dvizheniia i vvedenii al'fa-tokoferola. Farmakol Toksikol 53(5):47-8.

Pulsinelli W.A., Buchan A.M. (1988): The four-vessel occlusion rat model: method for complete occlusion of vertebral arteries and control of collateral circulation. Stroke. 19(7): 913-4.

Pumphrey C.W., Fuster V., DeWanjee M.K., Murphy K.P., Dietstra R.E., Kaye M.P. (1982). A new in vivo model of arterial thrombosis: the effect of administration of ticlopidine and verapamil in dogs. Thromb Res.28:663-75.

Purcell B., Richardson J., Radolf J., Hansen E. (1991). A temperature-dependent rabbit model for production of dermal lesions by Haemophilus ducreyi. J Infect Dis 164(2):359-67.

Purcell R.H., Satterfield W.C., Bergmann K.F., Smedile A., Ponzetto A., Gerin J.L. (1987). Experimental hepatitis delta virus infection in the chimpanzee. Prog Clin Biol Res. 234:27-36.

Purtilo D., Falk K., Pirruccello S., Nakamine H., Kleveland K., Davis J., Okano M., Taguchi Y., Sanger WG., Beisel KW. (1991). SCID mouse model of Epstein-Barr virus-induced lymphomagenesis of immunodeficient humans. Int J Cancer 47(4):510-7.

Puschel W., Stiehl P., Rosenkranz M., Geifer G., Wiesenhaken U., Richter R.F. (1982). Suitability of experimental antigen-induced arthritis in rabbits as a model of rheumatoid arthritis. Agents Actions [Supp]. 10:243-53.

Puskas E., Uher F., Gergely J., Bazin H. (1984). An experimental immuno- cytoma model in /LOU/M/Wsl X CFY/F1 rats: neoplastic cells as targets of the host's immune apparatus. Immunology. 52:547-54.

Qian C., Li T., Shen T.Y., Libertine-Graham L., Eckman J., Biftu T., Ip S. (1993). Epibatidine is a nicotinic analgesic. Eur J Pharmacol. 250:R13-R14.

Quan S., Witten M., Grad R., Ray CG., Lemen R. (1991). Changes in lung mechanics and histamine responsiveness after sequential canine adenovirus 2 and canine parainfluenza 2 virus infection in beagle puppies. Pediatr Pulmonol 10(4):236-43.

Quandt L., Hutz R. (1993). Induction by estradiol-17 beta of polycystic ovaries in the guinea pig. Biol Reprod 48(5):1088-94.

Quesada-Pascual F., Rojas-Espinosa O., Santos Argumendo L., Estrada-Parra S. (1987). A Mexican armadillo (Dasypus novemcinctus) colony for leprosy research. Int J Lepr Other Mycobact Dis. 55:716-8.

Quezada A., von Stowasser V., Murray G., Andreis M. (1983). Experimental model of hypersensitivity pneumonia in rats. Rev Med Chil. 111:389-96. (English Abstract). (Spanish)

Quinlan D., Gearhart J., Jeffs R. (1988). Abdominal wall defects and cryptorchidism: an animal model. J Urol 140(5 Pt 2):1141-4.

Quinn T.C., Taylor H.R., Schachter J. (1986). Experimental proctitis due to rectal infection with Chlamydia trachomatis in nonhuman primates. J Infect Dis. 154:833-41.

Qureshi M.A., Sajjad M., Vora M.M., Bakr S.A, Lambrecht R.M. et al. (1987). Production of iodine-124 an its incorporation in meta-iodobenzylguanidine. Proc. Ninth Australian Sym. on Analytical Chemistry, Sydney, 27 April - 1 May 1987. Analytical Chemistry Division of the Royal Australian Chemical Institute, North Ryde, Vol. 2:716-23.

Rabe A., Haddad R., Dumas R. (1985). Behavior and neurobehavioral teratology using the ferret. Lab Anim Sci. 35:256-67.

Raberger G. (1986). A model of transient myocardial dysfunction in conscious dogs. Regional shortening in the presence of impaired coronary flow reserve and treadmill exercise. J Pharmacol Methods. 16:23-37.

Racaniello V., Ren R., Bouchard M. (1993). Polio virus attenuation and pathogenesis in a transgenic mouse model for poliomyelitis. Dev Biol Stand 78:109-16.

Racz P., Letvin N.L., Gluckman J.C. (Ed.) (1993). Animal models of HIV and other retroviral infections. Basel; New York: Karger. 200 P.

Radl J., Croese J., Zurcher C., Van d. E. M., de L. A. (1988). Animal model of human disease. Multiple myeloma. Am J Pathol 132(3):593-7.

Radzinski C., McGuire E., Smith D., Wein AJ., Levin R., Miller L., Elbadawi A. (1991). Creation of a feline model of obstructive uropathy. J Urol 145(4):859-63.

Raghavan D., Debruyne F., Herr H., Jocham D., Kakizoe T., Okajima E. et al. (1986). Experimental models of bladder cancer: a critical review. Prog Clin Biol Res. 221:171-208.

Raine C.S., Traugatt U. (1984). Experimental autoimmune demyelination. Chronic relapsing models and their therapeutic implications for multiple sclerosis. Ann NY Acad Sci. 436:33-51.

Rajan T., Nelson F., Cupp E., Schultz L., Greiner D. (1992). Survival of Onchocerca volvulus in nodules implanted in immunodeficient rodents. J Parasitol 78(1):160-3.

Rajeswaran S., Jones W.F., Byars L.G. et al. (1992). Physical characteristics of a small diameter positron emission tomograph. IEEE Nucl Sci Symp Med Imaging Conference :985-7.

Rajkumar K., Schott P., Simpson CW. (1990). The rat as an animal model for endometriosis to examine recurrence of ectopic endometrial tissue after regression. Fertil Steril 53(5):921-5.

Rajs J., Isberg B., Paul C., Ahlberg N.E. (1982). Daunorubicin-induced chronic cardiomyopathy--an experimental model system for study of sudden death. Forensic Sci Int. 20:217-25.

Raju T. (1992). Some animal models for the study of perinatal asphyxia. Biol Neonate 62:202-14.

Rak J., Kusnierczyk H., StrzadaLa L., Radzikowski C. (1988). Transplantable mouse 16/C mammary adenocarcinoma as a model in experimental cancer therapy. I. Kinetics of growth and spread. Arch Immunol Ther Exp (Warsz) 36(3):325-34.

Ramos-Martinex E. (1988): Experimental models of chronic active hepatitis and its relation to hepatocellular carcinoma. Rev Gastroenterol Mex. 53(3):201-6. (English Abstract). (Spanish)

Rana S.V., Mehta S., Chopra J.S., Nain C.K., Dhand U.K., Mehta J. (1984). Lipid composition of the peripheral nerves in malnutrition: an experimental study in young rhesus monkeys. J Med Primatol. 13:205-17.

Ranasinghe A.W., Johnson N.W., Rountree R. (1983). Experimental iron deficiency in Syrian hamsters (Mesocricetus auratus). Lab Anim. 17:210-2.

Rangel M., Pontes J. (1989). Animal models of renal cell carcinoma. Semin Urol 7(4):237-46.

Rank R.G., Whitum-Hudson J.A. (1994). Animal models for ocular infections. Methods Enzymol. 235:69-83.

Rao G.A., Sankaran H., Larkin E.C. (1988): Rat models for chronic alcohol consumption. J Nutr. 118(6): 799-801.

Rapacz J., Hasler-Rapacz J., Taylor K.M., Cheocvich W.J., Attie A.D. (1986). Lipoprotein mutations in pigs are associated with elevated plasma cholesterol and atherosclerosis. Science. 234:1573-7.

Rashid V. (1991). [A comparative study of the efficacy of Vermox, albendazole and medamine in an experimental model of trichocephaliasis in mice] Sravnitel'noe izuchenie effektivnosti vermoksa, al'bendazola i medamina na eksperimental'noi modeli trikhotsefaleza myshei. Med Parazitol (Mosk) (5):44-6.

Raskova H. (1982). Transfer of data to man and pathological models. Cas Lek Cesk. 121:1087-90. (English Abstract). (Czechoslovakian)

Ratajczak M.Z., Kant J.M., Luger S.M. et al. (1992). In vivo treatment of human leukemia in a SCID mouse model with c-myb antisense oligonucleotides. Proc Natl Acad Sci USA 89:11823-7.

Ratech H., Hirschhorn R., Thorbecke G.J. (1985). Effects of deoxycoformycin in mice. III. A murine model reproducing multi-system pathology of human adenosine deaminase deficiency. Am J Pathol. 119:65-72.

Rattazzi M.C., Appel A.M., Baker H.J. (1982). Enzyme replacement in feline GM2 gangliosidosis: catabolic effects of human beta-hexosaminidase A. Prog Clin Biol Res. 94:213-20.

Ravingerova T., Ziegelhoffer A., Tribulova N., Slezak J., Tregerova V. (1989). [Methods in experimental models of heart damage using reactive forms of oxygen] Nase metodicke skusenosti s experimentalnym modelom poskodenia srdca reaktivnymi formami kyslika. Cesk Fysiol 38:513-6.

Reba R.C. (Ed.) (1995). Molecular nuclear medicine. J Nucl Med. 36(Suppl):1S-30S.

Reddy G.S., Wilcken D.E. (1982). Experimental homocysteinemia in pigs: comparison with studies in sixteen homocystinuric patients. Metabolism. 31:778-83.

Redha F., Uhlschmid G., Ammann R., Freiburghaus A. (1990). Injection of microspheres into pancreatic arteries causes acute hemorrhagic pancreatitis in the rat: a new animal model. Pancreas 5(2):188-93.

Regan T. (1983). The Case for Animal Rights. Routledge and Kegan Paul, London.

Rege R.V., Dawes L.G., Ostrow J.D. (1993). Animal models of pigment gallstones. Adv Vet Sci Comp Med. 37:257-87.

Rege R.V., Nahrwold D.L. (1987). Animal models of pigment gallstone disease. J Surg Res. 43:196-203.

Reichart B.A., Human P.A., Rose A.G., Novitzky D., Cooper D.K. (1987). Is pulmonary ischemia a factor in the reperfusion response? An experimental study in the chacma baboon. J Heart Transplant. 6:238-43.

Reichart E. (1986). Multiple stress of the lung: the emphysema model induced by elastase. Agressologie. 27:825-8. (English Abstract). (French)

Reichmann K., Twist J., McKenzie R. (1989). Inhibition of alpha-glucosidase in cattle by Castanospermum australe: an attempted phenocopy of Pompe's disease. Aust Vet J 66(3):86-9.

Reid L.M. (1980). Needs for animal models of human diseases of the respiratory system. Am J Pathol. 101:S89-S101.

Reigel C.E. (1986). The genetically epilepsy-prone rat: an overview of seizure-prone characteristics and responsiveness to anticonvulsant drugs. Life Sci. 39:763-74.

Reinoso-Suárez F. (1961). Topographischer Hirnatlas der Katze. Darmstadt: E. Merck AG , 74p.

Reitman J.S., Mahley R.W., Fry D.L. (1982). Ycatan miniature swine as a model for diet-induced atherosclerosis. Atherosclerosis. 43:119-32.

Reivich M., Alavi A. (1983). Pharmacokinteic models and positron emission tomography: Studies of physiologic and pathophysiologic conditions. In: Lambrecht R.M., Rescigno A. (Eds.). Tracer Kinetics and Physiologic Modelling - Theory to Practice. Lecture Note in Biomathematics, vol 48. Heidelberg: Springer Verlag, p 345-83.

Reivich M., Kuhl D. et al. (1979). The [^{18}F]fluorodeoxyglucose method for the measurement of local cerebral glucose utilization in man. Circ Res. 44:127-37.

Rekel' IuI. (1982). Method of modeling uterine tuberculosis and its potential use in phthisiogynecology. Probl Tuberk. 6:62-5.

Renaud A. (1988). [Animal models of depression] Modeles animaux de la depression. Soins Psychiatr (88):10-3.

Renkawek K. (1986). Experimental model of Parkinson disease induced by N-methyl-4-phenyl-1,2,3,6-tetrahydropyridine (MPTP). Neuropatol Pol. 24:1-8. (English Abstract). (Polish)

Rennie J.S., MacDonald D.G. (1982). Experimental iron deficiency in the Syrian hamster (Mesocricetus auratus). Lab Anim. 16:14-6.

Report (1993) of group B of the American Cancer Society Research Workshop on Cancer and Nutrition: panel on animal studies. Cancer Res, 53 (10 Suppl):2452s-2454s.

Resnick J.S. (1981). Experimental models of renal cystic disease. Nippon Jinzo Gakkai Shi. 23:989-98.

Resnick O., Morgane P.J. (1983). Animal models for small-for-gestational- age (SGA) neonates and infants-at-risk (IAR). Brain Res. 312:221-5.

Rest J.R. (1982). Cerebral malaria in inbred mice. I. A new model and its pathology. Trans R Soc Trop Med Hyg. 76:410-5.

Reuman P., Keely S., Schiff G. (1989). Assessment of signs of influenza illness in the ferret model. J Virol Methods 24(1-2):27-34.

Reuzel P.G., Immel H.R., Spit B.J., Feron V.J. (1984). Electrocoagulation as a method to induce local lesions in the tracheal wall of Syrian hamsters. Z Versuchstierkd. 26:211-6.

Rewers A., Redgate E., Deutsch M., Fisher ER., Boggs S. (1990). A new rat brain tumor model: glioma disseminated via the cerebral spinal fluid pathways. J Neurooncol 8(3):213-9.

Reyes M.P., Ho K.L., Smith F., Lenner A.M. (1981). A mouse model of dilated-type cardiomyopathy due to coxsackievirus B3. 144:232-6.

Rhodes G., Tapsall J., Lykke A. (1989). Alveolár epithelial responses in experimental streptococcal pneumonia. J Pathol 157(4):347-57.

Ribeiro A.B., Franco R.J., KohlMann O. Jr., Marson O., Ramos O.L. (1981). Etiopathogenesis of excess methylprednisolone arterial hypertension in the rat. Clin Exp Hypertens. 3:1219-37.

Riccardi V.M., Womack J.E., Jacks T. (1994). Neurofibromatosis and related tumors. Natural occurrence and animal models. Am J Pathol. 145(5):994-1000.

Richardson J. (1991). Animal models of depression reflect changing views on the essence and etiology of depressive disorders in humans. Prog Neuropsychopharmacol Biol Psychiatry 15(2):199-204.

Richardson S.H., Giles J.C., Kruger K.S. (1984). Sealed adult mice: new model for enterotoxin evaluation. Infect Immun. 43:482-6.

Riche D., Hantraye P., Guilbert B., Naquet R., Loc'h C., Maziere B., Maziere M. (1988). Anatomical atlas of the baboon's brain in the orbitomeatal plane used in experimental positron emission tomography. Brain Res Bull. 20:283-301.

Richter A., Loscher W., Loschmann P. (1993). The AMPA receptor antagonist NBQX exerts antidystonic effects in an animal model of idiopathic dystonia. Eur J Pharmacol 231(2):287-91.

Ridgway R.L., Oaks S.C. Jr., La Barre D.D. (1986). Laboratory animal models for human scrub typhus. Lab Anim Sci. 36:481-5.

Riegger A.J., Liebau G. (1982). The renin-angiotensin-aldosterone system, antidiuretic hormone and sympathetic nerve activity in an experimental model of congestive heart failure in the dog. Clin Sci. 62:465-9.

Rieke G.K., Scarfe A.D., Hunter J.F. (1984). L-pyroglutamate: an alternate neurotoxin for a rodent model of Huntington's disease. Brain Res Bull. 13:443-56.

Rissing J.P., Buxton T.B., Weinstein R.S., Shockley R.K. (1985). Model of experimental chronic osteomyelitis in rats. Infect Immun. 47:581-6.

Rissman E. (1990). The musk shrew, Suncus murinus, a unique animal model for the study of female behavioral endocrinology. J Exp Zool Suppl 4:207-9.

Roberts J.A. (1983). Vesicoureteral reflux in the monkey: a review. Urol Radiol. 5:211-7, 219.

Roberts R., Kier A., Walker S. (1989). The RHJ/Le rhino mutant: description of a unique murine model of autoimmunity. J Comp Pathol 100(4):391-404.

Robertson W.W. Jr., Janssen H.F. (1983). Hematoma formation after bone biopsy: a canine model. South Med J. 76:966-8.

Rock D.L., Reed D.E. (1982). Persistent infection with bovine herpesvirus type 1: rabbit model. Infect Immun. 35:371-3.

Roder J.C. (1982). Characterization of a murine model (beige) for a natural killer cell immunodeficiency in the Chediak-Higashi syndrome of man. Prog Clin Biol Res. 94:315-25.

Rodgers J.B., Monier-Faugere M.C., Malluche H. (1993). Animal models for the study of bone loss after cessation of ovarian function. Bone 14(3):369-77.

Rodolakis A. (1987): Experimental models in chlamydiosis. Ann Rech Vet. 18(4):345-54. (73 ref.). (English Abstract) (French)

Rodriguez M., Oleszak E., Leibowitz J. (1987). Theiler's murine encephalomyelitis: a model of demyelination and persistence of virus. CRC Crit Rev Immunol. 7:325-65.

Roe F.J. (1987): Liver tumors in rodents: extrapolation to man. Adv Vet Sci Comp Med. 31:45-68.

Rogatskii G.G. (1984). Interrelation of cardiodynamics and pulmonary gas exchange in an experimental model of the acute respiratory failure syndrome. Biull Eksp Biol Med. 98:273-5. (English Abstract) (Russian)

Rogers A.E., Nauss K.M. (1985). Rodent models for carcinoma of the colon. Dig Dis Sci. 30:87S-102S.

Rogers F., Baumgartner N., Robin A., Barrett J. (1991). Absorbable mesh splenorrhaphy for severe splenic injuries: functional studies in an animal model and an additional patient series. J Trauma 31(2):200-4.

Rohozkova D., Havelka S., Tranavsky K. (1990). [Experimental models and their importance in the study of osteoarthrosis] Experimentalni modely a jejich vyznam pro studium osteoartrozy. Cesk Fysiol 39(2):97-103.

Rojkind M., Greenwel P. (1993). Animal models of liver fibrosis. Adv Vet Sci Comp Med. 37:333-55.

Rolston D.D., Borodo M.M., Kelly M.J., Dawson A.M., Farthing M.J. (1987). Efficacy of oral rehydration solutions in a rat model of secretory diarrhea. J Pediatr Gastroenterol Nutr. 6:624-30.

Romanova T. (1989). [Method for modelling intracerebral hematomas in arterial hypertension] Sposob modelirovaniia vnutrimozgovykh gematom pri arterial'noi gipertenzii. Patol Fiziol Eksp Ter (3):80-1.

Roncoroni L., Violi V., Muri M., Moccia G., Mangoni L., De Bernardinis M., Monatanari M. (1982). Verification of a protocol for inducing hypersplenism in the rat by means of methylcellulose. Chir Patol Sper. 29:172-9. (Italian)

Roomi M.W., Ho P.K, Sarma D.S. et al. (1985). A common biochemical pattern in preneoplastic hepatocyte nodules generated in four different models in the rat. Cancer Res. 45:564-71.

Rooney S.A., Chu A.J., Gross I., Marino P.A., Schwartz R., Seghal P., Singer D.B., Susa J.B., Warsaw J.B., Wilson C.M. (1983). Lung surfactant in the hyperinsulinemic fetal monkey. Lung. 161:313-7.

Roos R.P., Wollmann R. (1984). DA strain of Theiler's murine encephalomyelitis virus induces demyelination in nude mice. Ann Neurol. 15:494-9.

Rordorf C., Pataki A., Nogues V., Schlager F., Feige U., Glatt M. (1987). Arthritis in MRL/LPR mice and in collagen II sensitized DBA-1 mice and their use in pharmacology. Int J Tissue React. 9:341-7.

Rose J. (1992). Virus-induced demyelination: from animal models to human diseases [editorial; comment]. Mayo Clin Proc 67(9):903-6.

Roselle G.A., Mendenhall C.L., Muhleman A.F., Chedid A. (1986). The ferret: a new model of oral ethanol injury involving the liver, bone marrow, and peripheral blood lymphocytes. Alcoholism (NY). 10:279-84.

Rosen F.S., Seligmann M. (Ed.) (1993). Immunodeficiencies. Chur, Switzerland; Philadelphia, Pa., USA: Harwood Academic Publishers. 761 P.

Rosenbaum J., Seymour B., Raymond W., Langlois L., Wu M., David L. (1988). Similar chemotactic factor for monocytes predominates in different animal models of uveitis. Inflammation 12(3):191-201.

Rosenberg L., Brown R.A., Dugrind W.P. (1983). A new approach to the induction of duet epithelial hyperplasia and nesidioblastosis by cellophane wrapping of the hamster pancreas. J. Surg. Res. 35: 63-72.

Rosenberg N.L. (1988): Neuromuscular histopathology in (New Zealand black x New Zealand white)F1 and MRL-1pr autoimmune mice: models for skeletal muscle involvement in connective tissue disease. Arthritis Rheum. 31(6):806-11.

Rosenberg N.L. (1993). Experimental models of inflammatory myopathies. Baillieres Clin Neurol. 2(3):693-715.

Rosenblum H.M., Haasler GB, Spotnitz WD, Lazar HL, Spotnitz HM. (1985). Effects of simulated clinical cardiopulmonary bypass and cardioplegia on mass of the canine left ventricle. Ann Thorac Surg. 39:139-48.

Rosenblum L.A., Paully G.S. (1987). Primate models of separation-induced depression. Psychiatr Clin North Am. 10:437-47.

Rosner I., Bellasai J., Schinini A., Rovira T., de A. A., Ferro E., Ferreira E., Velazquez G., Monzon M., Maldonado M., et al. (1989). Cardiomyopathy in Cebus apella monkeys experimentally infected with Trypanosoma cruzi. Trop Med Parasitol 40(1):24-31.

Ross D.S., Steele G. Jr. (1984). Experimental models in cancer immunotherapy. J Surg Res. 37:415-30.

Ross J., Sahenk Z., Hyser C., Mendell J., Alden C. (1988). Characterization of a murine model for human bismuth encephalopathy. Neurotoxicology 9(4):581-6.

Ross R., Agius L. (1992). The process of atherogenesis - cellular and molecular interaction: from experimental animal models to humans. Diabetologia 35Suppl 2:S34-40.

Rossan R.N., Harper J.S. 3d, Davidson D.E. Jr., Escajadillo A., Christensen H.A. (1985). Comparison of Plasmodium falciparum infections in Panamanian and Colombian owl monkeys. Am J Trop Med Hyg. 34:1037-47.

Rossi G.A., Hunninghake G.W., Kawanami O., Ferrans V.T., Hansen C.T., Crystal R.G. (1985). Motheaten mice - an animal model with an inherited form of interstitial lung disease. Am Rev Respir Dis. 131:150-8.

Rossle M., Deckert J., Jones E. (1989). Autoradiographic analysis of GABA-benzodiazepine receptors in an animal model of acute hepatic encephalopathy. Hepatology 10(2):143-7.

Rossotto P., Georgacopulo P., Franchella A., Riccipetitoni G., Morsianti E., Morsiani V. et al. (1982). Experimental intrauterine surgery: the creation of a congenital diaphragmatic hernia in a sheep fetus. Minerva Med. 73:1859-69 (English Abstract). (Italian)

Roth K., Carter B., Higgins E. (1991). Succinylacetone effects on renal tubular phosphate metabolism: a model for experimental renal Fanconi syndrome. Proc Soc Exp Biol Med 196(4):428-31.

Roth S.I., Conaway H.H. (1982). Animal model of human disease. Spontaneous diabetes mellitus in the New Zealand white rabbit. Am J Pathol. 109:359-63.

Rothwell T., Pope S., Rajczyk Z., Collins G. (1991). Haematological and pathological responses to experimental Trixacarus caviae infection in guinea pigs. J Comp Pathol 104(2):179-85.

Roux C., Rey F., Lyonnet S., Nizard S., Mulliez N., Munnich A. (1991). An animal model for maternal phenylketonuria. J Med Genet 28(10):718-9.

Rowland E., Lozykowski M., McCormick T. (1992). Differential cardiac histopathology in inbred mouse strains chronically infected with Trypanosoma cruzi. J Parasitol 78(6):1059-66.

Rozvadovskii V.D., Trenin S.O., Tel'pukhov V.I. (1985). A microsurgical model of cerebral ischemia. Biull Eksp Biol Med. 99:140-2. (English Abstract). (Russian)

Ruben Z., Miller J.E, Rohrbacher E., Walsh G.M. (1984). A potential model for a human disease: spontaneous cardiomyopathy-congestive heart failure in SHR/N-cp rats. Hum Pathol. 15:902-3.

Rubin E.M., Smith D.J. (1994). Atherosclerosis in mice: getting to the heart of a polygenic disorder. Trends Genet. 10(6):199-203.

Rubino G.J., Young W. (1988): Ischemic cortical lesions after permanent occlusion of individual middle cerebral artery branches in rats. Stroke. 19(7):870-7.

Rubinstein G. (1993). Schizophrenia, infection and temperature. An animal model for investigating their interrelationships. Schizophr Res. 10(2):95-102.

Rubio C.A., Wallin B., Sveander M., Duvander A. (1987). A model for the study of metastases from colonic tumors by autotransplantation. Dis Colon Rectum 30:884-7.

Rucker R., Opsahl W., Abbott U., Greve C., Kenney C., Stern R. (1986). Scoliosis in chickens. A model for the inherited form of adolescent scoliosis. Am J Pathol. 123:585-8.

Ruckert N., Schmidt W. (1993). The sigma receptor ligand 1,3-di-(2-tolyl)guanidine in animal models of schizophrenia. Eur J Pharmacol 233(2-3):261-7.

Rudolph R. (1983). Spontaneous keratoacanthoma--an animal model for the tumor in man?. DTW. 90:349-52. (German)

Rudzki E., Zawisza E., Rebandel P. (1982). Atopic eczema in dogs as a natural model of prurigo. Przegl Dermatol. 69:235-8 (English Abstract). (Polish)

Rueda C. J., Ortega M. L., Arguello d. A. J., Landa G., Balibrea C. J. (1991). [Experimental acute pancreatitis in the rat. The quantification of pancreatic necrosis after the retrograde ductal injection of sodium taurocholate] Pancreatitis aguda experimental en la rata. Cuantificacion de la necrosis pancreatica tras la inyeccion retrograda ductal de taurocolato sodico. Rev Esp Enferm Dig 80(3):178-82.

Rugarli E., Lutz B., Kuratani S., Wawersik S., Borsani G., Ballabio A., Eichele G. (1993). Expression pattern of the Kallmann syndrome gene in the olfactory system suggests a role in neuronal targeting. Nat Genet 4(1):19-26.

Ruiz-Palacios G.M., Escamilla E., Torres N. (1981). Experimental Campylobacter diarrhea in chickens. Infect Immun. 34:250-5.

Runyon B., Sugano S., Kanel G., Mellencamp M. (1991). A rodent model of cirrhosis, ascites, and bacterial peritonitis. Gastroenterology 100(2):489-93.

Rupniak N., Tye S., Iversen S. (1990). Drug-induced purposeless chewing: animal model of dyskinesia or nausea? Psychopharmacology (Berl) 102(3):325-8.

Ruprecht R.M., Fratazzi C., Sharma P.L., Greene M.F., Penninck D., Wyand M. (1993). Animal models for perinatal transmission of pathogenic viruses. Ann N Y Acad Sci. 693:213-28.

Russell K.H., Hagenmeyer-Houser S.H., Sanberg P.R. (1987). Haloperidol-induced emotional defecation: a possible model for neuroleptic anxiety syndrome. Psychopharmacology (Berlin). 91:45-9.

Russell M.L. (1983). The tight-skin mouse: is it model for scleroderma? J Rheumatol. 10:679-81.

Ruwe W.D. (1986). Alcohol dependence and withdrawal in the rat. An effective means of induction and assessment. J Pharmacol Methods. 15:225-34.

Ruzov V. (1990). [Experimental hypodynamia as a model of the disintegration of the main body hormonal systems] Eksperimental'naia gipodinamiia kak model' dezintegratsii osnovnykh gormonal'nykh sistem organizma. Vopr Kurortol Fizioter Lech Fiz Kult (4):55-6.

Ryder R.D. (1975). Victims of Science. The Use of Animals in Research. Davis-Poyntor Ltd., UK.

Ryder R.D. (1989). Animal Revolution; Changing Attitudes Towards Speciesism. Blackwell, Oxford.

Ryder R.D. (1991). Sentientism. The Psychologist 14(5):201.

Sackett G.P. (1984). A non-human primate model of risk for deviant develoment. Am J Ment Defic. 88:469-76.

Sackler A.M., Weltman A.S. (1985). Effects of methylphenidate on whirler mice: an animal model for hyperkinesis. Life Sci. 37:425-31.

Sado Y., Kagawa M., Rauf S., Naito I., Moritoh C., Okigaki T. (1992). Isologous monoclonal antibodies can induce anti-GBM glomerulonephritis in rats. J Pathol 168(2):221-7.

Sadowski W., Samkow R., Wilczynski J., Krus S., Kantoch M. (1987): The cotton rat (Sigmodon hispidus) as an experimental model for studying viruses in respiratory tract infections. II. Influenza viruses types A and B. Med Dosw Mikrobiol. 39:43-55 (English Abtract). (Polish)

Sadowski W., Semkow R., Wilczynski J., Krus S., Kantoch M. (1987): The cotton rat (Sigmodon hispidus) as an experimental model for studying viruses in human respiratory tract infections. I. Para-influenza virus type 1, 2 and 3, adenovirus type 5 and RS virus. Med Dosw Mikrobiol. 39:33-42 (English Abstract) (Russian)

Saetta M., Fabbri L., Danieli D., Picotti G., Allegra L. (1989). Pathology of bronchial asthma and animal models of asthma. Eur Respir J Suppl, 6:477s-482s.

Sagrada A., Turconi M., Bonali P., Schiantarelli P., Micheletti R., Montagna E., Nicola M., Algate D., Rimoldi EM., Donetti A. (1991). Antiemetic activity of the new 5-HT3 antagonist DAU 6215 in animal models of cancer chemotherapy and radiation. Cancer Chemother Pharmacol 28(6):470-4.

Sagstrom S., McMillan E., Marijianowski M., Mulders H., Roomans G. (1990). Changes in rat and mouse salivary glands and pancreas after chronic treatment with diuretics: a potential animal model for cystic fibrosis. Scanning Microsc 4(1):161-70; discussion 170.

Sagvolden T., Metzger M., Schiorbeck H., Rugland A., Spinnangr I., Sagvolden G. (1992). The spontaneously hypertensive rat (SHR) as an animal model of childhood hyperactivity (ADHD): changed reactivity to reinforcers and to psychomotor stimulants. Behav Neural Biol 58(2):103-12.

Sahlin C., Brismar J., Delgado T., Owman C., Salford L.G., Svendgaard N.A. (1987): Cerebrovascular and metabolic changes during the delayed vasospasm following experimental subarachnoid hemorrhage in baboons and treatment with a calcium antagonist. Brain Res. 403:313-32.

Sakai K., Tomoike H., Ootsubo H., Kikuchi Y., Nakamura M. (1982). Preocclusive perfusion area as a determinant of infarct size in a canine model. Cradiovasc Res. 16:408-16.

Sakamoto N., Hotta N., Uchida K. (Ed.) (1992). Current concepts of a new animal model: the NON mouse. Amsterdam; New York: Elsevier. 176 P.

Sakamoto Y. (1989). [The pathogenesis of trehalose dimycolate-induced hemorrhagic pneumonia induced in mice as animal model of human alveolar hemorrhagic syndrome]. Nippon Kyobu Shikkan Gakkai Zasshi 27(2):206-13.

Sakiyama T., Tsuda M., Kitagawa T., Fujita R., Miyawaki S. (1982). A lysosomal storage disorder in mice: a model Niemann-Pick disease. J Inherited Metab Dis. 5:239-40.

Sakly R., Zarrouk K., Hedhili A., Achour A., Mbazzaa A. (1991). [Study of anti-lithogenic action of zinc sulfate in experimental lithiasis in the rat] Etude sur l'action anti-lithogene de sulfate de zinc vis-a-vis de la lithiase experimentale chez le rat. Ann Urol (Paris) 25(5):246-9.

Saku K., Fujino M., Yamamoto K., Ying H., Tashiro N., Harada R. et al. (1990). Cardiac function of WHHL rabbit, an animal model of familial hypercholesterolemia. Artery 17(5):271-80.

Sakurada O., Kennedy C., Jehle J., Brown J.D., Garbin G.L., Sokoloff L. (1978). Measurement of local cerebral blood flow with iodo(^{14}C)antipyrine. Am J Physiol 234:H59-H66.

Salinas A., Triebling A., Toth L., Dreiling D.A. (1985). The pathogenesis of pancreatic pseudocysts--a canine experimental model. Am J Gastroenterol. 80:126-31.

Salzman L.A. (1986): Animal Models of Retrovirus Infection and Their Relationship to AIDS. Academic Press, New York.

Salzman S., Dabney K., Mendez A., Beauchamp J., Daley J., Freeman G. et al. (1988). The somatosensory evoked potential predicts neurologic deficits and serotonergic pathochemistry after spinal distraction injury in experimental scoliosis. J Neurotrauma 5(3):173-86.

Sambuco C.P. (1985). Miniature swine as an animal model in photodermatology: factors influencing sunburn cell formation. Photodermatol. 2:144-50.

Samosiuk I.Z. (1987). Experimental model of cerebral arachnoiditis. Vrach delo. (8):89-91 (English Abstract) (Russian)

Sampson D., Willner P., Muscat R. (1991). Reversal of antidepressant action by dopamine antagonists in an animal model of depression. Psychopharmacology (Berl) 104(4):491-5.

Samson H.H. (1986). Initiation of ethanol reinforcement using a sucrose-substitution procedure in food-and water-sated rats. Alcoholism (NY). 10:436-42.

Sanberg P., Emerich D. (1990). Neural basis of behavior: animal models of human conditions. Brain Res Bull 25(3):447-51.

Sanberg P., Giordano M., Henault MA., Nash D., Ragozzino M., Hagenmeyer-Houser S. (1989). Intraparenchymal striatal transplants required for maintenance of behavioral recovery in an animal model of Huntington's disease. J Neural Transplant 1(1):23-31.

Sanberg P.R., Wictorin K., Isacson O. (1994). Cell transplantation for Huntington's disease. Austin: R.G. Landes.

Sande M.A. (1981). Evaluation of antimicrobial agents in the rabbit model of endocarditis. Rev Infect Dis. 3 (Suppl):S240-9.

Sande R.D., Bingel S.A. (1983). Animal models of dwarfism. Vet Clin North Am [Small Animal Practice]. 1:71-89.

Sanders T., Sandaradura S. (1992). The cholesterol-raising effect of coffee in the Syrian hamster. Br J Nutr 68(2):431-4.

Sanders W.E., Read M.S., Reddick R.L., Garris J.B., Brinkhous K.M. (1988): Thrombotic thrombocytopenia with von Willebrand factor deficiency induced by botrocetin. An animal model. Lab Invest. 59(4):443-52.

Sandhar B., Niblett D., Argiras E., Dunnill M., Sykes M. (1988). Effects of positive end-expiratory pressure on hyaline membrane formation in a rabbit model of the neonatal respiratory distress syndrome. Intensive Care Med 14(5):538-46.

Santalo J., Badenas J., Calafell J., Catala V., Munne S., Egozcue J., Estop A. (1992). The genetic risks of in vitro fertilization techniques: the use of an animal model. J Assist Reprod Genet 9(5):462-74.

Sanyal S.C., Islam K.M., Neogy P.K., Islam M., Speelman P., Huq M.I.(1984). Campylobacter jejuni diarrhea model in infant chickens. Infect Immun. 43:931-6.

Sarter M.. (1987): Animal models of brain ageing and dementia. Compr Gerontol [A]. 1(1):4-15.

Sartoris D.J., Holmes R.E., Bucholz R.W., Resnick D. (1986). Coralline hydroxyapatite bone graft substitutes in a canine diaphyseal defect model: radiographic features of failed and successful union. Skeletal Radiol. 15:642-7.

Sarvetnick N. (1990). Transgenic models of diabetes. Curr Opin Immunol 2(4):604-6.

Satellite conference of the International Society of Neurochemists. (1984). Experimental allergic encephalomyelitis, a useful model for multiple sclerosis. Seattle, Washington, July 16-19, 1983. Prog. Clin. Biol. Res. 146:1-554.

Sato N., Sato T., Takhashi S., Kikuchik. (1986). Establishment of murine endothelial cell lines that develop angiosarcomas in vivo: brief demonstration of a proposed animal model for Kaposi's sarcoma. Cancer Res. 46:362-6.

Sato T., Kamiyama Y., Kamano T., Ruthowski J., Adams Cowley R., Trump B.F., Jones R.T. (1985) Pathophysiology of hemorrhagic shock. A model for studying the effects of acute blood loss in the rat. Virchows Arch [Cell Pathol]. 48:361-75.

Sato T., Nara Y., Note S., Yamori Y. (1987): Effect of calcium antagonists on hypertension and diabetes in new hypertensive diabetic models. J Cardiovasc Pharmacol. 10: S192-4.

Sato Y., Toma H. (1990). Strongyloides venezuelensis infections in mice. Int J Parasitol 20:57-62.

Satoh K. (1982). A study on experimental pleurisy. I. Animal model of experimetnal pleurisies. Sci Rep Res Inst Tohoku Univ [Med]. 29:42-56; Part II. Sci Rep Res Inst Tohoku Univ [Med]. 29:57-64; Part III. Sci Rep Res Inst Tohoku Univ [Med]. 29:65-76.

Satyaswaroop P.G., Zaino R.J., Mortel R. (1987). Steroid receptors and human endometrial carcinoma: studies in a nude mouse model. Cancer Metastasis Rev 6:223-41.

Sawtell N.M., Weiss M.A., Pesce A.J., Michael J.G. (1987). An immune complex glomerulopathy associated with glomerular capillary thrombosis in the laboratory mouse. A highly reproducible accelerated model utilizing cationized antigen. Lab Invest. 56:256-63.

Scanley B.E., Al-Tikriti M.S., Gandelmann M.S. et al. (1995). Comparison of [^{123}I]β-CIT and [^{123}I]-IPCT as single photon emission tomography radiotracers for the dopamine transporter in non-human primates. Eur J Nucl Med 22:4-11.

Scannapieco G., Pauletto P., Semplicini A., Dario C., Vescovo G., Mazzucato A., Pessina A.C., Angelini A.(1983). Evaluation of the efficacy of various hypotensive drugs in broad-breasted white turkeys as an experimental model of arterial hypertension with high catecholamine levels. Boll Soc Ital Biol Sper. 59:1265-71. (English Abstract) (Italian)

Schachter P., Buckley N., Oyama H., Christy M., Leight G. J., Lobaugh B. (1989). Primary hyperparathyroidism: a new experimental animal model. Surgery 106(6):997-1001.

Schackert G., Fidler I. (1988). Development of in vivo models for studies of brain metastasis. Int J Cancer 41(4):589-94.

Schackert H., Fidler I. (1989). Development of an animal model to study the biology of recurrent colorectal cancer originating from mesenteric lymph system metastases. Int J Cancer 44(1):177-81.

Schaffner A., Douglas H., Davis C.E. (1983). Models of T cell deficiency in listeriosis: the effects of cortisone and cyclosporin A on normal and nude BALB/c mice. J Immunol. 131:450-3.

Schalkwijk J., Joosten L., van d. B. W., van d. P. L. (1990). Antigen induced arthritis in beige (Chediak-Higashi) mice. Ann Rheum Dis 49(8):607-10.

Scheffel U., Carroll F.I., Kepler J.A., Taylor G.F., Stathis M., London E.D., Kuhar M.J. (1995). In vivo labeling of nicotinic acetylcholine receptors with (+) and (-) [H-3] norchloro-epibatidine. J Nucl Med. 36(5):253P.

Scheffel U., Goldfarb, Lever S.Z. et al. (1988). Comparison of technetium-99m aminoalkyl diaminodithiol (DADT) analogs as potential brain blood flow imaging agents. J Nucl Med. 29:73-82.

Scheinberg D., Strand M. (1990). Radioimmunotherapy in experimental animal models: principles derived from models. Cancer Res 50(3 Suppl):962s-963s.

Scheinberg D.A., Strand M. (1990). Radioimmunotherapy in experimental animal models: Principles derived from models. Cancer Research (Suppl) 50:962s-963s.

Scheld W.M. (1987). Therapy of streptococcal endocarditis: correlation of animal model and clinical studies. J Antimicrob Chemother. 20 (Supp A):71-85.

Scheper R., von B. B., de G. J., Goeptar AR., Lang M., Oostendorp R., Bruynzeel D., van T. R. (1990). Low allergenicity of clonidine impedes studies of sensitization mechanisms in guinea pig models. Contact Dermatitis 23(2):81-9.

Scher I. (1982). The CBA/N mouse strain: an experimental model illustrating the influence of the X-chromosome on immunity. Adv Immunol. 33:1-71.

Scherkl R., Voits M. (1991). Efficacy of anti-epileptic drugs in a rat petit mal epilepsy model during chronic treatment. Acta Vet Scand Suppl 87:185-7.

Scheuer J. (1985). Animal preparations relevant for study with positron emission tomography or nuclear magnetic resonance. Circulation 72:IV139-IV144.

Schiller G., Daws L., Overstreet D., Orbach J. (1991). Lack of anxiety in an animal model of depression with cholinergic supersensitivity. Brain Res Bull 26(3):433-5.

Schilsky M.L., Sternlieb I. (1993). Animal models of copper toxicosis. Adv Vet Sci Comp Med. 37:357-77.

Schimmel D. (1987). Results of experimental infections of SPF piglets with Pasteurella multocida-proposal for a reproducible infection model.Arch Exp Veterinarmed. 41:455-62 (English Abstract) (German)

Schirrmacher V. (1984). Cancer mestastasis and the use of animal model systems. Behring Inst Mitt. 74:195-200.

Schlaff W.D., Cooley B.C., Shen W., Gittlesohn A.M., Rock J.A. (1987). A rat uterine horn model of genital tract would healing. Fertil Steril. 48:866-72.

Schlemmer R.F. Jr., Davis J.M. (1983). A comparison of three psychotomimetic-induced models of psychosis in nonhuman primate social colonies. Prog Clin Biol Res. 131:33-78.

Schlenker E., Burbach J. (1991). The dystrophic hamster: an animal model of alveolar hypoventilation. J Appl Physiol 71(5):1655-62.

Schlitt M. (1986). A rabbit model of focal herpes simplex encephalitis. J Infect Dis. 153:732-5.

Schlosser M.J., Kapeghian J.C., Verlangieri A.J. (1984). Effects of streptozotocin in the male guinea pig: a potential animal model for studying diabetes. Life Sci. 35:649-55.

Schmajuk N.A. (1987). Animal models for schizophrenia: the hippocampally lesioned animal. Schizophr Bull. 13:317-27.

Schmale M.C., Hensley G., Udey L.R. (1983). Neurofibromatosis, von Rechlinghausen's disease, multiple schwannomas in the bicolor damselfish, Pomacentrus partitus (pisces, pomacentridae). Am J pathol. 112:28-41.

Schmidt J., Rattner D., Lewandrowski K., Compton C., Mandavilli U., Knoefel W., Warshaw A. (1992). A better model of acute pancreatitis for evaluating therapy. Ann Surg 215(1):44-56.

Schmidt W., Popham R.E., Israel Y. (1987). Dose-specific effects of alcohol on the lifespan of mice and the possible relevance to man. Br J Addict. 82:775-88.

Schoene R., Goldberg S. (1992). The quest for an animal model of high altitude pulmonary edema. Int J Sports Med 13 Suppl 1:S59-61.

Schoenecker P.L., Lesker P.A., Ogata K. (1984). A dynamic canine model of experimental hip dysplasia. Cross and histological pathology and the effect of position of immobilization on capital femoral epiphyseal blood flow. J.Bone Joint Surg [Am]. 66:1281-8.

Schold S.C. Jr., Friedman H.S., Bigner D.D. (1987). Therapeutic profile of the human glioma line D-54 MG in athymic mice. Cancer Treat Rep. 71:849-50.

Scholmerich J., Fabian M., Tauber R., Lohle E., Kottgen E., Grun M., Wietholtz H., Baumgartner U., Gerok W. (1991). Portacaval shunt as an experimental model of impaired hepatic release of vitamin A in liver disease. Gastroenterology 100(5 Pt 1):1379-84.

Schrek R. (1990). An animal model for intractable chronic lymphocytic leukemia. Med Hypotheses 33(3):175-6.

Schroder W., Wilkerson D., Zatina M. (1990). One hundred percent oxygen reverses muscle hypoxia in a rat hindlimb model of acute arterial occlusion. J Vasc Surg 12(6):667-74; discussion 674-5.

Schubiger P.A., Westera G. (Eds.) (1992). Progress in Radiopharmacy. In: P.H. Cox (Ed.). Series on Developments in Nuclear Medicine. Vol 22. Dordrecht: Kluwer Academic. ISBN 0-7923-1525-1.

Schuller H., Becker K., Witschi H. (1988). An animal model for neuroendocrine lung cancer. Carcinogenesis 9(2):293-6.

Schultz A.M., Hu S.L. (1993). Primate models for HIV vaccines. AIDS 7(Suppl 1):S161-70.

Schunior A., Zengel A., Mullenix P., Tarbell N., Howes A., Tassinari M. (1990). An animal model to study toxicity of central nervous system therapy for childhood acute lymphoblastic leukemia: effects on growth and craniofacial proportion. Cancer Res 50(20):6455-60.

Schuyler M., Subramanyan S., Hassan M.O. (1987). Prolonged exposure to M. faeni in strain II guinea-pigs: pulmonary interstitial inflammation. Br J Exp Pathol. 68:743-54.

Schwartz D., Deschryver-Kecskemeti K., Needleman P. (1984). Renal arachidonic acid metabolism and cellular changes in the rabbit renal vein constricted kidney: inflammation as a common process in renal injury models. Prostaglandins. 27:605-13.

Schwartz E.R., Leveille C., Oh W.H. (1981). Experimentally-induced osteoarthritis in guinea pigs: effect of surgical procedure and dietary intake of vitamin C. Lab Anim Sci. 31:683-7.

Schwartz G. (1991). Vasectomy and human immunodeficiency virus of mice and men [letter; comment]. Fertil Steril 55(3):650-1.

Schwartz P.J., Vanoli E. (1981). Cardiac arrhythmias elicited by interaction between acute myocardial ischemia and sympathetic hyperactivity: a new experimental model for the study of antiarrhythmic drugs. J Cardiovasc Pharmacol. 3:1251-9.

Schwartzkroin P.A. (Ed.) (1993). Epilepsy: models, mechanisms, and concepts. Cambridge, England; New York, N.Y.: Cambridge University Press. 544 P.

Schwarz M., Block F. (1993). Visual evoked potentials in the rat quinolinic acid model of Huntington's disease. Neurosci Lett 152(1-2):81-3.

Schwarz R.H. (1990). Animal research: A position statement. Science 244:1128.

Scivittaro V., Amore A., Emancipator S.N. (1993). Animal models as a means to study IgA nephropathy. Contrib Nephrol. 104:65-78.

Scott G.H., Williams J.C., Stephenson E.H. (1987). Animal models in Q fever: pathological responses of inbred mice to phase I Coxiella burnetii. J Gen Microbiol. 133 (Pt 3):691-700.

Scott S.M., Chou P.J., Fisher D.A. (1983) Nerve growth factor concentration in a congenitally hypothyroid mouse model (hyt/hyt) and its responsivity to thyroxine treatment. J Dev Physiol. 5:413-8.

Sebunya T.N., Saunders J.R., Osborne A.D. (1983). A model aerosol exposure system for induction of porcine Haemophilus pleuropneumonia. Can J Comp Med. 47:48-53.

Secrist R., Traynelis V., Schochet S. J. (1989). MR imaging of acute cortical venous infarction: preliminary experience with an animal model. Magn Reson Imaging 7(2):149-53.

Sedgwick A.D., Moore A.R., Al-Davij A.Y., Edwards J.C., Willoughbe D.A. (1985). The immune response to pertussis in the 6-day air pouch: a model of chronic synovitis. Br J Exp Pathol. 66:455-64.

See R., Ellison G. (1990). Comparison of chronic administration of haloperidol and the atypical neuroleptics, clozapine and raclopride, in an animal model of tardive dyskinesia. Eur J Pharmacol 181(3):175-86.

Segal R., Janetta P.J., Walfson S.K. Jr., Dujovny M., Cook E.E. (1982). Implanted pulsatile balloon device for simulation of neurovascular compression syndromes in animals. J Neurosurg. 57:646-50.

Segall M., Crnic L. (1990). An animal model for the behavioral effects of interferon. Behav Neurosci 104(4):612-8.

Seichter U. (1983). Effect of diphosphonate on inflammatory-resorptive horizontal bone destruction-an animal model. Dtsch Zahnarztl Z. 38:921-4. (English Abstract). (German)

Seller M.J., Beck S.E., Adinoki M. (1981):The curley-tail mouse: an experimental model for human neural tube defects. Life Sci. 29:1607-15.

Selve N. (1992). Chronic intrajejunal TNBS application in TNBS-sensitized rats: a new model of chronic inflammatory bowel diseases. Agents Actions Spec No:C15-7.

Sembrat R.F., Di Stazio J., Stremple J.F.(1979):The pony as a model for septic shock. Adv Shock Res. 2:137-51.

Senior P.V., Pritchett C.J., Sunter J.P., Appleton D.R., Watson A.J. (1985). Transplantation of a segment of ileum to the external abdominal wall: an animal model of intestinal mucosal hyperplasia. J Pathol. 146:39-49.

Serakovski S., Kukhazh E., Bernatska K. (1989). [Experimental models of systemic scleroderma] Eksperimenta'lnye modeli sistemnoi sklerodermii. Revmatologiia (Mosk) (3):36-46.

Serikawa T. (1992). [Review: development of the spontaneously epileptic rat]. Jikken Dobutsu 41(1):1-11.

Serikawa T., Ohno Y., Sasa M., Yamada J., Takaori S. (1987): A new model of petit mal epilepsy: spontaneous spike and wave discharges in tremor rats. Lab Anim, 21: 68-71.

Serio M. and Martini L. (Eds) (1980): Animal Models in Human Reproduction. Raven, New York, 500 pp.

Serizawa N. (1993). [Initial characterization of a new miniature animal model in the rat: studies on anatomy, pituitary hormones and GH mRNA in miniature rat Ishikawa]. Nippon Naibunpi Gakkai Zasshi 69(1):33-45.

Sershen H., Hashim A., Lajtha A. (1987). Behavioral and biochemical effects of nicotine in a MPTP-induced mouse model of Parkinson's disease. Pharmacol Biochem Behav, 28: 299-303.

Sethia K., Brading A., Smith J. (1990). An animal model of non-obstructive bladder instability. J Urol 143(6):1243-6.

Setnikar I., Pacini M., Revel L. (1991). Antiarthritic effects of glucosamine sulfate studied in animal models. Arzneimittelforschung 41(5):542-5.

Seto H., Ihara F., Kakishita M. (1989). Twenty-four-hour whole-body retention of 47Ca-chloride: an index of global bone metabolism in rat models. Int J Rad Appl Instrum [B] 16(8):799-804.

Shah K.R., West M. (1984). Behavioral changes in rat following perinatal exposure to ethanol. Neurosci lett. 47:145-8.

Shah S., Sands H. (1990). Preclinical models and methods for the study of radiolabeled monoclonal antibodies in cancer diagnosis and therapy. Cancer Treat Res 51:53-96.

Shakutsui S., Abe H., Chihara K. (1989). GHRH treatment: studies in an animal model. Acta Paediatr Scand Suppl 349:101-7; discussion 108.

Shanbhag A.B., Nevagi S.A., Nadkarni. (1984). Studies on polycystic ovaries of neonatally androgenized rats. Indian J Exp Biol. 22:18-24.

Sharkis S.J., Jedrzejczak W.W. (1984). The W/Wv mouse as a model of bone marrow failure. Prog Clin Biol Res. 148:211-8 (21 ref.).

Sharpe K., Zimmer R., Khan R., Penney L. (1992). Proliferative and morphogenic changes induced by the co-culture of rat uterine and peritoneal cells: a cell culture model for endometriosis. Fertil Steril 58(6):1220-9.

Shaw J.H., Wolfe R.R. (1984). A conscious septic dog model with hemodynamic and metabolic responses similar to responses of humans. Surgery. 95:553-61.

Shaywitz B.A., Wolf A., Shaywitz S.E., Loomis R., Cohen D.J. (1982). Animal models of neuropsychiatric disorders and their relevance for Tourette syndrome. Adv Neurol. 35:199-202.

Shear H.L. (1993). Transgenic and mutant animal models to study mechanisms and protection of red cell genetic defects against malaria. Experimentia 49(1):37-42.

Shelt D., Walton D., Sato P. (1982). Feasibility of using an isolated intestinal segment as an artificial organ for enzyme replacement therapy. Biomater Med Devices Artif Organs. 10:55-62.

Shelton G., Linenberger M., Grant C., Abkowitz J. (1990). Hematologic manifestations of feline immunodeficiency virus infection. Blood 76(6):1104-9.

Shelub I., van Grondelle A., McCullough R., Hofmeister S., Reeves J.T.(1984). A model of embolic chronic pulmonray hypertension in the dog. J Appl Physiol. 56:810-5.

Shen R., Lu L., Broxmeyer H. (1990). New therapeutic strategies in the treatment of murine diseases induced by virus and solid tumors: biology and implications for the potential treatment of human leukemia, AIDS, and solid tumors. Crit Rev Oncol Hematol 10(3):253-65.

Sherman A.D., Sacquitne J.L., Petty F. (1982). Specificity of the learned helplessness model of depression. Pharmacol Biochem Behav. 16:449-54.

Shestakova N.K., Danilov M.A., Onishchenko N.A. (1988): Dynamic activity of the splenic lymphocytes during the modelling of chronic denervation-delymphatization of the kidneys in mice. Biull Eksp Biol Med. 106(11):572-4. (English Abstract). (Russian)

Sheu C., Lee J., Arras C., Jones R., Lavappa K. (1990). The feasibility of using Chinese hamsters as an animal model for aneuploidy. Environ Mol Mutagen 16(4):320-3.

Shevrin D., Gorny K., Rosol T., Kukreja S. (1991). Effect of etidronate disodium on the development of bone lesions in an animal model of bone metastasis using the human prostate cancer cell line PC-3. Prostate 19(2):149-54.

Shi C.Q.X., Sinusas A.J., Dione D.P., Singer M.J., Young L.H., Heller E.N., Rinker B.D., Wackers F.J.T., Zaret B.L. (1995). Technetium-99m-nitroimidazole (BMS181321): A positive imaging agent for detecting myocardial ischemia. J Nucl Med. 36:1078-86.

Shibata M., Okkubo T., Takahashi H., Kudo T., Inoki R. (1986). Studies of inflammatory pain response: related pain producing substance and endogenous opioid system. Nippon Yakurigaku Zasshi. 87:405-15. (English Abstract). (Japanese)

Shibayama T., Tachibana M., Deguchi N., Jitsukawa S., Tazaki H. (1991). SCID mice: a suitable model for experimental studies of urologic malignancies. J Urol 146(4):1136-7.

Shibuya M., Ikegami K., Sakano T., Yokota J., Sugimoto H., Yoshioka T. et al. (1987). Development of an animal model of autonomic over-activity in tetanus. Nippon Geka Gakkai Zasshi. 88:14-9. (English Abstract) (Japanese)

Shields A.F., Mankoff D.A., Zheng M., Kozawa S.M., Graham M.M., Link J.M., Grierson J.R., Martin G.V., Caldwell J.M., Krohn K.A. (1995). Cardiac retention of labeled thymidine in human and primates. J Nucl Med 36:143P.

Shiga J., Mori W. (1985). Protracted histopathological change of the liver necrosis induced by Shwartzman reaction. An experimental animal model of liver cirrhosis? Acta Pathol Jpn. 35:103-7.

Shih J.C., Pullman E.P., Kao K.J. (1983). Genetic selection, general characterization, and history of atherosclerosis-susceptible and resistant Japanese quail. Atherosclerosis. 49:41-53.

Shimada K., Maeda S., Murakami T., Nishiguchi S., Tashiro F., Yi S., Wakasugi S. et al. (1989). Transgenic mouse model of familial amyloidotic polyneuropathy. Mol Biol Med 6(4):333-43.

Shimamura T., Tazume S., Hashimoto K., Sasaki S. (1981). Experimental cholera in germfree suckling mice. Infect Immun. 34:296-8.

Shimeld C., Hill T., Blyth W., Easty D. (1990). Reactivation of latent infection and induction of recurrent herpetic eye disease in mice. J Gen Virol 71(Pt 2):397-404.

Shimizu K., Maeda K., Shibata M., Ise M., Sugano M., Uehara Y. (1990). [Daunomycin rats. Second Report. Is it possible to use daunomycin rats as an experimental model of chronic renal failure?]. Nippon Jinzo Gakkai Shi 32(2):137-45.

Shimizu T. (1986). Analysis of lung metastasis using a transplantable stomach cancer of the rat - establishment of a new animal model of spontaneous metastasis. Nippon Geka Gakkai Zasshi. 87:1406-13.

Shimokawa I., Higami Y., Hubbard G., McMahan C., Masoro E., Yu B. (1993). Diet and the suitability of the male Fischer 344 rat as a model for aging research. J Gerontol 48(1):B27-32.

Shipilova L.D., Padeiskaia E.N., Kutchak S.N. (1982). Staphylococcal necrotic suppurative encephalomeningitis in mice as a chemotherapeutic model. Antibiotiki 27:353-6. (English Abstract). (Russian)

Shipley P., Shevrin D., Kukreja S. (1988). Increased renal calcium reabsorption in an animal model of hypercalcemia of human malignancy. J Bone Miner Res 3(5):555-60.

Shippenberg T., Stein C., Huber A., Millan M., Herz A. (1988). Motivational effects of opioids in an animal model of prolonged inflammatory pain: alteration in the effects of kappa- but not of mu-receptor agonists. Pain 35(2):179-86.

Shirai M., Izumi H., Yamagami T. (1991). Experimental transplantation models of mouse sarcoma 180 in ICR mice for evaluation of anti-tumor drugs. J Vet Med Sci 53(4):707-13.

Shiraishi N., Aono K., Taguchi T. (1988). Copper metabolism in the macular mutant mouse: an animal model of Menkes's kinky-hair disease. Biol Neonate 54(3):173-80.

Shiraishi N., Aono K., Taguchi T. (1988). Copper metabolism in the macular mutant mouse. An animal model of Menkes' kinky-hair disease. Biol Neonate 54:173-180.

Shiraishi N., Taguchi T., Kinebuchi H. (1991). Copper-induced toxicity in macular mutant mouse: an animal model for Menkes' kinky-hair disease. Toxicol Appl Pharmacol 110(1):89-96.

Shiroyama Y., Nagamitsu T., Yamashita K., Yamashita T., Abiko S., Ito H. (1991). Changes in brain stem blood flow under various grades of brain stem ischemia. Tohoku J Exp Med 164(3):237-46.

Shoenfeld Y. (1989). Experimental and induced animal models of systemic lupus erythematosus and Sjogren's syndrome. Curr Opin Rheumatol 1(3):360-8.

Shoenfeld Y., Mozes E. (1990). Pathogenic idiotypes of autoantibodies in autoimmunity: lessons from new experimental models of SLE. FASEB J 4(9):2646-51.

Shohami E., Evron S., Weinstock M., Soffer D., Carmon A. (1986). A new animal model for action myoclonus. Adv Neurol. 43:545-52.

Short B.L. (1983). Rat intraperitoneal sepsis--a clinically relevant model. Circ Shock. 10:351-9.

Shull R.M., Munger R.J., Spellacy E., Hall C.W. (1982). Canine alpha-L-iduronidase deficiency. A model of mucopolysaccharidosis I. Am J Pathol. 109:244-8.

Shultz L., Lane P., Coman D., Taylor S., Hall E., Lyons B., Wood BG. et al. (1991). Hairpatches, a single gene mutation characterized by progressive renal disease and alopecia in the mouse. A potential model for a newly described heritable human disorder. Lab Invest 65(5):588-600.

Shumiya S., Nagase S. (1984). Establishment of an albumin-deficient and fatty strain of rats. Jikken Dobutsu. 33:97-103.

Shvilkin A., Afonskaia N., Sadretdinov S., Cherpachenko N., Levitskii D., Ruda M. (1991). [Effects of verapamil and nitroglycerin on experimental occlusion- reperfusion-induced myocardial infarction in rabbits] Vliianie verapamila i nitroglitserina na eksperimental'nyi okkliuzionno-reperfuzionnyi infarkt miokarda u krolikov. Kardiologiia 31(1):15-7.

Sibley G.N. (1985). An experimental model of detrusor instability in the obstructed pig. Br J Urol. 57:292-8.

Siebelink K., Chu I., Rimmelzwaan G., Weijer K., van H. R., Knell P. et al. (1990). Feline immunodeficiency virus (FIV) infection in the cat as a model for HIV infection in man: FIV-induced impairment of immune function. AIDS Res Hum Retroviruses 6(12):1373-8.

Siegel R., Katsumata M., Komori S., Wadsworth S., Gill-Morse L., Jerrold-Jones S., Bhandoola A., Greene M., Yui K. (1990). Mechanisms of autoimmunity in the context of T-cell tolerance: insights from natural and transgenic animal model systems. Immunol Rev 118:165-92.

Sijtsma S., West C., Rombout J., Van d. Z. A. (1989). The interaction between vitamin A status and Newcastle disease virus infection in chickens. J Nutr 119(6):932-9.

Sillence D., Ritchie H., Dibbayawan T., Eteson D., Brown K. (1993). Fragilitas ossium (fro/fro) in the mouse: a model for a recessively inherited type of osteogenesis imperfecta. Am J Med Genet 45(2):276-83.

Sillevis S. P., de J. J., Troost D., Kuipers M. (1991). Muscular changes in the guinea pig caused by chronic ascorbic acid deficiency. J Neurol Sci 102(1):4-10.

Silverstein F., Buchanan K., Johnston M.V. (1984). Pathogenesis of hypoxic-ischemic brain injury in a perinatal rodent model. Neurosci Lett. 49:271-7.

Sima A.A., Garcia-Salinas R., Andrade Z.A. (1983). The BB Wistar rat: an experimental model for the study of diabetic retinopathy. Metabolism. 32(7 Suppl 1):136-40.

Simmons E., Grynpas M. (1990). Treatment of castration-induced osteoporosis by a capacitively coupled electric signal in rat vertebrae [letter; comment]. J Bone Joint Surg [Am] 72(2):307.

Simon M.R. (1984). The rat as an animal model for the study of senile idiopathic osteoporosis. Acta Anat (Basel). 119:248-50.

Simons R., Maier R., Chi E. (1991). Pulmonary effects of continuous endotoxin infusion in the rat. Circ Shock 33(4):233-43.

Simpson C.F., Boucek R.J. (1983). The B-aminopropionitrile-fed turkey: a model for detecting potential drug action on arterial tissue. Cardiovasc Res. 17:26-32.

Simpson J., Butterfield M., Lefferts P., Dyer E., Snapper J., Meyrick B. (1991). Role of pulmonary inflammation in altered airway responsiveness in three sheep models of acute lung injury. Am Rev Respir Dis 143(3):585-9.

Simpson K.J., Peters T.J. (1993). Animal models of alcoholic liver disease. Baillieres Clin Gastroenterol. 7(3):609-25.

Simson P., Weiss J. (1988). Altered activity of the locus coeruleus in an animal model of depression. Neuropsychopharmacology 1(4):287-95.

Singer G., Wallace M. (1984). Schedule-induced self injection of drugs. Prog Neuropsychopharmacol Biol Psychiatry. 8:171-8.

Singer P. (1975). Animal liberation. New York: Random House.

Singer P. (1980). Practical Ethics. Oxford University Press, Oxford.

Singh N.B., Srivastava A., Verma V.K., Kumar A., Gupta S.K. (1984).Mastomys natalensis: a new animal model for Myobacterium ulcerans research. Indian J Exp Biol. 22:393-4.

Singh S., Sharma S., Chatterjee P. (1990). Clinical and experimental mycotic keratitis caused by Aspergillus terreus and the effect of subconjunctival oxiconazole treatment in the animal model. Mycopathologia 112(3):127-37.

Sisodia S., Price D. (1992). Amyloidogenesis in Alzheimer's disease: basic biology and animal models. Curr Opin Neurobiol 2(5):648-52.

Sisson J.C., Wieland D.M., Koeppe R.A., Normolle D., Frey K.A., Bolgos G., Johnson J., van Dort M.E., Gildersleeve D.L. (1991). Scintigraphic portrayal of beta receptors in the heart. J Nucl Med. 32:1399-407.

Sisson J.C., Wieland D.M., Sherman P., Mangner T.J., Tobes M.C., Jacques S. (1987). Metaiodobenzylguanidine as an index of the adrenergic nervous system intensity and function. J Nucl Med. 28:1620-4

Skolnick P., Ninan P., Insel T., Crawley J., Paul S. (1984). A novel chemically induced animal model of human anxiety. Psychopathology. 17 (Suppl) 1: 25-36.

Skow L.C., Burkhart B.A., Johnson F.M., Popp D.M., Goldberg S.Z., Anderson W.F. et al. (1983). A mouse model for beta-thalessemia. Cell. 34:1043-52.

Slakter J.S., Spertus A.D., Weissman S.S., Henkind P. (1984). An experimental model of carotid artery occlusive disease. Am J Ophthalmol. 97:168-72.

Slaveikova O., Makaveeva V. (1986). Experimental model of chronic salpingitis and the histological changes as affected by sinusoidal modulated currents. Akush Ginekol (Soflia). 25:44-9. (English Abstract) (Bulgarian)

Slavin S., Weiss L., Morecki S., Bassat H.B., Leizerowitz R., Gamliel H., Korkesh A., Voss R., Polliack A. (1981). Ultrastructural, cell membrane, and cytogenetic characteristics of B-cell leukemia, a murine model of chronic lymphocytic leukemia. Can Res. 14:4162-6.

Slodzian G., Daigne B., Girard F., Boust F., Hillion F. (1992). Scanning secondary ion analytical microscopy with parallel detection. Biol Cell 74:43-50.

Smego R.A. Jr., Durack D.T. (1984). An experimetnal model for Naegleria fowleri-induced primary amoebic meningoencephalitis in rabbits. J Parasitol. 70:78-81.

Smiseth O.A., Mjos O.D. (1982). A reproducible and stable model of acute ischaemic left ventricular failure in dogs. Clin Physiol. 2:225-39.

Smith D., Wiegeshaus E. (1989). What animal models can teach us about the pathogenesis of tuberculosis in humans. Rev Infect Dis 11 Suppl 2:S385-93.

Smith D.A. (1987). Species variations in pharmacokinetics. In: Bedford D.J., Bridges J.W., Gibson G.G. (Eds.) Drug Metabolism - from Molecule to Man. London: Taylor & Francis, pp 330-51.

Smith D.A., Brown K., Neal M.G. (1985). Drug Metabolism Disp. 16:365.

Smith G. (1988): Animal models of Alzheimer's disease: experimental cholinergic denervation. Brain Res. 472(2):103-18.

Smith G. (1989). Animal models of human eating disorders. Ann N Y Acad Sci 575:63-72; discussion 72-4.

Smith H. (1989). Animal models of asthma. Pulm Pharmacol 2(2):59-74.

Smith H., Hansen C., Rose R., Canoso R. (1990). Autoimmune MRL-1 pr/1pr mice are an animal model for the secondary antiphospholipid syndrome. J Rheumatol 17(7):911-5.

Smith H., Sweet C. (1988). Lessons for human influenza from pathogenicity studies with ferrets. Rev Infect Dis 10(1):56-75.

Smith J.A., Boyd K.M. (Eds.) (1991). Lives in the Balance. The Ethics of Using Animals in Biomedical Research. Oxford University Press, Oxford.

Smith M.L., Bendek G., Dahlgren N., Rosen I., Wieloch T., Siesjo B.K. (1984). Models for studying long-term recovery following forebrain ischemia in the rat. 2. A 2-vessel occlusion model. Acta Neurol Scand. 69:385-401.

Smith R., Birndorf M., Gluck G., Hammond D., Moore W. (1992). The effect of low-energy laser on skin-flap survival in the rat and porcine animal models. Plast Reconstr Surg 89(2):306-10.

Smith R., Engelhardt J., Tajti J., Appel S. (1993). Experimental immune-mediated motor neuron diseases: models for human ALS. Brain Res Bull 30(3-4):373-80.

Smith S.B., Yielding K.L. (1986). Retinal degeneration in the mouse. A model induced transplacentally by methylnitrosourea. Exp Eye Res. 43:791-801.

Smithers S.R., Simpson A.J., Yi X., Omer-Ali P., Kelly C., McLaren D.J. (1987). The mouse model of schistosome immunity. Acta Trop (Basel), Jun; (44 Suppl) 12:21-30.

Smithies O. (1993). Animal models of human genetic diseases. Trends Genet 9(4):112-6.

Snead O. 3., Depaulis A., Vergnes M., Marescaux C. (1992). Effect of intranigral muscimol on animal models of generalized absence seizures. Epilepsy Res Suppl 8:345-9; discussion 349-50.

Snead O. 3., Hechler V., Vergnes M., Marescaux C., Maitre M. (1990). Increased gamma-hydroxybutyric acid receptors in thalamus of a genetic animal model of petit mal epilepsy. Epilepsy Res 7(2):121-8.

Snider G.L., Lucey E.C., Stone P.J. (1986). Animal models of emphysema. Am Rev Respir Dis. 133:149-69.

Snider T.G. 3d, Ochoa R., Williams J.C. (1983). Menetrier's disease. Pre-Type II and Type II ostertagiosis in cattle. Am J Pathol. 113:410-2.

Snoswell A., Fishlock R., Runciman W., Carapetis R. (1989). An animal model of systemic carnitine deficiency produced by haemodialysis of sheep. Comp Biochem Physiol [B] 93(4):741-5.

Snouwaert J.N., Brigman K.K., Latour A.M., Malouf N.N., Boucher R.C., Smithies O., Koller B.H. (1992). An animal model for cystic fibrosis made by gene targeting. Science 257:1083-8.

Snowden K., Hammerberg B. (1989). The lymphatic pathology of chronic Brugia pahangi infection in the dog. Trans R Soc Trop Med Hyg 83(5):670-8.

Snyder R.L., Tyler G., Summers J. (1982). Chronic hepatitis and hepatocellular carcinoma associated with woodchuck hepatitis virus. Am J Pathol. 107:422-5.

Sohmer H., Freeman S. (1991). Hypoxia induced hearing loss in animal models of the fetus in-utero. Hear Res 55(1):92-7.

Soifer S.J., Kaslow D., Roman C., Heymann M.A. (1987). Umbilical cord compression produces pulmonary hypertension in newborn lambs: a model to study the pathophysiology of persistent pulmonary hypertension in the newborn. J Dev Physiol, Jun; 9:239-52.

Soike K.F., Rangan S.R., Gerone P.J. (1984). Viral disease models in primates. Adv Vet Sci Comp Med. 28:151-99.

Sokoloff L. (1977). Relation between physiological function and energy metabolism in the central nervous system. J Neurochem. 29:3-26.

Sokoloff L. (1984). Animal models of rheumatoid arthritis. Int Rev Exp Pathol. 26:107-45.

Sokoloff L., Reivich M., Kennedy C., Des Rosiers M.H., Patlak C.S. et al. (1977). The [^{14}C]-deoxyglucose method for the measurement of local cerebral glucose utilization: Theory, procedure, and normal values in the conscious and anesthetized albino rat. J Neurochem. 28:897-916.

Sokoloff L., Smith C. (1983). Basic principles underlying radioisotopic methods for assay of biochemical processes in vivo. In: Lambrecht R.M., Rescigno A. (Eds.). Tracer Kinetics and Physiologic Modelling - Theory to Practice. Lecture Note in Biomathematics, vol 48. Heidelberg: Springer Verlag, p 202-34.

Soldaini E., Matteucci D., Lopez-Cepero M., Specter S., Friedman H., Bendinelli M. (1989). Friend leukemia complex infection of mice as an experimental model for AIDS studies. Vet Immunol Immunopathol 21(1):97-110.

Soliman A. (1990). Type II collagen-induced inner ear disease: critical evaluation of the guinea pig model. Am J Otol 11(1):27-32.

Solomon P., Beal M., Pendlebury W. (1988). Age-related disruption of classical conditioning: a model systems approach to memory disorders. Neurobiol Aging 9(5-6):535-46.

Solomon R.A., Antunes J.L., Chen R.Y., Bland L., Chien S. (1985). Decrease in cerebral blood flow in rats after experimental subarachnoid hemorrhage: a new animal model. Stroke. 16:58-64.

Someya S. (1984). Experimental tuberculosis in mice. Nippon Saikingaku Zasshi. 39:745-8.

Somova L., Machuganska A., Dashev G., Zlatareva N. et al. (1987): Model of myocardial infarct in rats for research on anti-infarct pharmacological preparations. Eksp Med Morfol. 26:50-5.

Somsen R., Molenaar P., Van d. M. M., Jennings J. (1991). Behavioral modulation patterns fit an animal model of vagus-cardiac pacemaker interactions. Psychophysiology 28(4):383-99.

Sonis S., Tracey C., Shklar G., Jenson J., Florine D. (1990). An animal model for mucositis induced by cancer chemotherapy. Oral Surg Oral Med Oral Pathol 69(4):437-43.

Sordat B., Wang W.R. (1984). Human colorectal tumor xenografts in nude mice: expression of malignancy. Behring Inst Mitt. 74:291-300.

Sorensen O., Coutter-Mackie M., Percy D., Dales S. (1981). In vivo and in vitro models of demyelinating diseases. Adv Exp Med Biol. 142:271-86.

Soskel N.T., Watanabe S., Hammond E., Sandberg L.B., Renzetti A.D. Jr., Crapo, J.D. (1982). A copper-deficient, zinc-supplemented diet produces emphysema in pigs. Am Rev Respir Dis. 126:316-25.

Soulez B., Riviere M., Richard J. (1988): The rabbit, experimental host of Pneumocystis carinii]. Ann Parasitol Hum Comp. 63(1):5-15. (English Abstract).

Spande T.F., Garaffo H.M., Edwards M.W., Yeh H.J.C., Pannell L., Daly J.W. (1992). Epibatidine: A novel (chloropyridyl)azabicycloheptane with potent analgesic activity from an Ecuadorian poison frog. J Am Chem Soc. 114:3475-8.

Spandow O., Hellstrom S. (1993). Animal model for persistent tympanic membrane perforations. Ann Otol Rhinol Laryngol 102(6):467-72.

Spear J.F., Michelson E.L., Moore E.N. (1982). The use of animal models in the study of the electrophysiology of sudden coronary deaths. Ann NY Acad Sci. 382:78-89.

Spears J.R., Crawford D.W., Serur J., Grossman w., Paulin S. (1983). A catheterization technique for reproduction of a human atherosclerotic lumen within the dog coronary artery in vivo. Cathet Cardiovasc Diagn. 9:219-29.

Spector E.B., Mazzocchi R.A. (1983). The sparse fur mouse: an animal model for a human inborn error of metabolism of the urea cycle. Prog Clin Biol Res. 127:85-96.

Speiser Z., Korczyn a.D., Teplitzky I., Gitter S. (1983). Hyperactivity in rats following postnatal anoxia. Behav Brain Res. 7:379-82.

Spence K.M., Graham M.M., O'Gorman L.A., Muzi M., Abbott G.L., Lewellen T.K. (1987). Regional blood-to-tissue transport in an irradiated rat glioma model. Radiat Res. 111:225-36.

Spertzel R. (1989). Animal models of human immunodeficiency virus infection. Public Health Service Animal Models Committee. Antiviral Res 12(5-6):223-30.

Spigelman M.K., Zappulla R.A., Malis L.I., Holland J.F., Goldsmith S.J., Goldberg J.D. (1983). Intracarotid dehydrocholate infusion: a new method for prolonged reversible blood-brain barrier disruption. Neurosurgery. 12:606-12.

Spindleruv Mlyn (1987). XXIIIrd International Symposium on Biological Models. April 21-24, 1986. CSSR Abstracts. Z Versuchstierkd, 30:37-73.

Spindleruv Mlyn. (1988): XXIVth International Symposium on Biological Models. Z Versuchstierkd. Abstracts. 31(4):155-201.

Spinnewyn B., Blavet N., Clostre F. (1986). Effects of Ginkgo biloba extract on a cerebral ischemia model in gerbils. Presse Med. 15:1511-5. (English Abstract). (French)

Spira W.M., Sack R.B. (1982). Kinetics of early cholera infection in the removable intestinal tie-adult rabbit diarrhea model. Infect Immun. 35:952-7.

Sponenberg D.P., de Lahunta A. (1981). Hereditary hypertrophic neuropathy in Tibetan Mastiff dogs. J Hered. 72:287.

Spreadbury C., Krausz T., Pervez S., Cohen J. (1989). Invasive aspergillosis: clinical and pathological features of a new animal model. J Med Vet Mycol 27(1):5-15.

Sprott R.L., Staats J. (1975). Behavioral studies using genetically defined mice - a bibliography. Behav Genet. 5(1).

Sprott R.L., Staats J. (1978). Behavioral studies using genetically defined mice - a bibliography. Behav Genet. 8(2).

Sprott R.L., Staats J. (1980). Behavioral studies using genetically defined mice - a bibliography. Behav Genet. 10(1).

Squire L., Zola-Morgan S., Chen K. (1988). Human amnesia and animal models of amnesia: Performance of amnesic patients on tests designed for the monkey. Behav Neurosci 102(2):210-21.

St. John RC., Mizer L., Weisbrode S., Dorinsky P. (1991). Increased intestinal protein permeability in a model of lung injury induced by phorbol myristate acetate. Am Rev Respir Dis 144(5):1171-6.

Stables J.N., Lees G.M., Rankin R. (1988): The potential of mice as animal models for antifilarial screening. Trop Med Parasitol. 39(1):25-8.

Stace N.H., Palmer T.J., Vaja S., Dowling R.H. (1987). Long term pancreaticobiliary diversion stimulates hyperplastic and adenomatous nodules in the rat pancreas: a new model for spontaneous tumour formation. Gut, 28 Suppl:265-8.

Stals F., Bosman F., van B. C., Bruggeman C. (1990). An animal model for therapeutic intervention studies of CMV infection in the immunocompromised host. Arch Virol 114(1):91-107.

Stanberry L. (1989). Animal model of ultraviolet-radiation-induced recurrent herpes simplex virus infection. J Med Virol 28(3):125-8.

Stanberry L. (1991). Evaluation of herpes simplex virus vaccines in animals: the guinea pig vaginal model. Rev Infect Dis 13(Suppl 11):S920-3.

Stanberry L.R., Bernstein D.I., Kit S., Myers M.G. (1985) . Recurrent genital herpes simplex virus infection in guinea pigs. Intervirology. 24:226-31.

Startsev V.G., Mamamtavrishvili S.K., Chirkova S.K., Chirkov A.M., Dzholiia T.M. (1986). Anti-stress and antineurotic action of psychotropic preparations in experiments on monkeys. Vestn Akad Med Nauk SSSR. 3:30-3. (English Abstract). (Russian)

Stefanovich V. (Ed) (1979):(Ed). Animal Models & Hypoxia: Proceedings of an International Symposium on Animal Models & Hypoxia, November 19, 1979. Weisbaden, (Advances in Bioscience Series, Vol. 30), Pergamon, New York.

Stefanski R., PaLejko W., Kostowski W., PLaznik A. (1992). The comparison of benzodiazepine derivatives and serotonergic agonists and antagonists in two animal models of anxiety. Neuropharmacology 31(12):1251-8.

Steffes M.W., Mauer S.M. (1984). Diabetic glomerulopathy in man and experimental animal models. Int Rev Exp Pathol. 26:147-75.

Stehbens W.E. (1981). Chronic vascular changes in the walls of experimental berry aneurysms of the aortic bifurcation in rabbits. Stroke. 12:643-7.

Stein C.A., Cheng Y.C. (1993). Antisense oligonucleotides as therapeutic agents. Is the bullet really magical? Science 261:1004-12.

Stein D.J., Dodman N.H., Borchelt P., Hollander E. (1994). Behavioral disorders in veterinary practice: relevance to psychiatry. Compr Psychiatry 35(4):275-85.

Stein J.H., Fried T.A. (1985). Experimental models of nephrotoxic acute renal failure. Transplant Proc. 17 (4 Suppl 1):72-80.

Stein-Streilein J., Lipscomb M.F., Fisch H., Whitney P.L. (1987): Pulmonary interstitial fibrosis induced in hapten-immune hamsters. Am Rev Respir Dis. 136:119-23.

Steinleitner A., Lambert H., Suarez M., Serpa N., Robin B., Cantor B. (1991). Periovulatory calcium channel blockade enhances reproductive performance in an animal model for endometriosis-associated subfertility. Am J Obstet Gynecol 164(4):949-52.

Steinman L., Sriram S., Adelman N.E., Zamvil S., McDevitt H.O., Urich H. (1982). Murine model for pertussis vaccine encephalopathy: linkage to H-2. Nature. 299 (5885):738-40.

Stepanov S.S., Gaonenko G.E., Semchenko V.V. (1983). Modeling the state of clinical death from acute blood loss and post-resuscitation disease in the rat]. Patol Fiziol Eksp Ter. 6:77. (Russian)

Stephanopoulos D., Myers M., Bernstein D. (1989). Genital infections due to herpes simplex virus type 2 in male guinea pigs. J Infect Dis 159(1):89-95.

Sterkers M., Larsen R.G. (1985). Experimental choroidal ischemia by vortex embolization in the monkey. Bull Mem Soc Fr Ophthalmol. 96:466-8.

Sternthal E., Like A.A., Sarantis K., Braverman L.E. (1981). Lymphocytic thyroiditis and diabetes in the BB/W rat. A new model of autoimmune endocrinopathy. Diabetes. 30:1058-61.

Stevens C.E., Argenzio R.A., Roberts M.C. (1986). Comparative physiology of the mammalian colon and suggestions for animal models of human disorders. Clin Gastroenterol. 15:763-85.

Stewart R., Brown S. (1990). Unilateral cryptorchidism: an animal model. Aust N Z J Surg 60(11):905-6.

Stewart-Phillips J.L., Lough J., Skamene E. (1988): Genetically determined susceptibility and resistance to diet-induced atherosclerosis in inbred strains of mice. J Lab Clin Med. 112(1):36-42.

Stobie P., Hansen C., Hailey J., Levine R. (1991). A difference in mortality between two strains of jaundiced rats. Pediatrics 87(1):88-93.

Stock E.L., Mendelsohn A.D., Lo G.G., Ghosh S., O'Grady R.B. (1985). Lipid keratopathy in rabbits. An animal model system. Arch Ophthalmol. 103:726-30.

Stöcklin G., Pike V.W. (Eds.) (1993). Radiopharmaceuticals for Positron Emission Tomography. Methodological Aspects. Dordrecht: Kluwer Academic Publisher. 178 p.

Stokes D.C., Gigliotti F., Rehg J.E., Snellgrove R.L., Hughes W.T. (1987): Experimental Pneumocystis carinii pneumonia in the ferret. Br J Exp Pathol. 68:267-76.

Stone W.H., Treichel R.C., VandeBerg J.L. (1987): Genetic significance of some common primate models in biomedical research. Prog Clin Biol Res. 229:73-93.

Storlien L., Oakes N., Pan D., Kusunoki M., Jenkins AB. (1993). Syndromes of insulin resistance in the rat. Inducement by diet and amelioration with benfluorex. Diabetes 42(3):457-62.

Storozhuk B.G. (1985). Antifibrillatory activity of anti-arrhythmia agents in maximally high ligation of the coronary artery and its reperfusion in cats. Farmakol Toksikol. 48:47-9. (English Abstract).

Stott D. (1990). Lessons about autoantibody specificity in systemic lupus erythematosus from animal models. Clin Exp Immunol 81(1):1-4.

Stott D.I., Hassman R., Neilson L., McGregor A.M. (1988): Analysis of the spectrotypes of autoantibodies against thyroglobulin in two rat models of autoimmune thyroiditis. Clin Exp Immunol. 73(2):269-75

Strassburger D., Carp H., Toder V. (1992). Immune reproductive failure: effect of nonspecific immunostimulation in mouse model. Am J Reprod Immunol 28(3-4):274-6.

Strauli P., Haemmerli G. (1984). The V2 carcinoma of the rabbit as an integrated model of tumor invasion. Bull Cancer (Paris). 71:447-52.

Strauss M., Griffith B. (1991). Guinea pig model of transplacental congenital cytomegaloviral infection with analysis for labyrinthitis. Am J Otol 12(2):97-100.

Strekalova V., Khachirov D., Dedenkov A., Suvorov I. (1991). [Characteristics of sodium metabolism in rats with experimental hypertension caused by chronic alimentary imbalance] Osobennosti obmena natriia u krys s eksperimental'noi gipertenziei, obuslovlennoi khronicheskim alimentarnym disbalansom. Vopr Pitan (3):35-8.

Strekalova V., Khachirov D., Dedenkov A., Suvorov I., Shvatsabaia I. (1989). [Modeling of experimental hypertension by chronic salt loading combined with a low-protein diet in Wistar rats] Modelirovanie eksperimental'noi gipertonii s pomoshch'iu khronicheskoi solevoi nagruzki v sochetanii s nizkobelkovoi dietoi u krys Vistar. Biull Vsesoiuznogo Kardiol Nauchn Tsentra AMN SSSR 12(1):48-51.

Strombeck D.R., Wheeldon E., Harrold D. (1984). Model of chronic pancreatitis in the dog. Am J Vet Res. 45:131-6.

Stromberg P., Grants I., Kociba G., Krakowka G., Mezza L. (1990). Serial syngeneic transplantation of large granular lymphocyte leukemia in F344 rats. Vet Pathol 27(6):404-10.

Stromberg P.C. (1985). Large granular lymphocyte leukemia in F344 rats. Model for human T gamma lymphoma, malignant histiocytosis, and T-cell chronic lymphocytic leukemia. Am J Pathol. 119:517-9.

Struhar D., Harbeck R., Gegen N., Kawada H., Mason RJ. (1989). Increased expression of class II antigens of the major histocompatibility complex on alveolar macrophages and alveolar type II cells and interleukin-1 (IL-1) secretion from alveolar macrophages in an animal model of silicosis. Clin Exp Immunol 77(2):281-4.

Strunin L., Harrison L.J., Davies J.M. (1983). Etiology of halothane hepato-toxicity [letter]. Anesthesiology. 58:391.

Strupp B.J., Levitsky D.A., Blumstein L. (1984). PKU, learning, and models of mental retardation. Dev Psychobiol. 17:109-20.

Stump K.C., Swindle M.M., Saudek C.D., Standberg J.D. (1988): Pancreatectomized swine as a model of diabetes mellitus. Lab Anim Sci. 38(4):439-43.

Sturrock R.F., Otieno F.M., Tarara R., Kimani R., Harrison R., Else J.G. (1984). Experimental Schistosoma mansoni infection in verve monkeys (Cercopithecus aethiops) in Kenya: I Susceptibility to a primary infection. J Helminthol. 58:79-92.

Stvolinskaia N.S., Gerasimova T.S.I., Korovkin B.F. (1988): Effect of hypoxia on a primary cardiomyocyte culture. Biull Eksp Biol Med. 160(11):607-9. (English Abstract). (Russian)

Su J.J. (1987). Experimental infection of human hepatitis B virus (HBV) in adult tree shrews. Chung-hua Ping Li Hsueh Tsa Chih, Jun; 16:103-6, 22 (English Abstarct)(Chinese)

Sucharit S., Harinasuta C., Choochote W. (1982). Experimental transmission of subperiodic Wuchereria bancrofti to the leaf monkey (Presbytis melalophos), and its periodicity. Am J Trop Med Hyg. 3 (Pt 1):599-601.

Suckling K.E., Jackson B. (1993). Animal models of human lipid metabolism. Prog Lipid Res. 32(1):1-24.

Suda T., Takahashi N., Shinki T., Yamaguchi A., Tanioka Y. (1986). The common marmoset as an animal model for vitamin D-dependent rickets type II. Adv Exp Med Biol. 196:432-35.

Suenaga I., Yamazaki T. (1984). Experimental Treponema hyodysenteriae infection of mice. Zentralbl Bakteriol Mikrobiol Hyg. 257:348-56.

Suga T., Kameyama T., Kinoshita T., Shimotohno K., Matsumura M., Tanaka H., Kushida S., Ami Y., Uchida M., Uchida K., et al. (1991). Infection of rats with HTLV-1: a small-animal model for HTLV-1 carriers. Int J Cancer 49(5):764-9.

Sugar A., Picard M. (1988). Experimental blastomycosis pneumonia in mice by infection with conidia. J Med Vet Mycol 26(6):321-6.

Sugio K., Horigome N., Sakaguchi T., Goto M. (1988): A model of bilateral hemispheric ischemia-modified four-vessel occlusion in rats. Stroke. 19(7):922.

Sugita T., Shiraki K., Ueda S., Iwa N., Shoji H., Ayata M., Kato S. (1984). Induction of acute myoclonic encephalopathy in hamsters by subacute sclerosing panencephalitis virus. J Infect Dis. 150:340-7.

Sugrobova N., Medvednik R., Efimova L., Katarzhnova T., Liubarev A., Shaposhnikov V., Obol'nikova E., Poznanskaia A. (1992). [The effect of ubiquinone-10 on the development of D-galactosamine-induced hepatitis in rats] Vliianie ubikhinona-10 na razvitie D-galaktozaminovogo gepatita u krys. Biull Eksp Biol Med 114(11):504-6.

Sulla I., Santa M., Marsala J. (1989). [Experimental model of ischemic injury of the spinal cord after temporary occlusion of the thoracic artery in the dog] Experimentelles Modell der ischämischen Schädigung des Rückenmarks nach zeitweiliger Okklusion der thorakalen Aorta beim Hund. Z Exp Chir Transplant Künstliche Organe 22(6):379-82.

Sullivan B.A., Hak L.J., Finn W.F. (1985). Cyclosporine nephrotoxicity: studies in laboratory animals. Transplant Proc. 17 (4 Suppl 1):145-54.

Sullivan D., Yue D., Capogreco C., McLennan S., Nicks J., Cooney G., Caterson I., Turtle J., Hensley WJ. (1990). The effects of dietary n - 3 fatty acid in animal models of type 1 and type 2 diabetes. Diabetes Res Clin Pract 9(3):225-30.

Sullivan J.P., Decker M.W., Brioni J.D., Donnelly-Roberts D., Anderson D.J., Bannon A.W. et al. (1994). (±)-epibatidine elicits a diversity of *in vitro* and *in vitro* effects mediated by nicotinic acetylcholine receptors. JPET 271:624-31.

Summerton J., Goeting N., Trotter G.A., Taylor I. (1985). Effect of deoxycholic acid on the tumour incidence, distribution, and receptor status of colorectal cancer in the rat model. Digestion. 31:77-81.

Sun G.X., Wang H.Y., Lin J.Z. (1988): A murine model of acute myocarditis infected by coxsackie virus B3m. Chin Med J. [England]. 101(1):7-12.

Sun M., Wang B., Annoni G., Degli E. S., Biempica L., Zern M. (1990). Two rat models of hepatic fibrosis. A morphologic and molecular comparison. Lab Invest 63(4):467-75.

Sunagawa K., Maughan W.L., Sagawa K. (1983). Effect of regional ischemia on the left ventricular end-systolic pressure-volume relationship of isolated canine hearts. Circ Res. 52:170-8.

Sundberg J.P. (Ed.) (1994). Handbook of mouse mutations with skin and hair abnormalities: animal models and biomedical tools. Boca Raton: CRC Press. 544 P.

Sunde D., Apfelberg D., Sergott T. (1990). Traumatic tattoo removal: comparison of four treatment methods in an animal model with correlation to clinical experience. Lasers Surg Med 10(2):158-64.

Sunderrajan E.V., McKenzie W.N., Lieske T.R., Kavanaugh J.L., Braun S.R., Walker S.E. (1986). Pulmonary inflammation in autoimmune MRL/Mp-lpr/lpr mice. Histopathology and bronchoalveolar lavage evaluation. Am J Pathol. 124:353-62.

Sundstrom E., Fredriksson A., Archer T. (1990). Chronic neurochemical and behavioral changes in MPTP-lesioned C57BL/6 mice: a model for Parkinson's disease. Brain Res 528(2):181-8.

Supance J.S. (1983). Antibiotics and steroids in the treatment of acquired subglottic stenosis. A canine model study. Ann Otol Rhinol Laryngol. 92(4 Pt 1):377-82.

Supance J.S., Marshak G., Doyle W.J., Cantekin E.I. (1982). Longitudinal study of the efficacy of ampicillin in the treatment of pneumococcal otitis media in a chinchilla animal model. Ann Otol Rhinol Laryngol. 91 (3 Pt 1):256-60.

Susskind H., Chanana A.D., Joel D.D., Brill A.B., Janaff A., Som P., Oster Z.H. (1984). Acute response to elastase in sheep lungs measured with Ga-67. J Nucl Med. 25:1310-6.

Suzuki H., Saruta T., Ferrario C.M., Brosnihan K.B. (1987). Characterization of neurohormonal changes following the production of the benign and malignant phases of two-kidney, two-clip Goldblatt hypertension. Jpn Heart J, 28:413-26.

Suzuki K. (1994). A genetic demyelinating disease globoid cell leukodystrophy: studies with animal models. J Neuropathol Exp Neurol. 53(4):359-63.

Suzuki K., Suzuki K. (1983). The twitcher mouse. A model of human globoid cell leukodystrophy (Krabbe's disease). 111:394-7.

Suzuki T., Futakata A., Shimada M., Yoshii T., Yanaura S. (1984). Comparison of three methods of inducing physical dependence to morphine in rats using short-term medication. Yakubutsu Seishin Kodo. 4:149-56. (English Abstract). (Japanese)

Suzuki T., Yoshii T., Yanaura S. (1984). Assessment of morphine-type physical dependence liability in mice using the drug-admixed food method. Nippon Yakurigaku Zasshi. 84:19-24. (English Abstract) (Japanese)

Swank R., Sweet H., Davisson M., Reddington M., Novak E. (1991). Sandy: a new mouse model for platelet storage pool deficiency. Genet Res 58(1):51-62.

Swenson C.E., Donegan E., Schacter J. (1983). Chlamdydia trachomatis- induced salpingitis in mice. J Infect Dis. 148;1101-7.

Swerdlow N., Geyer M. (1993). Clozapine and haloperidol in an animal model of sensorimotor gating deficits in schizophrenia. Pharmacol Biochem Behav 44(3):741-4.

Swerdlow N.R., Braff D.L., Taaid N., Geyer M.A. (1994). Assessing the validity of an animal model of deficient sensorimotor gating in schizophrenic patients. Arch Gen Psychiatry 51:139-54.

Swindle M., Spinale F., Smith A., Schumann R., Green C., Nakano K. et al. (1991). Anesthetic and postoperative protocols for a canine model of reversible left ventricular volume overload. J Invest Surg 4(3):339-46.

Swindle M.M., Moody D.C., Phillips L.D. (Ed.) (1992). Swine as models in biochemical research. Ames: Iowa State University Press. 312 P.

Szypryt E., Hardy J., Hinton C., Worthington B., Mulholland R. (1988). A comparison between magnetic resonance imaging and scintigraphic bone imaging in the diagnosis of disc space infection in an animal model. Spine 13(9):1042-8.

Tabakoff B. (1983). Current trends in biologic research on alcoholism. Drug Alcohol Depend. 11:33-7.

Tabakoff B., Culp S.G. (1984). Studies on tolerance development in inbred and heterogeneous stock National Institutes of Health rats. Alcoholism (NY). 8:495-9.

Tabbara K.F. and Cello R.M. (1984): Animal Models of Ocular Diseases. C C Thomas, Springfield, IL., 300 pp.

Tabor E., Purcell R.H., Gerety R.J. (1983). Primate animal models and titered inocula for the study of human hepatitis A, hepatitis B, and non-A, non-B hepatitis. J Med Primatol. 12 305-18.

Tada Y., Tabuchi Y., Saito Y. (1992). [Establishment of an experimental model with a high frequency of liver metastasis and recurrence from gastric VX2 cancer: histological analysis of the developmental process of primary and metastatic cancer lesions]. Nippon Geka Gakkai Zasshi 93(8):818-26.

Tadzhiev I., Podymova S., Tsodikov G. (1991). [Incidence of cholelithiasis after its experimental induction by various methods] Chastota kholelitiaza pri razlichnykh sposobakh ego induktsii v eksperimente. Vopr Pitan (2):46-9.

Tafuri W., de, L. M., Chiari E., Caliari M., Bambirra E., Rios-Leite V., Barbosa A. (1988). [Dogs as experimental models for the study of the natural course of Chagas disease] O cao como modelo experimental para o estudo da historia natural da doenca de Chagas. Rev Soc Bras Med Trop 21(2):77.

Takada M., Tani Y., Miyamoto M. (1984). Intraperitoneal transplantation derived from spontaneous colonic cancer of WF rat strain. Gan To Kagaku Ryoho. 11:487-91. (English Abstract) (Japanese)

Takagi H., Marmarou A., Lax F., Horoupian D.S. (1983). Study of brain edema by an infusion edema Model--the method and characteristics of the model. No Shinkei Geka. 11:957-64.

Takahashi H., Iqisu H., Suzuki K., Suzuki K. (1984). Murine globoid cell leukodystrophy: the twitcher mouse. An ultrastructural study of the kidney. Lab Invest. 50:42-50.

Takatsu H., Uno Y., Fujiwara H. (1995). Modulation of left ventricular iodine-125-MIBG accumulation in cardiomyopathic Syrian hamsters using the renin-angiotensin system. J Nucl Med. 36:1055-61.

Takeda T. (1989). [Experimental model of respiratory distress syndrome by lung lavage with fluorocarbon]. Nippon Sanka Fujinka Gakkai Zasshi 41(9):1417-22.

Takeda T., Hosokawa M., Higuchi K. (1991). Senescence-accelerated mouse (SAM): a novel murine model of accelerated senescence. J Am Geriatr Soc 39(9):911-9.

Takeichi N., Kobayashi H., Yoshida M., Sasaki M., Dempo K., Mori M. (1988). Spontaneous hepatitis in Long-Evans rats. A potential animal model for fulminant hepatitis in man. Acta Pathol Jpn 38(11):1369-75.

Takeuchi K., Furukawa O., Okabe S. (1986). Induction of duodenal ulcers in rats under water-immersion stress conditions. Influence of stress on gastric acid and duodenal alkaline secretion. Gastroenterology. 91:554-63.

Takiguchi K., Tashiro M., Nakamura K. (1990). Influenza C virus infection in rats. Microbiol Immunol 34(1):35-44.

Takizawa H., Ohta K., Horiuchi T., Suzuki N., Ueda T., Yamaguchi M. et al. (1992). Hypersensitivity pneumonitis in athymic nude mice. Additional evidence of T cell dependency. Am Rev Respir Dis 146(2):479-84.

Talacko A., Radden B. (1988). The pathogenesis of oral pulse granuloma: an animal model. J Oral Pathol 17(3):99-105.

Talalaenko A.N., Zin'Kovskaia L.Ia. (1988): Characteristics of the anxiolytic action of benzodiazepine and GABA derivatives on experimentally modelled anxiety states]. Farmakol Toksikol. 51(4):20-2. (English Abstract) (Russian)

Tallents R., Macher D., Rivoli P., Puzas JE., Scapino R., Katzberg R. (1990). Animal model for disk displacement. J Craniomandib Disord 4(4):233-40.

Talmadge E., Lenz B.F., Collins M.S., Uithoven K.A., Schneider M.A. (1984). Tumor models to investigate the therapeutic efficiency of immunomodulators. Behring Inst Mittr 74:219-29.

Talmadge J.E., Fidler I.J., Oldham R.K. (1984). The NCI preclinical screen of biological response modifiers. Behring Inst Mitt. 74:189-94.

Tamagawa K., Scheidt P., Friede RL. (1989). Experimental production of leptomeningeal heterotopias from dissociated fetal tissue. Acta Neuropathol (Berl) 78(2):153-8.

Tamura A., Gotoh O., Sano K. (1986). Focal cerebral infarction in the rat: I. Operative technique and physiological monitorings for chronic model. No to Shinkei. 38:747-51.

Tamura Y., Sakata Y., Tsushima K., Narushima S., Yamada Y., Ogasawara H., Ito T., Saitoh S., Suzuki H., Yoshida Y. (1990). A novel model of solitary hepatic tumor in rats using ascites hepatoma AH13: suitability for chemotherapeutic studies. Jpn J Cancer Res 81(10):1045-51.

Tan-Liu N.S., Sadigursky M., Andrade Z.A. (1982). Immunopathology of Schistosoma mansoni infection in rabbits. Mem Inst Oswaldo Cruz. 77:165-71.

Tanaka E., Katou M., Kuze F. (1988). [A murine model of chronic bronchial infection with Pseudomonas aeruginosa, mucoid strain]. Nippon Kyobu Shikkan Gakkai Zasshi 26(1):50-4.

Tanaka K., Okamoto Y., Nagaya Y., Nishimura F., Takeoka A., Hanada S., Kohno S., Kawai M. (1988). A nasal allergy model developed in the guinea pig by intranasal application of 2,4-toluene diisocyanate. Int Arch Allergy Appl Immunol 85(4):392-7.

Tanaka N., Christensen P., Ryden S., Klofver-stahl B., Bengmark S. (1985). A rat model for sepsis in chronic biliary obstruction. Acta Pathol Microbiol Immunol Scand [B]. 93:171-4.

Tani E.M., Franco M., Peracoli M.T., Montenegro M.R. (1987). Experimental pulmonary paracoccidioidomycosis in the Syrian hamster: morphology and correlation of lesions with the immune response. J Med Vet Mycol, 25:291-300.

Tani S., Okabayashi Y., Nakamura T., Fujii M., Itoh H., Otsuki M. (1990). Effect of a new cholecystokinin receptor antagonist loxiglumide on acute pancreatitis in two experimental animal models. Pancreas 5(3):284-90.

Tanigawa M., Akaike I., Adachi J., Shinkai H., Tokoi K., Uchiyama T., Ibaraki T., Mochizuki K. (1986). Gottingen miniature swine as a model for diet-induced atherosclerosis. Jikken Dobutsu. 35:47-57. (English Abstract). (Japanese)

Tanner M.S., Jackson D., Mowat A.P. (1981). Hepatic collagen synthesis in a rat model of cirrhosis, and its modification by colchicine. J Pathol. 135:179-87.

Tanoue K., Kitano S., Hashizume M., Wada H., Sugimachi K. (1991). A rat model of esophageal varices. Hepatology 13(2):353-8.

Tanswell A., Wong L., Possmayer F., Freeman B. (1989). The preterm rat: a model for studies of acute and chronic neonatal lung disease. Pediatr Res 25(5):525-9.

Taoka Y. (1985). Animal disease models-injury, death and various changes of liver cellsA. Nippon Rinsho. 43:1239-50. (Japanese)

Tarkka M., Uhari M., Koskinen M., Heikkinen. (1982). Experimental aortic coarctation in puppies. J Surg Res. 33:208-13.

Tarkowski A., Jonsson R., Klareskog L. (1986): Experimental Sjogren's syndrome: a review. Scand J Rheumatol [Suppl]. 61:274-9.

Tartaglione T., Taylor T., Opheim K., See W., Berger R. (1991). Antimicrobial tissue penetration in a rat model of E. coli epididymitis. J Urol 146(5):1413-7.

Tartakovskii TsSh., Barkhatova O.I., Prozorovskii E.V. (1984). Models for the study of the toxic action of Legionella pneumophila. Zh Mikrobiol Epidemiol Immunobiol. 5:52-5. (English Abstract) (Russian)

Tashiro T., Inaba M., Kobayashi T., Sakurai Y., Maruo K., Ohnishi Y., Ueyama Y., Nomura T. (1989). Responsiveness of human lung cancer/nude mouse to antitumor agents in a model using clinically equivalent doses. Cancer Chemother Pharmacol 24(3):187-92.

Tateishi J. (1989). [Review: experimental studies on Creutzfeldt-Jakob disease]. Jikken Dobutsu 38(4):289-92.

Tatematsu M., Ho R.H., Kaku T., Ekem, J.K., Farber E. (1984). Studies on the proliferation and fate of oval cells in the liver of rats treated with 2-acetylaminofluorene and partial hepatectomy. Am J Pathol. 114:418-30.

Tauber M.G. (1986). Experimental models of CNS infections. Contributions to concepts of disease and treatment. Neurol Clin. 4:249-64.

Taurog J. (1990). Immunology, genetics, and animal models of the spondyloarthropathies. Curr Opin Rheumatol 2(4):586-91.

Taylor G., Scott E.J., Hughes M., Collins A.P. (1984). Respiratory syncytial virus infection in mice. Infect Immun. 43:649-55.

Taylor P., Dowling R., Palmer T., Hanley D., Murphy G., Mason R., McColl I. (1989). Induction of pancreatic tumours by longterm duodenogastric reflux. Gut 30(11):1596-600.

Taylor-Robinson D., Furr P.M., Tully J.G., Barile M.F., Maller B.R. (1987). Animal models of Mycoplasma genitalium urogenital infection. Isr J Med Sci, Jun; 23:561-4.

Teixeira A.R. (1986). Chagas disease in inbred III/J rabbits. Am J Pathol. 124:363-5.

Tel L.Z., Roitshtein M.B., Lysenkov S.P. (1987). A new model of hemodynamic edema of the lungs. Patol Fiziol Eksp Ter, Sept-Oct; 85-6. (Russian)

Tel' L., Roitshtein M., Sharipova N. (1991). [Novel methods for modelling unilateral pulmonary edema] Novye sposoby modelirovaniia inlateral'nogo oteka legkikh. Patol Fiziol Eksp Ter 2:59-60.

Tel' L.Z., Lysenkov S.P., Velichko A.N. (1985). Pulmonary edema in the rat, guinea pig, rabbit, cat and dog after various actions on the vagus nerves ("vagal edema"). Fiziol Zh. 31:707-11. (English Abstract)

Telner J.I., Singhal R.L. (1984). Psychiatric progress. The learned helplessness model of depression. J Pscyhiatr Res. 18:207-15.

Temes R., Kauten R., Schwartz M. (1991). Nuclear magnetic resonance as a noninvasive method of diagnosing intestinal ischemia: technique and preliminary results. J Pediatr Surg 26(7):775-9.

Tenenbaum J. (1984). Experimental models of osteoarthritis: a reappraisal [editorial]. J Rheumatol. 11:120-2.

Terpstra O.T., Reuvers C.B., Kooy P.P., TenKate F.J., Jeekel J. (1983). Auxiliary transplantation of a partial liver graft in the dog and the pig. Neth J Surg. 35:188-91.

Terribile Wiel Marin V., Baroni A., Zitelli A., Zanon G., Balzan M. (1982). An experimental model for hemorrhagic shock-induced lesions in the rat. Agressologie. 23:309-16.

Terriere D., Abi-Dargham A., Laruelle M., Innes R. et al. (1995). Preliminary evaluation of a new ^{123}I-labeled 5HT$_{2A}$ receptor tracer in baboon with SPECT. Eur J Nucl Med. 22:833.

Terris J.M., Simmonds R.C. (1982). The Yucatan miniature swine: an improved pig model for the study of dexosycorticosterone-acetate (DOCA) and aldosterone hypertension. Proc Soc Exp Biol Med. 171:79-82.

Teschner M., Schaefer R., Paczek L., Heidland A. (1992). Effect of disease on glomerular proteinases. Przegl Lek 49(1-2):1-5.

Testa N.G., Orions D.E., Lord B.I. (1988): A feline model for the myelodysplastic syndrome pre-leukaemic abnormalities caused in cats by infection with a new/isolate of feline leukaemia virus (FeLV). AB/GM1. Haematologica (Pavia). 73(4):317-20. (12 ref.).

Teuscher C., Wild G.C., Tung K.S. (1983). Experimental allergic orchitis: the isolation and partial characterization of an aspermatogenic polypeptide (AP3) with an apparent sequential disease-inducing determinant(s). J Immunol. 130:2683-8.

Thakur M.L., Park C.H., Fazio F. et al. (1984). Preparation and evaluation of ^{99m}Tc-DEPE as a cardiac perfusion agent. Int J Appl Radiat Isot. 35:507-15.

Thatcher C.D., Keith J.C. Jr. (1986). Pregnancy-induced hypertension: development of a model in the pregnant sheep. Am J Obstet Gynecol. 155:201-7.

Theofilopoulos A.N., Dixon F.J. (1985). Murine models of systemic lupus erythematosus. Adv Immunol. 37:269-390.

Thiebot M.H. (1983). Behavioral models of anxiety in animals. Encephale. 9 (4 Suppl 2):167B-176B. (English Abstract). (French)

Thomas D., Merton R., Gray E., Barrowcliffe T. (1989). The relative antithrombotic effectiveness of heparin, a low molecular weight heparin, and a pentasaccharide fragment in an animal model. Thromb Haemost 61(2):204-7.

Thomas G., Varma R. (1991). Isolated paced guinea pig left atrium: a new ouabain-induced arrhythmia model. Methods Find Exp Clin Pharmacol 13(7):459-62.

Thomas J.A., Hamm Jr. T.E., Perkins P.L., Raffin T.A., and the Stanford University Medical Center Commitee on Ethics. (1988). Animal reseacrh at Stanford Universitsy - principles, policies and practice. New England Journal of Medicine 318:1630-2.

Thomas S., Dave P.K. (1985). Experimental scoliosis in monkeys. Acta Orthop Scand. 56:43-6.

Thompson H. (1993). Diet, nutrition, and cancer: development of hypotheses and their evaluation in animal studies. Cancer Res 53(10 Suppl):2442s-2445s.

Thompson J.P., Crandall R.B., Crandall C.A. (1985). Brugia malayi: intravenous injection of microfilariae in ferrets as an experimental method for occult filariasis. Exp Parasitol. 60:181-94.

Thompson R. J., Oegema T. J., Lewis J., Wallace L. (1991). Osteoarthrotic changes after acute transarticular load. An animal model. J Bone Joint Surg [Am] 73(7):990-1001.

Thompson T.C., Truong L.D., Timme T.L., Kadmon D., McCune B.K., Flanders K.C. et al. (1993). Transgenic models for the study of prostate cancer. Cancer 71(Suppl 3):1165-71.

Thorgeirsson S. (1992). The LEC rat - an animal model for human hepatitis and hepatocellular carcinoma. Jpn J Cancer Res 83(10):inside front cover.

Thormar H., Mehta P.D., Barshatzky M.R., Brown H.R. (1985). Measles virus encephalitis in ferrets as a model for subacute sclerosing panencephalitis. Lab Anim Sci. 35:299-32.

Thorner P., Baumal R., Binnington A., Valli V., Marrano P., Clarke H. (1989). The NC1 domain of collagen type IV in neonatal dog glomerular basement membranes. Significance in Samoyed hereditary glomerulopathy. Am J Pathol 134(5):1047-54.

Thorp J.M. (1987). Drug design: Role of laboratory animals. Laboratory Animals 21:164-72.

Tibaldi J.M., Surks M.I. (1985). Animal models of non-thyroidal disease. Endocr Rev. 6:87-102.

Tierno P.M Jr., Malloy V., Matias J.R., Hanna B.A. (1987): Effects of toxic shock syndrome Staphylococcus aureus, endotoxin and tampons in a mouse model. Clin Invest Med. 10:64-70.

Tilton G.D., Buja L.M., Bilheimer D.W., Apprill P., Ashton J., McNaatt J., Kita T., Willerson J.T. (1985). Failure of a slow channel calcium antagonist, verapamil, to retard atherosclerosis in the Watanabe heritable hyperlipidemic rabbit: an animal model of familial hypercholesterolemia. J Am Coll Cardiol. 6:141-4.

Tilton R.G., Larson K.B., Udell J.R., Sobel B.E., Williamson J.R. (1983). External detection of early microvascular dysfunction after no-flow ischemia followed by reperfusion in isolated rabbit hearts. Circ Res. 52:210-25.

Timchenko N.F., Isachkova L.M., Shipacheva E.A., Garshkava R.P., Sidorova V.E. (1983). Pathogenic properties of Yersinia pseudotuberculosis in different biological models. Zh Mikrobiol Epidemiol Immunobiol. 5:43-6. (English Abstract). (Russian)

Timsit J., Savino W., Boitard C., Bach J. (1989). The role of class II major histocompatibility complex antigens in autoimmune diabetes: animal models. J Autoimmun 2 Suppl:115-29.

Timson B. (1990). Evaluation of animal models for the study of exercise-induced muscle enlargement. J Appl Physiol 69(6):1935-45.

Tissi L., Marconi P., Mosci P., Merletti L., Cornacchione P., Rosati E., Recchia S., von H. C., Orefici G. (1990). Experimental model of type IV Streptococcus agalactiae (group B streptococcus) infection in mice with early development of septic arthritis. Infect Immun, 58 (9):3093-100.

Tissot R.G., Beattie C.W., Amoss M.S. Jr. (1987). Inheritance of Sinclair swine cutaneous malignant melanoma. Cancer Res, 47:5542-5.

Tita B., Bolle P., Martinoli L., Mazzanti G., Silvestrini B. (1988). A comparative study of Atropa belladonna and atropine on an animal model of urinary retention. Pharmacol Res Commun 20 Suppl 5:55-8.

Tobin B., Finegood D. (1993). Reduced insulin secretion by repeated low doses of STZ impairs glucose effectiveness but does not induce insulin resistance in dogs. Diabetes 42(3):474-83.

Todd M.M., Dunlop B.J., Shapiro H.M., Chadwick N.C., Powell H.C. (1981). Ventricular fibrillation in the cat: a model for global cerebral ischemia. Stroke. 12:808-15.

Todd N.V., Crockard H.A., Russel R.W., Picozzi P. (1984). Cerebral blood flow in the four-vessel occlusion rat model. Stroke. 15:579.

Todd N.V., Picozzi P., Crokard H.A., Ross Russell R.W. (1986). Recirculation after cerebral ischemia. Simultaneous measurement of cerebral bloodflow, brain edema, cerebrovascular permeability and cortical EEG in the rat. Acta Neurol Scand. 74:269-78.

Toivanen A., Merilahti-Palo, Gripenberg C., Lahesmaa-Rantala R., Soderstrom K.O., Jaakkola U.M. (1986): Yersinia-associated arthritis in the rat; experimental model for human reactive arthritis? Acta Pathol Microbiol Immunol Scand [C]. 94:261-9.

Tokuriki M., Takeuchi A., Sawazak H. (1981). Idiopathic neurologic diseases in dogs and cats in Japan from the viewpoint of animal models of human disease. Jikken Dobutsu. 30:233-40. (English Abstract) (Japanese)

Tomida S., Nowak T.S., Vass K., Lohr J.M., Klatzo I. (1987). Experimental model for repetitive ischemic attacks in the gerbil: the cumulative effect of repeated ischemic insults. J Cereb Blood Flow Metab, 7:773-82.

Tomino Y., Shimizu M., Koide H., Abe M., Shirai T. (1993). Effect of monoclonal antibody CD4 on glomerulonephritis of ddY mice, a spontaneous animal model of IgA nephropathy. Am J Kidney Dis 21(4):427-32.

Tomita S., Myones B., Shulman,ST. (1993). In vitro correlates of the L. casei animal model of Kawasaki disease. J Rheumatol 20(2):362-7.

Tompkins D.S., Wyatt J.I., Rathbone B.J., West A.P. (1988): The characterization and pathological significance of gastric Campylobacter-like organisms in the ferret: a model for chronic gastritis? Epidemoil Infect. 101(2):269-78.

Tonkin N., Popkhristova E. (1982). Experience in developing an animal model of acute diffuse alopecia using cyclophosphamide. Vestn Dermatol Venerol. 7:74-6. (English Abstract) (Russian)

Toplian S.L., Ziegler M.M. (1984). Necrotizing enterocolitis: a review of animal models. J Surg Res. 37:320-36.

Torikata C., Kijimoto C., Koto M. (1991). Ultrastructure of respiratory cilia of WIC-Hyd male rats. An animal model for human immotile cilia syndrome. Am J Pathol 138(2):341-7.

Toth J., Svoboda P., Halouzka R., Haluza Z., Doubek J. (1991). [Experimental liver cirrhosis in laboratory rats] Experimentalni jaterni cirhoza u laboratorniho potkana. Cesk Fysiol 40(3):293-8.

Townsend C.M. Jr., Franklin R.B., Gelder F.B., Glass E., Thompson J.C. (1982). Development fo a transplantable model of pancreatic duct adenocarcinoma. Surgery. 92:72-8.

Traupe H., Kruse E., Heiss W.D. (1982). Reperfusion of focal ischemia of varying duration: postischemic hyper-and-hypo-perfusion. Stroke. 13:615-22.

Trautmann M., Bruckner O., Hofstoetter T., Seiler F.R., Hahn H. (1982). Protective action of various antibody preparations in experimental bacterial sepsis]. Beitr Infusionther Klinis Ernähr. 9:155-65. (German)

Traverso L.W., Moore C.C., Tillman F.J. (1984). A clinically applicable exsanguination shock model in swine. Circ Shock. 12:1-7.

Trcka V., Siblikova O. (1985). Substance-induced liver injury as a model for evaluating hepatoprotective drugs. Cas Lek Cesk. 124:161-4. (English Abstract) (Czechoslovakian)

Trechsel U., Stutzer A., Fleisch H. (1987). Hypercalcemia induced with an arotinoid in thyroparathyroidectomized rats. New model to study bone resorption in vivo. J Clin Invest, 80:1679-86.

Treit D. (1985). Animal models for the study of anti-anxiety agents: a review. Neurosci Biobehav Rev. 9:203-22.

Treit D., Pesold C. (1990). Septal lesions inhibit fear reactions in two animal models of anxiolytic drug action. Physiol Behav 47(2):365-71.

Trentham D.E. (1987). Clues provided by animal models of arthritis. Rheum Dis Clin North Am, 13:307-18.

Tripathi R.M. (1986). A simple method for the the production of ventricular tachycardia in the rat and guinea pig. J Pharmacol Methods. 15:279-82.

Trivedi P., Mowat A.P. (1983). Carbon tetrachloride-induced hepatic fibrosis and cirrhosis in the developing rat: an experimental model of cirrhosis in childhood. Br J Exp Pathol. 64:25-33.

Tron F. (1990). [Contribution of murine models of spontaneous lupus to the analysis of genetic factors in human disease] Apport des modeles murins spontanes de lupus a l'analyse des facteurs genetiques de la maladie humaine. Ann Med Interne (Paris) 141(3):217-21.

Troncone R., Ferguson A. (1991). Animal model of gluten induced enteropathy in mice. Gut 32(8):871-5.

Trott K.R., Huczkowski J. (1987). Experimental animal model for late post-radiation reaction of the large intestine. Nowotwory, 37:114-21 (English Abstract). (Polish)

Trotter J.L., Clark H.B., Collins K.G., Wegeschiede C.L., Scarpellini J.D. (1987). Myelin proteolipid protein induces demyelinating disease in mice. J Neurol Sci, Jun; 79:173-88.

Trouillas J., Girod C. (1988). Animal models of human pituitary tumors. Pathol Res Pract 183(5):638-41.

Trouillas J., Girod C., Claustrat B., Joly-Pharaboz M., Chevallier P. (1990). Spontaneous prolactin transplantable tumor in the Wistar/Furth rat (SMtTW): a new animal model of human prolactinoma. Cancer Res 50(13):4081-6.

Troyer D.A. (1987). Models of ischemic acute renal failure: do they reflect events in human renal failure? [editorial]. J Lab Clin Med, 110:379-80.

Trzepacz P., Leavitt M., Ciongoli K. (1992). An animal model for delirium. Psychosomatics 33(4):404-15.

Tsinzerling V.A., Popova E.D., Avtushenko S.S., Soldatova V.M. (1981). Experimental model of respiratory mycoplasmosis]. Arkh Patol. 43:95. (Russian)

Tsuboi R., Shi C., Rifkin D., Ogawa H. (1992). A wound healing model using healing-impaired diabetic mice. J Dermatol 19(11):673-5.

Tsuji M., Matsumoto K. (1982). Animal models with models receptor deficiencies--mice and rats as testicular feminization. Jikken Dobutsu. 31:303-9. (Japanese)

Tsuji S. (1981). Animal models for a deficiency of myelin formation of the central nervous system. Jikken Dobutsu. 30:353-8. (Japanese)

Tsukada N., Koh C.S., Yanagisawa N., Okano A., Behan W.M., Behan P.O. (1987). A new model for multiple sclerosis: chronic experimental allergic encephalomyelitis induced by immunization with cerebral endothelial cell membrane. Acta Neuropathol (Berl), 73:259-66.

Tsuno K., Terasaki H., Hashiguchi A., Nakamura M., Tanoue T., Okamoto T., Sadanaga M., Higashi K., Yano T., Saito Y. (1987). Extracorporeal lung assist on premature sheep and goat delivered by cesarean-section used as an experimental model of infant respiratory failure. Masui. 36:909-13 (English Abstract) (Japanese)

Tsurufuji S., Yoshimo S., Ohuchi K. (1982). Induction of an allergic air-pouch inflammation in rats. Int Arch Allergy Apply Immunol. 69:189-98.

Tu L.H. (1988). Experimental rabbit model of myasthenia gravis produced with acetylcholine receptor of nicotinic type from the 'generating organ' of electric ray. Chung Hua Shen Ching Ching Shen Ko Tsa Chih. 14:16-8. (Chinese)

Tufveson G., Gannedahl G., Johnsson C., Olausson M., Wamders A., Ekberg H. (1993). New immunosupressants: testing and development in animal models and the clinic: with special reference to DSG. Immunol Rev. 136:99-109.

Tung K.S., Ellis L., Teuscher C., Meng A., Blaustein J.C., Kohno S., Howell R. (1981). The black mink (Mustela vison). A natural model of immunologic male infertility. J Exp Med. 154:1016-32.

Tur J., Prieto R., Grases F. (1991). An animal model to study the effects of diet on risk factors of calcium stone formation. Scand J Urol Nephrol 25(4):311-4.

Turi Z., Rezkella S., Campbell C., Kloner R. (1990). Left main percutaneous transluminal coronary angioplasty with the autoperfusion catheter in an animal model. Cathet Cardiovasc Diagn 21(1):45-50.

Turnbull B.W., Mitchell T.J. (1984). Non-parametric estimation of the distribution of time to onset for specific diseases in survival/sacrifice experiments. Biometrics. 40:41-50.

Turner J.H., Claringbold P.G., Klemp P.F.B., Cameron P.J., Martindale A.A., Glancy R.J., Norman E.L., Hetherington E.L., Najdovski L., Lambrecht R.M. (1994). Holmium-166 microsphere liver radiotherapy. A preclinical SPECT dosimetry study in the pig. Nucl Med Commun. 15:545-53.

Turusov V.S. (1985). Experimental models of 2-stage carcinogenesis. Eksp Onkol. 7:5-12. (English Abstract) (Russian)

Tutrone R. J., Ball R., Ornitz D., Leder P., Richie J. (1993). Benign prostatic hyperplasia in a transgenic mouse: a new hormonally sensitive investigatory model. J Urol 149(3):633-9.

Tuxen A., Kirkeby S. (1990). An animal model for human masseter muscle: histochemical characterization of mouse, rat, rabbit, cat, dog, pig, and cow masseter muscle. J Oral Maxillofac Surg 48(10):1063-7.

Tuxen A., Rostrup E. (1993). Histochemical characterization of pig masseter muscle: an animal model. Scand J Dent Res 101(1):57-61.

Tzipori S., Robins-Browne R.M., Gonis G., Hayes J., Withers M., McCartney E. (1985). Enteropathogenic Escherichia coli enteritis: evaluation of the gnotobiotic piglet as a model of human infection. Gut. 26:570-8.

Ubatuba F. (1989). An animal model for the study of arterial thrombosis. Braz J Med Biol Res 22(8):993-1000.

Uchida M., Yano S., Watanabe K. (1991). A reliable method for the production of antral gastric ulcer by a combination of 2-deoxy-D-glucose, aspirin and ammonia in rats. Jpn J Pharmacol 56(4):475-81.

Uchida T., Soe S., Suzuki K., Komatsu K., Shikata T., Iida F., Rikihisa T., Mizuno K. (1988). [Epidemic non-A, non-B viral hepatitis - animal model and causative virus]. Nippon Rinsho 46(12):2589-95.

Udelsman R., Bacher J., Gallucci W.T., Gold P.W., Morin M.L., Renquist D., Loriaux D.L., Chrousos GP. (1984). Hemodynamic and endocrine parameters in the anesthetized cynomolgus monkeys: a primate model. J Med Primatol. 13:327-38.

Udintsev S., Fomina T., Razina T. (1992). [An experimental model of metastatic liver involvement by using Ehrlich's ascitic cancer] Eksperimental'naia model' metastaticheskogo porazheniia pecheni s ispol'zovaniem astsitnogo raka Erlikha. Vopr Onkol 38(6):723-6.

Ugriumov E.P., Barinskiii I.F., Bezprozvannyi B.K., Shubladze A.K., Melik-Andreasian G.G. (1982). Experiment in infecting the green monkey Cercopithecus aethiops with a leukocyte virus isolated in hepatitis A. Vopr Virusol. 27:190-2. (English Abstract) (Russian)

Ullrich S.J., Zeng Z.Z., Jay G. (1994). Transgenic mouse models of human gastric and hepatic carcinomas. Semin Cancer Biol. 5(1):61-8.

Umemura K., Kohno Y., Matsuno H., Uematsu T., Nakashima M. (1990). A new model for photochemically induced thrombosis in the inner ear microcirculation and the use of hearing loss as a measure for microcirculatory disorders. Eur Arch Otorhinolaryngol 248(2):105-8.

Umemura K., Nakashima M. (1993). [A new model of middle cerebral artery thrombosis in rats]. Yakubutsu Seishin Kodo 13(1):9-17.

Ungar B., Burris J., Quinn C., Finkelman F. (1990). New mouse models for chronic Cryptosporidium infection in immunodeficient hosts. Infect Immun 58(4):961-9.

Unverferth D.V., Croskery R.W., Leier C.V., Allschuld R., Pipers F.S., Thomas J., Magorien R.D., Hamlin R.L. (1983) Canine cobalt cardiomyopathy: a model for the study of heart failure. Am J Vet Res. 44:989-95.

Urbain J.L., Shore S., Vekemans M.C., Manzone T., Shea F., Charkes N.D. et al. (1995). Does scintigraphic imaging of antisense probe making sense? Eur J Nucl Med. 22:499-504.

Uren N.G., Marraccini P., Gistri R., De Silva R., Camici P. (1993). Altered coronary vasodilator reserve and metabolism in myocardium subtended by normal arteries in patients with CAD. J Am Coll Cardiol. 22:650-8.

Valentine B., Cooper B., de L. A., O'Quinn R., Blue J. (1988). Canine X-linked muscular dystrophy. An animal model of Duchenne muscular dystrophy: clinical studies. J Neurol Sci 88(1-3):69-81.

Valentine B., Winand N., Pradhan D., Moise N., de L. A., Kornegay J., Cooper B. (1992). Canine X-linked muscular dystrophy as an animal model of Duchenne muscular dystrophy: a review. Am J Med Genet 42(3):352-6.

Vales N., Barron B., Padilla J., Sandoval H., Sotelo J. (1991). Effect of dsRNA from phi 6 bacteriophage on herpetic infection in cell culture and an animal model. J Interferon Res 11(5):271-4.

Valette H., Deleuze P., Syrota A., Delforge J., Crouzel C., Fuseau C., Loisance D. (1995). Canine myocardial beta-adrenergic, muscarinic receptor densities after denervation: A PET study. J Nucl Med. 36:140-6.

Valette H., Loc'h C., Mardon K., Bendriem B., Merlet P., Fuseau C., Sabry S., Raffel D., Maziere B., Syrota A. (1993). Bromine-76-metabromobenzylguanidine: a PET radiotracer for mapping sympathetic nerves of the heart. J Nucl Med. 34:1739-44.

Valji K., Bookstein J.J. (1987). Fibrinolysis with intra-thrombic injection of urokinase and tissue-type plasminogen activator. Results in a new model of subacute venous thrombosis. Invest Radio. 22:23-7.

Valtin H. (1982). The discovery of the Brattleboro rat, recommended nomenclature, and the question of proper controls. Ann NY Acad Sci. 394:1-9.

Van Alphen H., Gao Y., Kamphorst W. (1990). An acute experimental model of saccular aneurysms in the rat. Neurol Res 12(4):256-9.

Van Aswegen A., Van Wijk A.J., Roodt J.P. et al. (1985). Evaluation of (o)-[^{77}Br]-bromohippuran as renal tubular function agent. Int J Appl Radiat Isot. 36:727-32.

Van den Bosch de Aguilar, P., Langhendries-Weverberg C., Gaemaere-Vanneste J., Flament-Duvand J., Brion J.P., Couck A.M. (1984). Transplantation of human cortex with Alzheimer's disease into rat occipital cortex; a model for the study of Alzheimer disease. Experientia 40:402-3.

Van der Giessen W.J., Mooi W., Rutteman A.M., van Vliet H.H., Verdouw P.P. (1983). A new model for coronary thrombosis in the pig: preliminary results with thrombolysis. Eur Heart J. 4 (Suppl) C:69-76.

Van der Kraan P., Vitters E., van B. H., van d. P. L., van d. W. (1990). Degenerative knee joint lesions in mice after a single intra-articular collagenase injection. A new model of osteoarthritis. J Exp Pathol (Oxford) 71(1):19-31.

Van Etten R.A. (1993). Disease progression in a murine model of bcr/abl leukemogenesis. Leuk Lymphoma 11(Suppl 1):239-42.

Van Herck H., Van W.J., Veldhuizen M., Baumans V., Stafleu F., Beynen A. (1989). Clinical examination of weanling rats with early zinc deficiency. Lab Anim 23(4):328-32.

Van Iperen H., Beijersbergen v. H. G. (1992). An animal model for extracorporeal photochemotherapy based on contact hypersensitivity. J Photochem Photobiol B 15(4):361-6.

Van Leeuwen F. (1992). Animal models for osmoregulatory disturbances. Prog Brain Res 93:273-82.

Van Wijk A.J., Bekker P., Niemann D., Roesch H. et al. (1983). Development and bioevaluation of (o)-^{82}Br [^{77}Br]-bromohippuran. Int J Appl Radiat Isot. 34:1019-21.

Vandendris M., Dumont P., Hermann R. et al. (1983). Development and characterization of a new murine renal tumor model. Chemotherapeutic results. Cancer Chemother Pharmacol. 11:182-7.

Vandendris M., Dumont P., Semal P., Heimann R., Atassi G. (1985). Investigation of a new murine model of regional lymph node metastasis: characteristics of the model and applications. Clin Exp Metastasis. 3:7-19.

Vandeputte M., Sobis H. (1988): Experimental rat model for human yolk sac tumor. Eur J Cancer Clin Oncol. 24(3): 551-8.

Vaneerdeweg W., Buyssens N., De W. T., Sebrechts M., Babloyan A., Arakelian S., De B. M. (1992). A standardized surgical technique to obtain a stable and reproducible chronic renal failure model in dogs. Eur Surg Res 24(5):273-82.

Varakis J.N., Kase C.S., Wilborn W.H., Cheshire L.B., Peterson R.D. (1981). Pathogenesis of an experimental meningeal leukemia model. Clin Immunol Immunopathol. 23:400-7.

Varastet M., Brouillet E., Chavoix C., Prenant C., Crouzel C., Stulzaft O., Bottlaender M., Cayla J., Maziere B., Maziere M. (1992). In vivo visualization of central muscarinic receptors using [^{11}C]quinuclidyl benzilate and positron emission tomography in baboons. Eur J Pharmacol. 213:275-84

Vargas K.J., Stephens L.C. (1983). Resistance of Rowett athymic (nude) rats to casein-induced amyloidosis. Am J Vet Res. 44:1597-9.

Varma K.J., Powers T.E., Powers J.D., Spurlock S.L. (1984). Standardization of an experimental disease model of Streptococcus zooepidemicus in the equine. J Vet Pharmacol Ther. 7:183-8.

Varshney A., Singh H., Gupta R., Singh S. (1989). Experimental model of staphylococcal osteomyelitis in dogs. Indian J Exp Biol 27(9):816-9.

Varsos V.G., Liszczak T.M., Han D.H., Kistler J.P., Vielma J., Black P.M., Heros R.C., Zervas N.T. (1983). Delayed cerebral vasospasm is not reversible aminophylline, nifedipine, or papaverine in a 'two-hemorrhage' canine model. J Neurosurg. 58:11-7.

Vas R., Elkayam U., Meerbaum S. (1981). A closed chest animal model for the study of reversible ischemia. Cardiology. 67:133-47.

Vatner D.E., Lee D.L., Schwarz K.R. et al. (1988). Impaired cardiac muscarinic receptor function in dogs with heart failure. J Clin Invest. 81:1836-42.

Vediaev F.P. (1984). Prolonged electrostimulation of the negative emotiogenic areas of the brain as a model of chronic emotional stress. Fiziol Zh SSSR. 70:1280-5. (English Abstract) (Russian)

Velasquez M., Kimmel P., Michaelis O. 4. (1990). Animal models of spontaneous diabetic kidney disease. FASEB J 4(11):2850-9.

Velazquez M., Haller J., Amundsen T., Schuster DP. (1991). Regional lung crater measurements with PET: Accuracy, reproducibility, and linearity. J Nucl Med. 32:719-25.

Verbalis J.G. (1984). An experimental model of syndrome of inappropriate antidiuretic hormone secretion in the rat. Am J Pathol. 247:E540-53.

Verdier F., Chazal I., Descotes J. (1994). Anaphylaxis models in the guinea-pig. Toxicology 93(1):55-61.

Verdouw P.D., Wolffenbuttel B.N., van der Giessen W.J. (1983). Domestic pigs in the study of myocardial ischemia. Eur Heart J. 4 (Suppl C):61-7.

Vergnes M., Marescaux C., Micheletti G., Reis J., Depaulis A., Ramback L., Warter J.M. (1982). Spontaneous paroxysmal electroclinical patterns in rat: a model of generalized non-convulsive epilepsy. Neurosci Lett. 33:97-101.

Vergona R.A., Herratt C., Garippa R., Hirkaler G. (1984). Mechanisms of methacholine-induced coronary vasospasm in an experimental model of variant angina in the anesthetized rat. Life Sci. 35:1877-84.

Verheul H.A., Schot C.P., Schuurs A.H. (1986). Effects of sex, gonadectomy and several steroids on the development of insulin-dependent diabetes mellitus in the BB rat. Clin Exp Immunol. 63:656-62.

Vertelkin V.A., Golofeevskii VIu, Stefaniuk N.F., Saltykov A.A. (1987). Cryogenic method of creating an experimental stomach ulcer. Pathol Fiziól Eksp Ter. 2:77-8. (Russian)

Vertes C., Gonczy S., Lendvay N., Debreczeni L.A. (1987). A model for experimental asthma: provocation in guinea-pigs immunized with Bordetella pertussis. Bull Eur Physiopathol Respir. (23 Suppl), 10:111s-113s. (Russian)

Vesselinovitch D. (1988): Animal models and the study of atherosclerosis. Arch Pathol Lab Med. 112(10):1011-7.

Vesselinovitch S.D., Negri S. (1988): Induction of focal and nodular liver lesions in rodents as an indication of human carcinogenic risk. Ann N Y Acad 534:99-105.

Vesvres M., Doutremepuich F., Lalanne M., Doutremepuich C. (1993). Effects of aspirin on embolization in an arterial model of laser-induced thrombus formation. Haemostasis 23(1):8-12.

Vezeridis M., Doremus C., Tibbetts L., Tzanakakis G., Jackson B. (1989). Invasion and metastasis following orthotopic transplantation of human pancreatic cancer in the nude mouse. J Surg Oncol 40(4):261-5.

Via C., Morse H. 3., Shearer G. (1990). Altered immunoregulation and autoimmune aspects of HIV infection: relevant murine models. Immunol Today 11(7):250-5.

Via C.S., Shearer G.M. (1988): Murine graft-versus-host disease as a model for the development of autoimmunity. Relevance of cytotoxic lymphocytes. Ann N Y Acad Sci 532:44-50

Vidal C., Jacob J. (1986). Hyperalgesia induced by emotional stress in the rat: an experimental animal model of human anxiogenic hyperalgesia. Ann NY Acad Sci. 467:73-81.

Vignaud J.M., Duprez A., Bene M.C., Leclere J., Faure G., Danchin N., Burlet C. (1984). Transplantation of human hyperthyroid tissue to the nude mouse. An experimental model. Am J Pathol. 117:355-9.

Villemagne V.L., Dannals R.F., Sánchez-Roa P.M., Ravert H.T., Vazquez S., Wilson A.A., Natarjan T.K., Wong D.F., Yanai K., Wagner H.N.Jr. (1991). Imaging histamine H1 receptors in the living human brain with carbon-11-pyrilamine. J Nucl Med. 32:308-11.

Virganskii A., Banin V., Klevtsov V., Rogulenko R., Strupin I., Tverskaia M., Tikhvinskaia E. (1990). [The systemic and regional changes in the modelling of a massive pulmonary artery embolism] Sistemnye i regionarnye izmeneniia pri modelirovanii massivnoi embolii legochnoi arterii. Fiziol Zh SSSR 76(10):1355-60.

Vishnevetskii F.E., Iushin M.I.U., Aiupova A.K., Urliapova N. G. (1988): Reproduction of experimental leprous infection in mice with a preliminary modelling of a failure of the mononuclear phagocyte system. Biull Eksp Biol Med. 106(11):574-8. (English Abstract) (Russian)

Visvesvara G.S., Dickenson J.W., Hearly G.R. (1988): Variable infectivity of human-derived Giardia lamblia cysts for Mongolian gerbils (Meriones unguiculatus). J Clin Microbiol. 26:837-41.

Vivaldi E., Macinelli s., Gunther B. (1983). Experimental hemorrhage shock in dogs: standardization. Res Exp Med (Berl). 182:127-37.

Vladutiu A.O. (1993). The severe combined immunodeficient (SCID) mouse as a model for the study of autoimmune diseases. Clin Exp Immunol. 93(1):1-8.

Vogel G., Meuleman D., Bourgondien F., Hobbelen P. (1989). Comparison of two experimental thrombosis models in rats effects of four glycosaminoglycans. Thromb Res 54(5):399-410.

Vogel G., Neill D., Hagler M., Kors D. (1990). A new animal model of endogenous depression: a summary of present findings. Neurosci Biobehav Rev 14(1):85-91.

Vogelweid C., Vogt D., Besch-Williford C., Walker S. (1993). New Zealand white mice: an experimental model of exencephaly. Lab Anim Sci 43(1):58-60.

Vol'pert E.L., Ganelina I.E., Kukui L.M., Ianushkene T.S., Borisova IIu. (1984). Modification of a model of ventricular fibrillation by a combination of ligation of the interventricular artery and ultraviolet irradiation autoblood. Kardiologiia. 24:66-9. (English Abstract) (Russian)

Volk M., Ershler W. (1991). The influence of immunosenescence on tumor growth and spread: lessons from animal models. Cancer Cells 3(1):13-8.

Volkow N.D., Fowler J.S., Logan J., Gatley S.J., Dewey S.L., MacGregor R.R., Schlyer D.J., Pappas N., King P., Wang G.J., Wolf A.P. (1995). Carbon-11-cocaine binding compared at subpharmacological and pharmacological doses: A PET study. J Nucl Med. 36:1289-97.

Volpe R., Akasu F., Morita T., Yoshikawa N., Resetkova E., Arreaza G., Mukuta T. (1993). New animal models for human autoimmune thyroid disease. Xenografts of human thyroid tissue in severe combined immunodeficient (SCID) and nude mice. Horm Metab Res. 25(12):623-7.

Volpe R., Kasuga Y., Akasu F., Morita T., Yoshikawa N., Resetkova E., Arreaza G. (1993). The use of the severe combined immunodeficient mouse and the athymic "nude" mouse as models for the study of human autoimmune thyroid disease. Clin Immunol Immunopathol 67(2):93-9.

Voltenko G.N., Hipkan G.N., Zapadniuk v.I. Bezverkhaia I.S. (1984). Experimental dystrophy of the stomach in rats of different ages. Patol Fiziol Eksp Ter. 2:51-2. (English Abstract) (Russian)

von Glass W., Kasler M., Lang T. (1992). Mode of action of photodynamic therapy with sulfonated aluminum phthalocyanine in induced squamous cell carcinomas in animal models. Eur Arch Otorhinolaryngol 249(6):309-12.

Vorob'eva T., Geiko V. (1990). [Experimental analysis of the neurobiological basis of genetically determined alcohol addiction in the progeny] Eksperimental'nyi analiz neirobiologicheskikh osnov vlecheniia k alkogoliu u potomstva, otiagoshchennogo alkogolizmom. Zh Nevropatol Psikhiatr 90(8):79-83.

Vorob'eva T., Gordienko Z., Paikova L. (1990). [Neurophysiologic and pathomorphologic characteristics of the development of alcoholism (experimental study)] Neirofiziologicheskie i patomorfologicheskie osobennosti formirovaniia alkogolizma (exkperimental'noe issledovanie). Zh Nevropatol Psikhiatr 90(2):77-84.

Voss G., Hunsmann G. (1993). Cellular immune response to SIVmac and HIV-2 in macaques: model for the human HIV-1 infection. J Acquir Immune Defic Syndr. 6(9):969-76.

Votiakov V.I., Kolomiets N.D., Kolomiets A.G., Luchko V.P. (1986). Modeling amyotrophic leukospongiosis in laboratory animals. Vestn Akad Med Nauk SSSR. 9:71-6. (English Abstract) (Russian)

Votiakov V.I., Kolomiets N.D., Kuacheva Z.B., Kalamiets A.B., Rytick P.G. (1985) Physiochemical and biological properties of the agents isolated from a patient with amyotrophic leukospongiosis and monkeys with experimentally reproduced disease. Vopr Virusol. 30:58-64. (English Abstract) (Russian)

Votiakov V.I., Kolomiets N.D., Luchko V.P., Kolomiets A.G. (1987): Biochemical and immunological changes in guinea pigs with experimentally reproduced amyotrophic leukospongiosis. Biull Eksp Biol Med. 103:292-4 (English Abstract) (Russian)

Votto J.J., Barton R.W., Gionfriddo M.A., Cole S.R., McCormick J.R., Thrall R.S. (1987): A model of pulmonary granulomata induced by beryllium sulfate in the rat. Sarcoidosis. 4:71-6

Voyles N.R., Powell A.M., Timmers K.I., Wilkins S.D., Bhathena S.J., Hansen C., Michaelis O.E 4th., Recant L. (1988): Reversible impairment of glucose-induced insulin secretion in SHR/N-cp rats. Genetic model of type II diabetes. Diabetes. 37(4): 398-404.

Vracko R., Thorning D. (1985). Freze-thaw injury of rat heart across an intact diaphrgm: a new model for the study of the response of myocardium to injury. Cardiovasc Res. 19:76-84

Wackers F.J., Klay J.W., Laks H., Schnitzer J., Zaret B.L., Geha A.S. (1981). Pathophysiologic correlates of right ventricular thallium-201 uptake in a canine model. Circulation. 64:1256-64.

Wada Y., Okuda H., Yoshida K., Hasegawa H., Jibiki I., Kido H., Yamaguchi N. (1987). A new experimental model for drug studies: effects of phenobarbital and phenytoin on photosensitivity in the lateral geniculate-kindled cat. Epilepsia, 28:667-72.

Wagland B., Abeydeera L., Rothwell T., Ouwerkerk D. (1989). Experimental Haemonchus contortus infections in guinea pigs. Int J Parasitol 19(3):301-5.

Wagner E.F., Theuring F. (Ed.) (1993). Transgenic animals as model systems for human diseases. Berlin; New York: Springer Verlag. 151 P.

Wagner H.N. Jr. (1991). Molecular medicine: From science to service. J Nucl Med. 32:11N-23N.

Wagner H.N. Jr., Burns H.D., Dannals R.F., Wong D.F., Langstrom B., Duelfer T., Frost J.J., Ravert H.T., Links J.M., Rosenbloom S.B., Lukas S.E., Kramer A.V., Kuhar M.J. (1983). Imaging dopamine receptors in the human brain by positron emission tomography. Science 221:1264-6.

Wagner H.N. Jr., Szabo Z., Buchanan J. (Eds.) (1995). Principles of Nuclear Medicine. 2nd ed. Philadelphia: W.B. Saunders. (in Press).

Wagner T., Swierczynska Z., Stankiewicz C., Bujalska H., Kosowska E. (1981). A new model of experimental amyloidosis? Z Rheumatol. 40:234-5.

Wainstein M., Tannhauser M., Barros H. (1990). Lack of tolerance to imipramine or mianserine in two animal models of depression. Pharmacology 41(6):327-32.

Wakefield T., Wrobleski S., Sarpa M., Taylor F. J., Esmon C., Cheng A., Greenfield L. (1991). Deep venous thrombosis in the baboon: an experimental model. J Vasc Surg 14(5):588-98.

Waldorf A.R., Halde C., Vedros N.A. (1982). Murine model of pulmonary mucormycosis in cortisone-treated mice. Sabouraudia. 20:217-24.

Walker D.H., Johnson K.M., Lange J.V., Gardner J.J., Kiley M.P., McCormick J.B. (1982). Experimental infection of rhesus monkeys with Lassa virus and a closely related arenavirus, Mozambique virus. J Infect Dis. 146:360-8.

Walker H.L., McLeod C.G. Jr., McManus W.F. (1981). Experimental inhalation injury in the goat. J Trauma. 21:962-4.

Walker K.Z., Boniface G.R., Phippard A.F., Harwood W. et al. (1991). Preclinical evaluation of ^{99m}Tc-labeled DD 3B6/22 Fab' for thrombus detection. Thromb Res. 64:691-701.

Wall C. 3., Casselbrant M. (1992). System identification of perilymphatic fistula in an animal model. Am J Otol 13(5):443-8.

Wallace J. (1988). Release of platelet-activating factor (PAF) and accelerated healing induced by a PAF antagonist in an animal model of chronic colitis. Can J Physiol Pharmacol 66(4):422-5.

Wallace J., Braquet P., Ibbotson G., MacNaughton W., Cirino G. (1989). Assessment of the role of platelet-activating factor in an animal model of inflammatory bowel disease. J Lipid Mediat 1(1):13-23.

Walovitch R.C., Cheesman E.H., Maheu L.J., Hall K.M. (1994). Studies of the retention mechanism of the brain perfusion imaging agent ^{99m}Tc-bicisate (^{99m}Tc-ECD). J Cereb Blood Flow Metab. 14(Suppl):S4-S11.

Walsh T.J., Bacher J., Pizzo P.A. (1988): Chronic silastic central venous catherization for induction, maintenance and support of persistent granulocytopenia in rabbits. Lab Anim Sci. 38(4):467-71.

Walvoort H.C. (1983). Glycogen storage diseases in animals and their potential value as models of human disease. J Inherited Metab Dis. 6:3-16.

Walvoort H.C., Dormans J.A., Van den Ingh T.S. (1985). Comparative pathology of the canine model of glycogen storage disease type II (Pompe's disease). J Inherited Metab Dis. 8:38-46.

Walzer P.D., Rutledge M.E., Yoneda K. (1983). Experimental Pneumocystis carinii pneumonia in C3H/HeJ and C3HeB/FeJ mice. J Reticuloendothel Soc. 33:1-9.

Walzer P.D., Young L.S. (1984). Clinical relevance of animal models of Pneumocystis carinii pneumonia. Diagn Microbiol Infect Dis. 2:1-6.

Wang S.J., Lin W.Y., Hsieh B.T., Shen L.H., Tsai Z.T., Knapp F.F. (1995). Rhenium-188 sulflur colloid as a radiation synovectomy agent. Eur J Nucl Med. 22:505-7.

Wang Z. (1988): Establishment of a model of human tongue squamous cell carcinoma in nude mice. Chung Hua Kou Chiang Hsueh Tsa Chih. 23(1):17-9, 62. (English Abstract). (Chinese)

Wang Z., Wang Z., Liu Z., Tan Y. (1990). [Experiment study of adriamycin-induced nephrotic syndrome in rats]. Hua Hsi I Ko Ta Hsueh Hsueh Pao 21(4):430-2.

Wanless R.B., Anand I.S., Poole-Wilson P.A., Harris P. (1987). An experimental model of chronic cardiac failure using adriamycin in the rabbit: central haemodynamics and regional blood flow. Cardiovasc Res, Jan; 21:7-13.

Wanner A. (1990). Utility of animal models in the study of human airway disease. Chest 98(1):211-7.

Wanner A., Abraham W., Douglas J., Drazen J., Richerson H., Ram J. (1990). NHLBI Workshop Summary. Models of airway hyper-responsiveness. Am Rev Respir Dis 141(1):253-7.

Wanner A., Abraham W.M. (1982). Experimental models of asthma. Lung. 160:231-43.

Ward R., Florence A., Baldwin D., Abiaka C., Roland F., Ramsey MH., Dickson D., Peters T., Crichton R. (1991). Biochemical and biophysical investigations of the ferrocene-iron-loaded rat. An animal model of primary haemochromatosis. Eur J Biochem 202(2):405-10.

Warren B.F., Watkins P.E. (1994). Animal models of inflammatory bowel disease. J Pathol. 172(4):313-6.

Warren I.F., Tanner M.S., McNeish A.S. (1982). A model of jejunal injury and recovery in the rat. Scand J Gastroenterol [Suppl]. 74:171-2.

Warren J., Dolatshahi M. (1992). Worldwide survey of AIDS vaccine challenge studies in non-human primates: vaccines associated with active and passive immune protection from live virus challenge. J Med Primatol 21(2-3):139-86.

Warren K.S. (1982). The secret of the immunopathogenesis of schistosomiasis: in vivo models. Immunol Rev. 61:189-213.

Wascher T., Dittrich P., Kukovetz W. (1991). Antiarrhythmic effects of two new propafenone related drugs. A study on four animal models of arrhythmia. Arzneimittelforschung 41(2):119-24.

Watanabe M., Uchida H., Okada H. et al. (1992). A high-resolution PET animal studies. IEEE Trans Med Imaging 11:577-80.

Watanabe Y., Ito T., Shiomi M. (1985). The effect of selective breeding on the development of coronary atherosclerosis in WHHL rabbits. An animal model for familial hypercholesterolemia. Atherosclerosis. 56:71-9.

Watson B.D., Prado R., Dietrich W.D., Ginsberg M.D., Green B.A. (1986). Photochemically induced spinal cord injury in the rat. Brain Res. 367:296-300.

Watson R. (1989). Murine models for acquired immune deficiency syndrome. Life Sci 44(3):iii-xv.

Watson R.R., Prabhala R.H., Darban H.R., Yahya M.D., Smith T.L.. (1988): Changes in lymphocyte and macrophage subsets due to morphine and ethanol treatment during a retrovirus infection causing murine AIDS. Life Sci. 43(6):v-xi.

Watson T. (1993). Animal regulations overturned. Science 259:1389.

Waynforth H.B., Hunter-Craig C.J. (1981). The Eker renal tumor rat. Tumor transplantability and a re-evaluation of tumor histology. Neoplasma. 28:309-15.

Webb G.P., Jagot S.A., Jakobson M.E. (1982). Fasting-induced torpor in Mus musculus and its implications in the use of murine models for human obesity studies. Comp Biochem Physiol [A]. 72:211-9.

Weber W.W., Tannen R.H. (1981). Pharmacokinetic studies on the drug-related lupus syndrome. Differences in antinuclear antibody development and drug-induced DNA damage in rapid and slow acetylator animal models. Arthritis Rheum. 24:979-86.

Wechsler-Jentzsch K., Huepfel H., Schmidt W., Wandl E., Kahn B. (1993). Failure of hyperfractionated radiotherapy to reduce bone growth arrest in rats. Int J Radiat Oncol Biol Phys 26(3):427-31.

Wedderburn N., Edwards J.M., Desgranges C., Fontaine C., Cohen B., de The G. (1984). Infectious mononucleosis-like response in common marmosets infected with Epstein-Barr virus. J Infect Dis. 150:878-82.

Wedderburn N., Mitchell G.H., Davies D.R. (1985). Plasmodium brasilianum in the common marmoset Callithrix jacchus Parasitology. 90 (Pt 3):573-8.

Wege H., Koga M., Wegen H., ter Meulen V. (1981). JHM infections in rats as a model for acute and subacute demyelinating disease. Adv Exp Med Biol. 142:327-40.

Wehling P., Pak M., Georgescu H. (1990). Intrathecal injection of a specific enzyme in rats as a model for chemically induced spinal cord injury. Acta Orthop Belg 56(3-4):539-44.

Wehner R.W., Smith R.G. (1983). Progressive cytomegalovirus glomerulonephritis - An experimental model. Am J Pathol. 112:313-25.

Weihe W.H. (1982). The problem of alternatives to scientific animal experimentation. Fortschr Med. 100:2162-5. (German)

Weil G., Chandrashekar R., Liftis F., McVay CS., Bosshardt S., Klei T. (1990). Circulating parasite antigen in Brugia pahangi-infected jirds. J Parasitol 76(1):78-84.

Weinberg A., Xie H., Hardy B., Skinner D. (1990). A juvenile animal model to study the growth potential of bowel segments in the urinary tract [see comments]. J Urol 143(2):377-80.

Weindruch R., Masoro E. (1991). Concerns about rodent models for aging research [editorial]. J Gerontol 46(3):B87-8.

Weingand K. (1989). A model of postprandial hyperinsulinemia in miniature swine. Lab Anim Sci 39(5):394-9.

Weinstein P.R. (1986). Neurological deficit and cerebral infarction after temporary middle cerebral artery occlusion in unanesthetized cats. Stroke. 17:318-24.

Weiss M.L., Kubat K. (1983). Plasmodium berghei: a mouse model for the 'sudden death' and 'malarial lung' syndromes. Exp Parasitol. 56:143-51.

Wekerle H., Kojima K., Lannes-Vieira J., Lassmann H., Linigton C. (1994). Animal models. Ann Neurol. 36(Suppl.):S47-53.

Welkos S.L. (1984). Experimental gastroenteritis in newly-hatched chicks infected with Campylobacter jejuni. J Med Microbiol. 18:233-48.

Wen R.Q., Wong P.Y. (1988): Reserpine treatment increases viscosity of fluid in the epididymis of rats. Biol Reprod. 38(5):969-74.

Wenk G.L. (1993). A primate model of Alzheimer's disease. Behav Brain Res. 57(2):117-22.

Wennberg R.P. (1993). Animal models of bilirubin encephalopathy. Adv Vet Sci Comp Med. 37:87-113.

Werner H., Herbertson M., Seear M. (1993). Operating characteristics of pediatric continuous arteriovenous hemofiltration in an animal model. Pediatr Nephrol 7(2):189-93.

Werner P. (1984). Animals as natural models for drug testing. A Arztl Fortbild (Jena). 78:293-6. (German)

Weseloh G., Liebig K., Kah-Kallnbach M. (1983). Experimental animal model for assaying cartilage-protective substances. Z Rheumatol. 42:206-9. (German)

West J., Goodlett C., Bonthius D., PierceD. (1989). Manipulating peak blood alcohol concentrations in neonatal rats: review of an animal model for alcohol-related developmental effects. Neurotoxicology 10(3):347-65.

Wetstein L., Mark R., Kelliher G.J., Friehling T., O'Connor K.M., Kowey P.R. (1985). Arrhythmia inducibility and ventricular vulnerability in a chronic feline infarction model. Am Heart J. 110:955-60.

Wetzel H., Wiedemann K., Holsboer F., Benkert O. (1991). Savoxepine: invalidation of an "atypical" neuroleptic response pattern predicted by animal models in an open clinical trial with schizophrenic patients. Psychopharmacology (Berl) 103(2):280-3.

Wexler B.C., McMurtry J.P. (1985). Anti-opiate (naloxone) suppression of Cushingoid degenerative changes in obese/SHR. Int J Obes. 9:77-91.

White E.J., Clark J.B. (1988): Menadione-treated synaptosomes as a model for post-ischaemic neuronal damage. Biochem J. 15;253(2):425-33.

White F.C., Roth D.M., Bloor C.M. (1986). The pig as a model for myocardial ischemia and exercise. Lab Anim Sci. 36:351-6.

White M., Chapman W. J., Hanson W. (1989). A comparison of experimental visceral leishmaniasis in the opossum, armadillo and ferret. Lab Anim Sci 39(1):47-50.

White M., Chapman W. J., Hanson W., Latimer K., Greene C. (1989). Experimental visceral leishmaniasis in the opossum. Vet Pathol 26(4):314-21.

Whiteley H.E., Everitt J.I., Kakoma I., James M.A., Ristic M. (1987): Pathologic changes associated with fatal Plasmodium falciparum infection in the Bolivian squirrel monkey (Saimiri sciureus boliviensis). Am J Trop Med Hyg. 37:1-8.

Whiting P.H., Thomson A.W., Simpson J.G. (1985). Cyclosporine: toxicity, metabolism, and drug interactions--implications from animal studies. Transplant Proc. 17 (4 Suppl 1):134-44.

Whitney J.B. 3d, Popp R.A. (1984). Animal model of human disease: thalassemia: alpha-thalassemia in laboratory mice. Am J Pathol. 116:523-5.

Wians F. J., Strickland D., Hankins G., Snyder R. (1990). The effect of hypermagnesemia on serum levels of osteocalcin in an animal model. Magnes Trace Elem 9(1):28-35.

Wicher K., Baughn R., Wicher V., Nakeeb S. (1992). Experimental congenital syphilis: guinea pig model. Infect Immun 60(1):271-7.

Wick G. (1986). Globular domain of basement membrane collagen induces autoimmune pulmonary lesions in mice resembling human Goodpasture disease. Lab Invest. 55:308-17.

Wick G., Boyd R.L., Muller P.U. (1982). Effect of cyclosporin A on spontaneous autoimmune thyroiditis of Obese strain (OS) chickens. Eur J Immunol. 12:877-81.

Wick G., Brezinschek H., Hala K., Dietrich H., Wolf H., Kroemer G. (1989). The obese strain of chickens: an animal model with spontaneous autoimmune thyroiditis. Adv Immunol 47:433-500.

Wiebe L.I. (1983). Small animal oncological models for screening diagnostic radiotracers. In: Lambrecht R.M., Eckelman W.C. (Eds). Animal models in radiotracer design. Heidelberg: Springer Verlag. pp 107-148.

Wiebe L.I. (1995). Radiopharmaceuticals to monitor gene therapy of cancer. 6th Eur. Symp. Radiopharmacy and Radiopharmaceuticals. Graz, Austria, 5-8 March. Abstract. Also see: (1994) Eur J Nucl Med Suppl. 21:489.

Wiebe L.I., Turner J.A., Franko A., Kanclerz A. (1991). Animal Tumor Models for the Evaluation of In-Vivo Diagnostic Radiotracers. Amer J Physiologic Imaging 6:133-149.

Wiebers D., Adams H. J., Whisnant J. (1990). Animal models of stroke: are they relevant to human disease? [editorial] [see comments]. Stroke 21(1):1-3.

Wienhard K., Dahlbom M., Eriksson L. et al. (1994). The ECAT EXACT HR: Performance of a new high-resolution positron scanner. J Comput Assist Tomogr. 18:110-8.

Wild G., Murray D. (1992). Alterations in quantitative distribution of Na,K-ATPase activity along crypt-villus axis in animal model of malabsorption characterized by hyperproliferative crypt cytokinetics. Dig Dis Sci 37(3):417-25.

Wilder R., Case J., Crofford L., Kumkumian G., Lafyatis R., Remmers EF., Sano H., Sternberg E., Yocum D. (1991). Endothelial cells and the pathogenesis of rheumatoid arthritis in humans and streptococcal cell wall arthritis in Lewis rats. J Cell Biochem 45(2):162-6.

Wilhelmi G., Maier R. (1983). Test of potential antiarthritic drugs on spontaneous arthritis of mice. Z Rheumatol. 42:203-5.   (German)

Williams G.H., Braley L.M., Menachery A. (1982). Decreased adrenal responsiveness to angiotensin II: a defect present in spontaneously hypertensive rats. A possible model of human essential hypertension. J Clin Invest. 69:31-7.

Williams L., Jodelis K., Donald M. (1989). Regional stimulation of cholinergic function by nerve growth factor in an animal model of Alzheimer's disease. Prog Clin Biol Res 317:1179-92.

Williams P.D., Bennett D.B., Comereski C.R. (1988): Animal model for evaluating the convulsive liability of beta-lactam antibiotics. Antimicrob Agents Chemother. 32(5):758-60.

Williams S.S., Alosco T.R., Croy B.A., Bankert R.B. (1993). The study of human neoplastic disease in severe combined immunodeficient mice. Lab Anim Sci. 43(2):139-46.

Willner P. (1984). The validity of animal models of depression. Psychopharmacology (Berlin). 83:1-16.

Willner P. (1986). Validation criteria for animal models of human mental disorders: learned helplessness as a paradim case. Prog Neuropsychopharmacol Biol Psychiatry. 10:677-90.

Willner P. (1991). Animal models as simulations of depression. Trends Pharmacol Sci 12:131-6.

Wilpizeski c.R., Lowry L.D. (1987): A two-factor model of rotation-induced motion sickness syndrome in squirrel monkeys. Am J Otolaryngol. 8:7-12.

Wilson C.B., Snook D.E., Dhokia B., Taylor C.V.J., Watson I., Lammertsma A.A., Lambrecht R.M., Waxman J., Jones T., Epenetos A.A. (1991). Quantitative measurement of monoclonal antibody distribution and blood flow using positron emission tomography and iodine in patients with breast cancer. Int J Cancer 47:344-7.

Wilson J.D., Dhall D.P., Simeonovic C.J., Lafferty K.J. (1986): Induction and management of diabetes mellitus in the pig. Aust J Exp Biol Med Sci. 64(Pt 6):489-500.

Wilson J.F., Cantor M.B. (1987). An animal model of excessive eating: schedule-induced hyperphagia in food-satiated rats. J Exp Anal Behav, May. 4:335-46.

Wilson J.R., Douglas P., Hickey W.F., Lanoce V., Ferraro N., Muhammad A., Reichek N. (1987): Experimental congestive heart failure produced by rapid ventricular pacing in the dog: cardiac effects. Circulation. 75:857-67.

Winkenmann R.K. (1986). Nicotinate white response of monkeys sexual skin-- a model for atopic reactivity. Clin Exp Dermatol 11:641-2.

Winn W.C. Jr., Davis G.S., Gump D.W., Craighead J.E., Beaty A.N. (1982). Legionnaires' pneumonia after intratracheal inoculation of guinea pigs and rats. Lab Invest. 47:568-78.

Winwood P., Arthur M. (1993). Kupffer cells: their activation and role in animal models of liver injury and human liver disease. Semin Liver Dis 13(1):50-9.

Wiranowska M., Wilson T., Bencze K., Prockop L. (1988). A mouse model for the study of blood-brain barrier permeability. J Neurosci Methods 26(2):105-9.

Wise W., Cook J., Tempel G., Reines H., Halushka P. (1989). The rat in sepsis and endotoxic shock. Prog Clin Biol Res 299:243-52.

Wohlhieter J. (1992). Summary report: workshop on animal models of human immunodeficiency virus infections in humans. Armed Forces Retrovirus Research Group. Mil Med 157(12):662-4.

Wojcicki J., Samochorwiec L., Jaworska M., Hinek A. (1985). A search for a model of experimental atherosclerosis: comparative studies in rabbits, guinea pigs and rats. Pol J Pharmacol Pharm. 37:11-21.

Wolf R.H., Gormus B.J., Martin L.N., Baskin G.B., Walsh G.P., Meyers W.M., Binford C.H. (1985). Experimental leprosy in three species of monkeys. Science. 227:529-31.

Wolfson L.I., Thal L.J., Brown L.L. (1986). Serotonin models of myoclonus in the guinea pig and rat. Adv Neurol. 43:519-27.

Wolkowski-Tyl R., Chin T.Y., Popp J.A., Heck H.D. (1982). Chemically induced urolithiasis in weanling rats. Am J Pathol. 107:419-21.

Wolman S.R., McMorrow L.E., Cohen M.W. (1982). Animal model of human disease: myelogenous leukemia in the RF mouse. Am J Pathol. 107:280-4.

Wolthuis O. (1991). Some animal models and their probability of extrapolation to man. Neurosci Biobehav Rev 15(1):25-34.

Womble J.R., Larson D.F., Copeland J.G., Russell D.H. (1982). A model of delayed aortic coarctation employing arterial and venous catheters for chronic blood sampling in conscious dogs. J Pharmacol Methods. 8:135-44.

Wonnacott S., Irons J., Rapier C., Thorne B., Lunt G.G. (1990). Presynaptic modulation of transmitter release by nicotinic receptors. In: Nordberg A., Fuxe K., Holmstedt B., Sundwall A. (Eds). Progress in Brain Research. Amsterdam: Elsevier. p 157-63.

Wood J.D., Brann C.R., Vermillon D.L. (1986). Electrical and contractile behavior of large intestinal musculature of piebald mouse model for Hirschsprung's disease. Dig Dis Sci. 31:638-50.

Woodland R.M., Johnson A.P., Tuffrey M. (1983). Animal models of chlamydial infection. Br Med Bull. 39:175-80.

Woodruff M.L., Nonneman A.J. (Ed.) (1994). Toxin-induced models of neurobiological disorders. New York: Plenum Press. 344 P.

Woodside J.R., Dail W.G., McGuire E.J., Wagner F.C. Jr. (1982). The Manx cat as an animal model for neurogenic vesical dysfunction associated with myelodysplasia. J Urol. 127:180-3.

Woolsey T.A. (1988). The domination of knowledge by ignorance: Politics and regulation of animal research for diagnosis and treatment of disease. Circulation 77:1197-202.

Working Group (1987) Pancreas Cancer. Evaluation and utilization of transgenic animal models in studies of pancreatic cancer. Pancreas. 2:470-2.

Working P.K. (1988): Male reproductive toxicology: comparison of the human to animal models. Environ Health Perspect 77:37-44 (49 ref.)

Workshop (1982). The Juvenile Diabetes Foundation Workshop on the spontaneously diabetes BB rat: its potential for insight into human juvenile diabetes. Banff, Alberta, Canada, Sept. 8-10. Metabolism. 32 (7 Suppl):1-166.

Workshop. (1983). Physiological and biochemical characteristics of animal models of nutritional dependent disease. Nahrung. 29:547-627.

Worlock P., Slack R., Harvey L., Mawhinney R. (1988): An experimental model of post-traumatic osteomyelitis in rabbits. Br J Exp Pathol. 69(2):235-44.

Wozniczko-Orlowska G. (1983). A model of polyarthritis in rats immunized with collagen. Reumatologia. 21:5-13 (English Abstract) (Polish)

Wright E. (1991). Experimental studies of radiation-induced leukaemia. Radiat Environ Biophys 30(3):209-11.

Wright J., Rang M. (1990). The spastic mouse. And the search for an animal model of spasticity in human beings. Clin Orthop (253):12-9.

Wu R.S., Zhang S.M., Ma J.W. (1985). Rat model of passive lung anaphylasis induced by trichosanthin. Chung Kuo Yao Li Hsueh Pao. 6:68-71. (English Abstract) (Chinese)

Wultz B., Sagvolden T., Moser E., Moser M. (1990). The spontaneously hypertensive rat as an animal model of attention-deficit hyperactivity disorder: effects of methylphenidate on exploratory behavior. Behav Neural Biol 53(1):88-102.

Wynne J.W. (1982). Aspiration pneumonitis. Correlation of experimental models with clinical disease. Clin Chest Med. 3:25-34.

Xiong L., Rauch R., Hagino N., Jinkins J. (1993). An animal model of corpus callosum impingement as seen in patients with normal pressure hydrocephalus. Invest Radiol 28(1):46-50.

Xu S. (1989). [Establishment of a transplantable human rectal mucoid adenocarcinoma model in nude mice and study of its biological characteristics]. Chung-hua Ping Li Hsueh Tsa Chih 18(1):47-9.

Yaes R.J., Kalend A. (1988): Local stem cell depletion model for radiation myelitis. Int J Radiat Oncol Biol Phys. 14(6):1247-59.

Yamada T., Sartor R., Marshall S., Specian RD., Grisham MB. (1993). Mucosal injury and inflammation in a model of chronic granulomatous colitis in rats. Gastroenterology 104(3):759-71.

Yamaguchi T., Kato M., Fukui M., Akazawa K. (1992). Rolling mouse Nagoya as a mutant animal model of basal ganglia dysfunction: determination of absolute rates of local cerebral glucose utilization. Brain Res 598(1-2):38-44.

Yamamoto H., Komatsuzaki T. (1987). Pathological study of Streptococcus faecalis antigen-induced arthritis in New Zealand white rabbits. Jikken Dobutsu. 36:17-25. (English Abstract) (Japanese)

Yamamoto K. (1985). Cerebral ischemia in rabbit: a new experimental model with immunohistochemical investigation. J Cereb Blood Flow Metab. 5:529-36.

Yamamoto K., Sargent P.A., Fisher M.M., Youson J.H. (1986). Periductal fibrosis and lipocytes (fat-storing cells or Ito cells) during biliary atresia in the lamprey. Hepatology. 6:54-9.

Yamamura K. (1988): Production of human disease models using transgenic mice. Nippon Rinsho. 46(5):1177-85. (Japanese)

Yamashiki M., Kosaka Y., Sakaguchi S., Ichida F. (1990). Simultaneous production of hepatic lesions and circulating antimitochondrial antibody in an experimental animal model of primary biliary cirrhosis. Gastroenterol Jpn 25(1):132.

Yamashita T., Ito J. (1988). [A new animal model for intravesical chemotherapy of bladder cancer]. Gan To Kagaku Ryoho 15(7):2087-92.

Yamori Y. (1991). Overview: studies on spontaneous hypertension-development from animal models toward man. Clin Exp Hypertens [A] 13(5):631-44.

Yamori Y., Horie R., Akiguchi I., Kihara M., Nara Y., Lovenberg W. (1982). Symptomatological classification in the development of stroke in stroke-prone spontaneously hypertensive rats. Jpn Circ J. 46:274-83.

Yamori Y., Horie R., Nara Y., Kohara M., Igawa T., Kanbe T., Mori K., Ikeda K. (1981). Genetic markers in spontaneously hypertensive rats. Clin Exp Hypertens. 3:713-25.

Yamori Y., Kitamura Y., Nara Y., Iritani N. (1981). Mechanism of hypercholesterolemia in arteriolipidosis-prone rats (ALR). Jpn Circ J. 45 1068-73.

Yan H.J. (1988): Experimental model of regional cerebral ischemia induced by occlusion of the middle cerebral artery in the rat. Chung Hua Shen Ching Ching Shen Ko Tsa Chih. 21(1):3-6, 61. (English Abstract) (Chinese)

Yang C., Niu C., Bodo M., Gabriel E., Notbohm H., Wolf E., Muller PK. (1993). Fulvic acid supplementation and selenium deficiency disturb the structural integrity of mouse skeletal tissue. An animal model to study the molecular defects of Kashin-Beck disease. Biochem J 289(Pt 3):829-35.

Yang S. (1992). [Chondronecrosis induced in rhesus monkeys fed with grains and water of Kaschin-Beck's disease endemic area]. Chung Hua I Hsueh Tsa Chih 72(6):361-2, 383.

Yao C.Z. (1987). Establishment of an animal model for the study of epidemic hemorrhagic fever]. Chung Hu I Hsueh Ts Chih, 67:243-6 (English Abstract).(Chinese)

Yapor W., Jafar J., Crowell R. (1991). One-stage construction of giant experimental aneurysms in dogs. Surg Neurol 36(6):426-30.

Yarom R., Sapoznikov D., Havivi Y., Avraham K., Schickler M., Groner Y. (1988). Premature aging changes in neuromuscular junctions of transgenic mice with an extra human CuZnSOD gene: a model for tongue pathology in Down's syndrome. J Neurol Sci 88(1-3):41-53.

Yasumura S., Jones K., Spanne P., Schidlovsky G., Wielopolski L., Ren X., Glaros D., Xatzikonstantinou Y. (1993). In vivo animal models of body composition in aging. J Nutr 123(2 Suppl):459-64.

Yates F.E., Kugler P.N. (1986). Similarity, principles and intrinsic geometries: Contrasting approaches to interspecies scaling. J Pharm Science 75:1019-27.

Yazawa Y., Yoo T.J., Isnibe T., Tomoda K. (1985). Type II collagen induced tympanosclerosis model in guinea pigs. Auris Nasus Larynx. 1:S200-2.

Yealy D. (1993). How much "significance" is significant? The transition from animal models to human trials in resuscitation research. Ann Emerg Med 22(1):11-6.

Yehuda R., Antelman S.M. (1993). Criteria for rationally evaluating animal models of posttraumatic stress disorder. Biol Psychiatry 33(7):479-86.

Yokoyama E., Nambu Z., Uchiyama I., Kyono H. (1987): An emphysema model in rats treated intratracheally with elastase. Environ Res. 42:340-52.

Yokoyama M., Sakamoto S., Kawashima S., Okada T., Fukuzaki H. (1985). Myocardial ischaemia produced by ergonovine-induced vasoconstriction during preexisting coronary stenosis: experimental conditions for the geometric theory. Cardiovasc Res. 19:237-48.

Yonas H., Wolfson S.K. Jr., Dujouny M., Boehnke M., Cook E. (1981). Selective lenticulostriate occlusion in the primate. A highly focal cerebral ischemia model. Stroke. 12:567-72.

Yong Z., Hill J.L., Hirofuji T., Mander M., Yu D.T. (1988): An experimental mouse model of Yersinia-induced reactive arthritis. Microb Pathog. 4(4):305-10.

Yoshida T., Shimizu K., Ushio Y., Hayakawa T., Kato A., Moganie H., Sakamoto Y. (1986). Development of experimental meningeal gliomatosis models using nude mice. Gan To Kagaku Ryoho. 13:2745-50. (English Abstract) (Japanese)

Yoshida T., Ushio Y., Hayakawa T., Arita N., Yamada K., Mogami H. (1984). Meningeal gliomatosis: development of experimental models. No Shinkei Geka. 12:1141-8. (English Abstract). (Japanese)

Yoshida T.O., Wilson J.M. (Ed.) (1992). Molecular approaches to the study and treatment of human diseases: proceedings of the International Symposium on Genetic Intervention in Diseases with Unkown Etiology, Tokyo, Japan, 30 November - 1 December 1990. Amsterdam; New York: Excerpta Medica. 455 P.

Yoshikawa T., Furukawa Y., Murakami M., Takemura S., Kondo M. (1981). Experimental model of disseminated intravascular coagulation induced by sustained infusion of endotoxin. Res Exp Med (Berl). 179:223-8.

Yoshikawa T., Murakami M. (1983). Effect of dipyridamole on experimental disseminated intravascular coagulation in rats. Thromb Res. 29:619-25.

Yoshikawa T., Murakami M., Furukawa Y., Takemura S., Kondo M. (1983). Effects of ticlopidine and aspirin on endotoxin-induced disseminated intravascular coagulation in rats. Thromb Haemost. 49:190-2.

Yoshikawa Y., Yamasaki K. (1991). Renal lesions of hyperlipidemic Imai rats: a spontaneous animal model of focal glomerulosclerosis. Nephron 59(3):471-6.

Yoshino S., Bacon P.A., Blake D.R., Scott D.L., Wainwright A.C. et al. (1984). A model of persistent antigen-induced chronic inflammation in the rat air pouch. Br J Exp Pathol. 65:201-14.

Yoshino S., Cromartie W.J., Schwal J.H. (1985). Inflammation induced by bacterial cell wall fragments in the rat air pouch. Comparison of rat strains and measurement of arachidonic acid metabolites. Am J Pathol. 121:327-36.

Young P.H., Fischer V.W., Guity A., Young P.A. (1987). Mural repair following obliteration of aneurysms: production of experimental aneurysms. Microsurgery, 8:128-37.

Young P.H., Yasargil M.G. (1982). Experimental carotid artery aneurysms in rats: a new model for microsurgical practice. J Microsurg. 3:135-46.

Yuan X.Q., Wu Z.G., He L.J., Cai Z.H. (1984). Natural course of septic shock in a canine model. Cardiorespiratory and metabolic parameters. Chin Med J [English]. 97:197-204.

Yurdaydin C., Gu Z., Nowak G., Fromm C., Holt AG., Basile A. (1993). Benzodiazepine receptor ligands are elevated in an animal model of hepatic encephalopathy: relationship between brain concentration and severity of encephalopathy. J Pharmacol Exp Ther 265(2):565-71.

Yutrzenka G.J., Patrick G.A., Rosenberger W. (1985). Continuous intraperitoneal infusion of pentobarbital: a model of barbiturate dependence in the rat. J Pharmacol Exp Ther. 232:111-8.

Zager R.A. (1987). Partial aortic ligation: a hypoperfusion model of ischemic acute renal failure and a comparison with renal artery occlusion.J Lab Clin Med,Oct; 110:396-405.

Zaino R.J., Satyaswaroop P.G., Mortel R. (1985). Hormonal therapy of human endometrial adenocarcinoma in a nude mouse model. Cancer Res. 45:539-41.

Zallone A.Z., Jet A. (1993). Animal models of bone physiology. Curr Opin Rheumatol. 5:363-7.

Zalups, R. (1993). The Os/+ mouse: a genetic animal model of reduced renal mass. Am J Physiol, 264 (1 Pt 2):F53-60.

Zamma T. (1983). Adjuvant-induced arthritis in the temporomandibular joint of rats. Infect Immun. 39:1291-9.

Zana J., Thomas D., Muffat-Joly M., de B. J., Pocidalo J., Orfila J., Carbon C., Salat-Baroux J. (1990). An experimental model for salpingitis due to Chlamydia trachomatis and residual tubal infertility in the mouse. Hum Reprod 5(3):274-8.

Zawirski M., Jakubowski J., Symon L., Bell A.B., Watson A. (1985). [Changes in the time of central neural conduction and of the amplitude of the potential N10 of the somatosensory evoked potentials in a model of subarachnoid hemorrhage in baboons]. Neurol Neurochir Pol. 19:241-6. (English Abstract) (Polish)

Zelter M., Dougvet D. (1986). Experimental permeability edemas. Bull Eur Physiopathol Respir. 22:281-314. (English, French)

Zhan, M., Ji, Q., Xu, Z., Li, H., Liu, J., Zhang, J., Huo, W., & Liu, J. (1989). Paraplegia caused by local spinal cord ischemia. An animal spinal cord ischemia model. Chin Med J (Engl), 102 (1):28-33.

Zhang G., Liu J. (1989). An experimental animal model of Kashin-Beck disease. Ann Rheum Dis 48(2):149-52.

Zhang J.X., Huang W.Z., Ye X.Y., Pan Y.R., Luo M.Z. (1982). Establishment of monkey model of Plasmodium cynomolgi-Anopheles stephensi system and its use for tissue shizontocide test. Chung Kuo I Hsueh Ko Hsueh Yuan Hsueh pao. 4:119-23. (English Abstract) (Chinese)

Zhang K. (1990). [An animal model of human laryngeal carcinoma and its biological characteristics]. Chung Hua Erh Pi Yen Hou Ko Tsa Chih 25(1):25-7, 62-3.

Zhang W. (1989). [Establishment of an animal model of intrauterine growth retardation (IUGR)]. Chung Hua I Hsueh Tsa Chih 69(11):629-30, 44.

Zhao D.Y., Feng G.J., Wu X.R., Zuo Q.H. (1985). Seizures induced by intraventricular microinjection of ionized cobalt in the rat- a new experimental model of epilepsy. Brain Res. 342:323-9.

Zhao D.Y., Wu X.R., Pei Y.Q., Zuo Q.H. (1985). Kindling phenomenon of hyperthermic seizures in the epilepsy-prone versus the epilepsy-resistant rat. Brain Res. 358:390-3.

Zhao N.K. (1985). Establishment of a model of transplantable myelocytic leukemia (L801) in LACA mice. Sci Sin [B]. 28:736-44.

Zhu Z.Y., Tang H.Y., Fu G.M., Weng J.Q., Yao S.R. (1986). Animal model of rabbits for researching epidemic hemorrhagic fever. Chin Med J [England]. 99:253-8.

Zia S., Hyde D., Giri S. (1992). Development of a bleomycin hamster model of subchronic lung fibrosis. Pathology 24(3):155-63.

Zierhut M. (1994). New findings on HSV-induced retinitis in the von Szily model. Boston: Butterworth-Heinemann; Buren, Netherlands: AEolus Press. 95 P.

Zigmond M., Stricker E. (1989). Animal models of parkinsonism using selective neurotoxins: clinical and basic implications. Int Rev Neurobiol 31:1-79.

Zigmond M.J., Stricker E.M. (1984). Parkinson's disease: studies with an animal model. Life Sci. 35:5-18.

Zimmerli W. (1993). Experimental models in the investigation of device-related infections. J Antimicrob Chemother. 31(Suppl D):97-102.

Zivin J., Grotta J. (1990). Animal stroke models. They are relevant to human disease. Stroke 21(7):981-3.

Zochodne D., Ward K., Low P. (1988). Guanethidine adrenergic neuropathy: an animal model of selective autonomic neuropathy. Brain Res 461(1):10-6.

Zovakia A., Chalon S., Kung H.F., Dognon A.M., Saliba E., Besnard J.C., Gilloteau D. (1994). Radioiodinated tracers for the evaluation of dopamine receptors in the neonatal rat brain after hypoxic-ischemic injury. Eur J Nucl Med. 21:488-92.

Zovickian J., Youle R. (1988). Efficacy of intrathecal immunotoxin therapy in an animal model of leptomeningeal neoplasia. J Neurosurg 68(5):767-74.

Zubova O., Batalova I., Oknina N. (1991). [Functional inactivation of the hippocampus by controlled neuroimmunization] Funktsional'naia dezaktivatsiia gippokampa putem napravlennogo neiroimmunnogo vozdeistviia. Biull Eksp Biol Med 111(1):57-9.

Zuccato E., Bertolo C., Colombo L., Mussini E. (1992). Indomethacin-induced enteropathy: effect of the drug regimen on intestinal permeability in rats. Agents Actions, Spec No:C18-21.

Zuziak P. (1992). Non-human primates hold clues to search for AIDS vaccine [news]. J Am Vet Med Assoc 201(11):1670-1.

GLOSSARY OF ABBREVIATIONS

AAAS	American Association for Advancement of Sciences
AEEC	Animal Experiment and Ethics Commission
AIDS	Acquired Immune Deficiency Syndrome
AMA	American Medical Association
ARG	Autoradiography
ASIH	American Society of Ichthiologists and Herpetologists
ASPCA	American Humane Society for the Care and Protection of Animals
BGO	Bismuth Germanate Crystals
CAD	Coronary Artery Stenosis
CBF	Cerebral Blood Flow
CBV	Cerebral Blood Volume
CMR_{glc}	Cerebral Glucose Metabolic Rate
$CMRO_2$	Cerebral Oxygen Metabolic Rate
DNA	Deoxyribonucleic Acid
ECAT	PET Scanner, Siemens
FDG	Fluorodeoxyglucose
FOV	Field Of View
HSV	Herpes Simplex Virus
ILAR	Institution of Laboratory Animal Resources
LAD	Left Anterior Descending Artery Disease
LAL	Limulus Amebocyte Lysate
mAChR	Muscarinic Cholinergic Receptor
MBBG	Metabromobenzylguanidine
MCA	Middle Cerebral Artery
MEDLINE	Medical Library Database Service
MIBG	Metaiodobenzylguanidine
MPTP	I-Methyl-4-phenyl-1,2,3,6-tetrahydropyridine
mRNA	messenger Ribonucleic Acid
nAChR	Nictonic Acetylcholase Receptor
NIH	National Institute of Health
NIMH	National Institute of Mental Health
OEF	Oxygen Enhancement Fraction
PET	Positron Emission Tomography
SCID	Severe Combined Immune Deficiencies
SIMS	Secondary Ion Mass Spectrometry
SPECT	Single Photon Emission Computer Tomography
SPET	Single Photon Emission Tomography
SPF	Specific Pathogen Free
UFAW	Universities Federation for Animal Welfare

Developments in Nuclear Medicine

1. P.H. Cox (ed.): *Cholescintigraphy.* 1981   ISBN 90-247-2524-0

2. P.H. Cox (ed.): *Progress in Radiopharmacology.* Selected Topics. Proceedings of the 3rd European Symposium (Noordwijkerhout, The Netherlands, April 1982). 1982
ISBN 90-247-2768-5

3. M.H. Jonckheer and F. Deconinck (eds.): *X-Ray Fluorescent Scanning of the Thyroid.* 1983   ISBN 0-89838-561-X

4. K. Kristensen and E. Nørbygaard (eds.): *Safety and Efficacy of Radiopharmaceuticals.* 1984   ISBN 0-89838-609-8

5. A. Bossuyt and F. Deconinck: *Amplitude/Phase Patterns in Dynamic Scintigraphic Imaging.* With a Foreword by A. Bertrand Brill. 1984   ISBN 0-89838-641-1

6. M.R. Hardeman and Y. Najean (eds.): *Blood Cells in Nuclear Medicine, Part I.* Cell Kinetics and Bio-distribution. 1984   ISBN 0-89838-653-5

7. G.F. Fueger (ed.): *Blood Cells in Nuclear Medicine, Part II.* Migratory Blood Cells. 1984   ISBN 0-89838-654-3

8. H.J. Biersack and P.H. Cox (eds.): *Radioisotope Studies in Cardiology.* 1985
ISBN 0-89838-733-7

9. P.H. Cox, G. Limouris and M.G. Woldring (eds.): *Progress in Radiopharmacology 1985.* 1985   ISBN 0-89838-745-0

10. P.H. Cox, S.J. Mather, C.B. Sampson and C.R. Lazarus (eds.): *Progress in Radiopharmacy.* 1986   ISBN 0-89838-823-6

11. H. Deckart and P.H. Cox (eds.): *Principles of Radiopharmacology.* 1987
ISBN 0-89838-774-4

12. W.-D. Heiss, G. Pawlik, K. Herholz and K. Wienhard (eds.): *Clinical Efficacy of Positron Emission Tomography.* 1987   ISBN 0-89838-898-8

13. G.B. Gerber, H. Métivier and H. Smith (eds.): *Age-related Factors in Radionuclide Metabolism and Dosimetry.* 1987   ISBN 0-89838-953-4

14. K. Kristensen and E. Nørbygaard (eds.): *Safety and Efficacy of Radiopharmaceuticals 1987.* 1987   ISBN 0-89838-986-0

15. C. Beckers, A. Goffinet and A. Bol (eds.): *Positron Emission Tomography in Clinical Research and Clinical Diagnosis.* Tracer Modelling and Radioreceptors. 1989
ISBN 0-7923-0254-0

16. M. De Schrijver: *Scintigraphy of Inflammation with Nanometer-sized Colloidal Tracers.* 1989   ISBN 0-7923-0272-9

17. Ch. Kessler, M.R. Hardeman, H. Henningsen and J.-N. Petrovici (eds.): *Clinical Application of Radiolabelled Platelets.* 1990   ISBN 0-7923-0729-1

18. H.J. Biersack and P.H. Cox (eds.): *Nuclear Medicine in Gastroenterology.* 1991
ISBN 0-7923-1074-8

19. R.P. Baum, P.H. Cox, G. Hör and G.L. Buraggi (eds.): *Clinical Use of Antibodies.* Tumours, infection, infarction, rejection and in the diagnosis of AIDS. 1991
ISBN 0-7923-1424-7

Developments in Nuclear Medicine

Kluwer Academic Publishers - Dordrecht / Boston / London